Martindale's Drugs Restricted in Sport Pocket Companion 2008

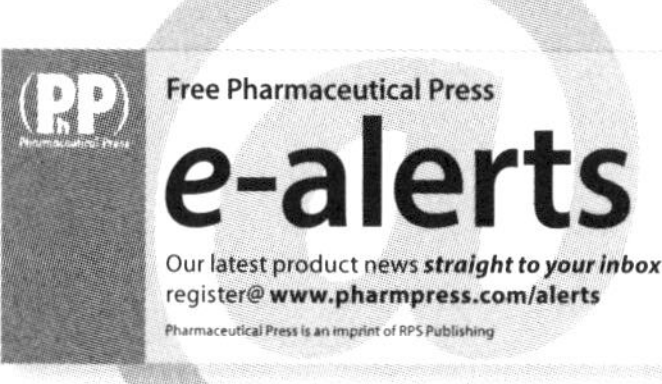

Martindale's Drugs Restricted in Sport Pocket Companion 2008

Editor

Sean C Sweetman, BPharm, FRPharmS

Project Team

Julie M McGlashan, BPharm, DipInfSc, MRPharmS

Elizabeth D King, DipBTECPharmSc

London • Chicago

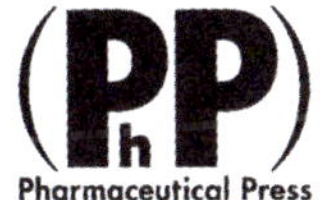

Published by the Pharmaceutical Press
An imprint of RPS Publishing

1 Lambeth High Street, London SE1 7JN, UK
100 South Atkinson Road, Suite 200, Grayslake, IL 60030-7820, USA

RPS Publishing is the publishing organisation of the Royal Pharmaceutical Society of Great Britain

First published 2008

Printed in Slovenia by 1010 Printing Ltd, Ljubljana

ISBN 978 0 85369 825 8

A catalogue record for this book is available from the British Library

Martindale Staff

Editor

Sean C Sweetman, BPharm, FRPharmS

Senior Assistant Editor

Paul S Blake, BPharm, GradDipHealthInformatics, FRPharmS

Assistant Editors

Alison Brayfield, BPharm, MRPharmS

Julie M McGlashan, BPharm, DipInfSc, MRPharmS

Gail C Neathercoat, BSc, MRPharmS

Anne V Parsons, BPharm, MRPharmS

Staff Editors

Catherine RM Cadart, BPharm, GradDipHospPharm, MRPharmS

Kathleen Eager, BPharm, MRPharmS

Prakash Gotecha, BSc, MRPharmS

Susan L Handy, BPharm, DipClinPharm, MRPharmS

Fauziah T Hashmi, BSc, MSc, MRPharmS

Sue W Ho, BPharm, MRPharmS

Joanna A Humm, MPharm, MRPharmS

Jean Macpherson, BSc, MRPharmS

Melissa TA Siew, BPharm, CertPharmPractice, MRPharmS, Cert Hum(Open)

Sandra C Sutton, BPharm, MSc Med, Cert Proj Mngt, SAPC (SA)

Gerda W Viedge, BPharm, MRPharmS, DO

Senior Editorial Assistant

Chloë SAJ Hitch, BSc, MRes

Editorial Assistants

Elizabeth D King, DipBTECPharmSc

James O'Reilly, BSc, MSc

Knowledge Systems Administrator

Michael C Evans, BSc

Editorial Secretarial Assistant

Christine L Iskandar

Contents

Preface

What is *Martindale's Drugs Restricted in Sport Pocket Companion?*

Martindale's Drugs Restricted in Sport Pocket Companion is a guide to drugs and medicines that may be restricted in or out of competition in some or all sports, either in their own right, or because they are a derivative of a restricted substance or a member of a prohibited group.

The information about drugs is taken from monographs in the full work, *Martindale: The Complete Drug Reference*. This renowned reference book, published continuously since the first edition in 1883, is a trusted source of reliable, unbiased, and evaluated information on drugs and medicines used throughout the world. The names given are based on the British Approved Names, the International Nonproprietary Names (in English, French, Latin, Spanish, and Russian), the US Adopted Names, names used in other European, Baltic, and Scandinavian countries, common synonyms, and manufacturers codes. Trade names for single- and multi-ingredient proprietary products, mainly for prescribable medications, are included from 40 countries worldwide.

The guidance given in this book on restrictions to the use in sport is based on the prohibited list of the *World Anti-doping Code 2008*. An updated code is issued annually by the World Anti-Doping Agency (WADA). In listing the drugs and medicines that may be interpreted as covered by these regulations, we have not omitted drugs usually applied topically — under certain circumstances enough may enter the body to produce a positive test result. Our aim is to alert the athlete to the potential of a problem and it is up to the individual to check with a competent authority about a specific circumstance.

If an athlete requires treatment for an illness or condition with a drug that falls under the prohibited list, a Therapeutic Use Exemption (TUE) may be granted to authorise the athlete to take the needed medication. WADA has issued an international standard for granting TUEs. Applications for TUEs are made to the appropriate International Federation (IF) or National Anti-Doping Organization (NADO) by the athlete.

In addition to the drugs and medicines listed, all intravenous infusions are prohibited at all times. In an acute medical situation where this method of administration is deemed necessary, a retroactive Therapeutic Use Exemption will be required.

How to use this book

The best way to find out whether there may be restrictions to the use of a particular drug or medicine is to look up the name in the index at the back of the book. The index includes ingredient (generic) names, synonyms, codes, or proprietary (trade; brand) names to help you find any relevant entries.

The main entries in the book are in the form of drug monographs, described in the section on Structure, below. Drug monographs are arranged alphabetically by generic name. If you know the generic name of the drug or medicine in question, you can quickly turn to the appropriate entry by using the alphabetical group tabs on the edges of the pages. However, the generic name of a drug may vary from country to country so the safest way to locate a drug is through the index.

Proprietary products sometimes include different active ingredients in different countries and may change from time to time, so it is always wise to check the ingredients listed on the packaging against the entry in the book.

The drug monograph indicates which class in the WADA prohibited list the drug belongs to and gives a summary of any exemptions or special circumstances that may apply. Full details can be found in the WADA prohibited list.

The omission of a monograph should not be taken as confirmation that the substance may legitimately be taken by a competitor. For further advice on a specific circumstance, please consult a healthcare professional, sports medicine specialist, or a representative of the appropriate national or international sporting body.

Disclaimer

The regulations issued by the World Anti-Doping Agency (WADA—see www.wada-ama.org) are subject to interpretation and therapeutic exemption, and may vary from sport to sport; particular sporting authorities may also issue additional restrictions, and competitors should always check with the appropriate body. Some drugs restricted by the WADA regulations are not the subject of monographs in *Martindale: The Complete Drug Reference* and thus do not appear in this publication. The rules are constantly evolving and the omission of a monograph or the absence of any indication of restriction in *Martindale's Drugs Restricted in Sport Pocket Companion* should not be taken as confirmation that the substance may legitimately be taken by a competitor.

Proprietary (trade) names are covered for 40 countries worldwide. However, the lists are not exhaustive and athletes should carefully check the ingredients listed for unfamiliar products. The same proprietary name may be used for products containing different ingredients in different countries, and athletes obtaining proprietary products outside their own country should be especially vigilant even if they have used a product of the same name in the past.

In general, herbal medicines have been omitted. However, some herbal medicines may have biological effects similar to prohibited substances and therefore may fall within the regulations.

Coverage

Martindale's Drugs Restricted in Sport Pocket Companion 2008 contains over 450 monographs pertaining to individual drug substances that may be restricted in some or all sports, either in or out of competition. These include many prescribed and over-the-counter medicines as well as unlicensed and illicit drugs of abuse.

The information on each drug or medicine includes nationally and internationally approved names, synonyms, and codes, a brief profile of the actions and properties of the drug, the WADA class(es) under which it may be restricted, and lists of international proprietary (trade) names for single- and multi-ingredient preparations, mainly for prescribable medications.

For this edition we have covered proprietary names from Argentina, Australia, Austria, Belgium, Brazil, Canada, Chile, Czech Republic, Denmark, Finland, France, Germany, Greece, Hong Kong, Hungary, India, Indonesia, Ireland, Israel, Italy, Malaysia, Mexico, the Netherlands, New Zealand, Norway, Philippines, Poland, Portugal, Russia, Singapore, South Africa, Spain, Sweden, Switzerland, Thailand, Turkey, the United Arab Emirates, UK, USA, and Venezuela. We have also included some proprietary preparations from Japan.

Please note that street names for drugs liable to abuse are not included. These names are subject to local variation and rapid change, and the same name may be applied to several related substances. Many commonly abused substances are prohibited under the WADA regulations.

Structure

Martindale's Drugs Restricted in Sport Pocket Companion is arranged alphabetically by drug substance. The International Nonproprietary Name (INN), where one exists, is used in preference for the title. For convenience, related derivatives and salts are listed together.

Other synonyms listed include British Approved Names, the French, Latin, Spanish, and Russian variants of International Nonproprietary Names, US Adopted Names, names used in other European, Baltic, and Scandinavian countries, common synonyms, and manufacturers codes.

The ***clinical profile*** is based on the full text of *Martindale: The Complete Drug Reference* and describes the basic actions and uses of the substance.

The ***WADA status*** indicates whether the substance is prohibited in or out of competition.

The ***WADA class*** gives an indication of the reason for the prohibition and gives more information about the range of substances covered in that class, plus any special circumstances.

Names of ***preparations*** are listed by country and are separated into single- and multi-ingredient preparations.

A comprehensive ***index*** of over 15200 entries is to be found at the back of the book, and includes all names, synonyms, and proprietary (trade) names found in the text. Cyrillic names are listed at the end of the index.

In addition a ***glossary*** providing a brief explanation of some of the pharmaceutical and medical terms used in the clinical profile and the WADA regulations is included at the start of the publication.

Acknowledgements

The Editor is grateful to the many organisations that have helped in providing information, including the World Anti-Doping Agency, the World Health Organization, the British Pharmacopoeia Commission, the Czech Pharmacopoeia Commission, the EDQM/European Pharmacopoeia, and our Spanish colleagues at Grupo Ars XXI.

Thanks are also due to Paul Weller, Charles Fry and the staff of the Pharmaceutical Press for their support. The contents of this edition were planned, written, checked, indexed, keyed, proofed, and processed by the Martindale staff. The Editor is pleased to acknowledge the skills and commitment of all the Martindale staff and to record his gratitude to them. Special thanks are due to Paul Blake for the original idea for this publication and to Julie McGlashan and Lisa King for their work on classifying substances according to the WADA regulations and maintaining the database on drugs restricted in sport.

Contact Details

We are always very pleased to receive feedback from those using our products. Anyone wishing to comment can contact us at the following e-mail address: martindale@rpsgb.org

Abbreviations

Arg.	Argentina
Austral.	Australia
Belg.	Belgium
Br.	British
Braz.	Brazil
Canad.	Canada
CNS	central nervous system
Cz.	Czech Republic
Denm.	Denmark
FDA	Food and Drug Administration of USA
Fin.	Finland
Fr.	France
FSH	follicle-stimulating hormone
g	gram(s)
Ger.	Germany
Gr.	Greece
Hung.	Hungary
Irl.	Ireland
Indon.	Indonesia
Ital.	Italy
Jpn	Japan
L	litre(s)
LH	luteinising hormone
Mex.	Mexico
mL	millilitre(s)
Neth.	The Netherlands
ng	nanogram(s)
Norw.	Norway
NZ	New Zealand
Philipp.	Philippines
Pol.	Poland
Port.	Portugal
q.v.	*quode vide* which see
Rus.	Russia
S. Afr.	South Africa
Swed.	Sweden
Switz.	Switzerland
Thai.	Thailand

Turk.	Turkey
UAE	United Arab Emirates
UK	United Kingdom
US and USA	United States of America
Venez.	Venezuela

Glossary

adjunct	a substance that enhances the effect of other treatment
adrenergic receptors	a type of receptor (q.v.) that binds adrenaline and related substances
adrenoceptors	a type of receptor (q.v.) that binds adrenaline and related substances
agonist	a substance that mimics the action or effects of another
allergic rhinitis	nasal hay fever
alopecia androgenetica	male-pattern baldness
alpha adrenoceptors	one of the 2 main classes of adrenergic receptors (q.v.)
alpha-reductase inhibitor	inhibitor of the enzyme responsible for converting testosterone to its active form, thus producing anti-androgenic effects
anabolic	promoting tissue growth and repair
anaemia	an abnormally low red blood cell count or haemoglobin concentration
analgesic	a drug used to relieve pain
analogue	molecule with a similar chemical structure and similar biological effects
androgenic	producing male sexual characteristics
angina pectoris	chest pain caused by a lack of oxygen supply to heart muscles
anorectic	a substance that reduces the appetite
antagonist	a substance that counteracts the actions or effects of another
antiemetic	a drug that reduces nausea and vomiting
anti-inflammatory	a drug that reduces inflammation
apnoea	the absence or cessation of breathing
aromatase inhibitor	a drug that inhibits the conversion of androgens to oestrogens in the body
auricular	relating to the ear
beta adrenoceptors	one of the 2 main classes of adrenergic receptors (q.v.)
beta-2 agonist	a bronchodilator (q.v.) that acts on the beta-2 class of adrenoceptors (q.v.) in the airways

beta blocker	a class of drugs that block the beta adrenoceptors (q.v.)
bronchodilator	a medicine that opens the airways, used in diseases like asthma
buccal	relating to the inside of the cheek
carbonic anhydrase inhibitor	a type of diuretic (q.v.) that is mainly used to reduce pressure in the eye
cardiac arrhythmia	irregular heart beats
cardioselective	acting selectively on the heart
cardiovascular	relating to the heart and blood vessels
corticosteroid	a class of steroid hormones, produced in the body by the adrenal cortex, and their derivatives
dermatological	relating to the skin
diuretic	a substance that increases the production of urine
drug	a substance administered to cause a change in physiological functions of the body for therapeutic, diagnostic, recreational, or other purposes
dyspnoea	difficult or laboured breathing
enantiomer	a particular type of isomer (q.v.)
endogenous	occurring naturally in the body
epidural drug administration	injection into the epidural space that surrounds the spinal cord
estrogenic	*see under* oestrogenic
exogenous	originating outside the body
gingival	relating to the gums
glaucoma	increased pressure in the eye that can lead to permanent loss of vision
glucocorticoid	a type of corticosteroid (q.v.) mainly used for their anti-inflammatory (q.v.) and immunosuppressive (q.v.) effects
glucocorticosteroid	a type of corticosteroid (q.v.) mainly used for their anti-inflammatory (q.v.) and immunosuppressive (q.v.) effects
haemostatic	a substance that promotes blood clotting
hormone	an endogenous (q.v.) substance involved in the regulation of the activity of specific organs or tissues – a "chemical messenger"
hypertension	high blood pressure (also used of raised pressure in the eye)
hyperthyroidism	overactivity of the thyroid gland

hypotension	low blood pressure
immunosuppression	suppression of the immune system
inhalation [drug administration]	delivery of a drug to the lungs as a vapour or powder
intraarticular	injection into a joint
intradermal	injection into the skin
intramuscular	injection into a muscle
intravenous	injection into the bloodstream via a vein
iontophoresis	a method of delivering a substance into the body through the skin by applying a low electrical current
isomers	substances with the same chemical formulae but differences in molecular structure
medicine	a drug (q.v.) used for therapeutic or diagnostic purposes
mineralocorticoid	a type of corticosteroid (q.v.) with actions on the fluid and electrolyte balance of the body
mucous membrane	the moist layer of tissue lining many body cavities, particularly those opening to the outside like the digestive and respiratory tracts
mydriatic	a drug used to dilate the pupil of the eye
myocardial infarction	damage to the heart muscle due to lack of blood supply, commonly known as a "heart attack"
narcolepsy/narcoleptic syndrome	a condition characterised by sudden or overwhelming attacks of sleepiness
narcotic	a drug that causes insensibility, but the term has specific legal connotations. See also opioids
nasal	relating to the nose
nootropic	a drug claimed to protect the brain against low oxygen levels
oedema	accumulation of fluid in the tissues
oestrogen	a naturally occurring hormone that controls female sexual characteristics, but having some effects on metabolic processes
oestrogenic	having the actions of oestrogen (q.v.)
oliguria	reduced urine production
ophthalmic	relating to the eye

opioids	substances derived from opium and their derivatives, commonly used as analgesics (q.v.)
orally	by mouth (swallowed)
perianal	relating to the region around the anus
periarticular drug administration	injection close to a joint
peritendinous drug administration	injection close to a tendon
phonophoresis	a method of delivering a substance into the body through the skin by applying ultrasound
plasma expander	a substance that increases the blood plasma volume
precursor	a substance from which another substance is formed
prodrug	a substance that is converted to an active form of the drug within the body
progesterone	a naturally occurring hormone, particularly associated with the menstrual cycle and pregnancy, but having some androgenic properties (q.v.)
progestogenic	having the actions of progesterone (q.v.)
prophylactic	a preventative measure
pruritus	itch
receptor	a structure in a cell (usually) that selectively binds a specific substance and allows it to act in the body
rectal	relating to the rectum
selective (o)estrogen receptor modulators	a class of drugs mainly given for their anti-oestrogenic effects but can also mimic the effects of oestrogen in some tissues
sympathomimetic	a substance that mimics the effects of adrenaline
symptomatic	relating to symptoms
systemic	throughout the body
topical/topically	applied to the skin or mucous membranes
vasoconstrictor	a substance that causes narrowing of the blood vessels

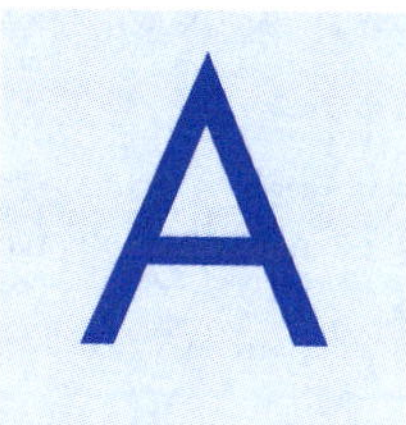

Acebutolol

Other names: Acébutolol; Acebutololum; Asebutolol; Asebutololi.
Ацебутолол

Acebutolol Hydrochloride

Other names: Acébutolol, chlorhydrate d'; Acebutolol-hidroklorid; Acebutolol-hydrochlorid; Acebutololhydroklorid; Acebutololi hydrochloridum; Acebutololio hidrochloridas; Acebutololu chlorowodorek; Asebutololihydrokloridi; Hidrocloruro de acebutolol; IL-17803A; M&B-17803A.

Ацебутолола Гидрохлорид

Clinical profile: Acebutolol is a cardioselective beta blocker used in the management of hypertension, angina pectoris, and cardiac arrhythmias.

WADA Status: Banned in and out of competition as specified below

WADA Class: Beta-Blockers

Unless otherwise specified, beta-blockers are prohibited *In-Competition* only in the following sports.

- Aeronautics (FAI)
- Archery (FITA, IPC) (also prohibited *Out-of-Competition*)
- Automobile (FIA)
- Billiards (WCBS)
- Bobsleigh (FIBT)
- Boules (CMSB, IPC bowls)
- Bridge (FMB)
- Curling (WCF)
- Gymnastics (FIG)
- Motorcycling (FIM)
- Modern Pentathlon (UIPM) for disciplines involving shooting
- Nine-pin bowling (FIQ)
- Powerboating (UIM)
- Sailing (ISAF) for match race helms only
- Shooting (ISSF, IPC) (also prohibited *Out-of-Competition*)
- Skiing/Snowboarding (FIS) in ski jumping, freestyle aerials/halfpipe and snowboard halfpipe/big air
- Wrestling (FILA)

WADA Class: Specified Substances

Also listed as a specified substance.

"The prohibited List may identify specified substances which are particularly susceptible to unintentional anti-doping rule violations because of their general availability in medicinal products or which are less likely to be successfully abused as doping agents."

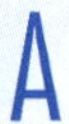

A doping violation involving such substances may result in a reduced sanction provided that the "...*Athlete can establish that the Use of such a specfied substance was not intended to enhance sport performance*..."

Preparations
Single ingredient: ***Belg.:*** Sectral; ***Canad.:*** Monitan; Rhotral; Sectral; ***Chile:*** Beloc; Grifobutol; ***Cz.:*** Acecor; Sectral; ***Denm.:*** Diasectral; ***Fin.:*** Diasectral; Espesil; ***Fr.:*** Sectral; ***Ger.:*** Prent; ***Hong Kong:*** Sectral; ***Israel:*** Sectral; ***Ital.:*** Prent; Sectral; ***Malaysia:*** Sectral; ***Neth.:*** Sectral; ***NZ:*** ACB; ***Pol.:*** Abutol; Sectral; ***Port.:*** Prent; ***S.Afr.:*** Butobloc; Sectral; ***Singapore:*** Sectral; ***Turk.:*** Prent; ***UK:*** Sectral; ***USA:*** Sectral.
Multi-ingredient: ***Belg.:*** Sectrazide; ***Ger.:*** Sali-Prent; Tredalat; ***Indon.:*** Sectrazide.

Acetazolamide

Other names: Acetazolam; Acetazolamid; Acetazolamida; Acetazolamidas; Acétazolamide; Acetazolamidum; Asetatsoliamidi; Asetazolamid.

Ацетазоламид

Acetazolamide Sodium

Other names: Acetazolamida sódica; Acétazolamide Sodique; Natrii Acetazolamidum; Sodium Acetazolamide.

Натрий Ацетазоламид

Clinical profile: Acetazolamide is an inhibitor of carbonic anhydrase with weak diuretic activity and is used mainly in the management of glaucoma. It is also used in some forms of epilepsy and in high-altitude disorders.

WADA Status: Banned in and out of competition

WADA Class: Diuretics and Other Masking Agents

Includes diuretics or substances with a similar chemical structure or similar biological effect(s).

Preparations
Single ingredient: ***Arg.:*** Diamox; ***Austral.:*** Diamox; ***Austria:*** Diamox; ***Belg.:*** Diamox; ***Braz.:*** Diamox; Zolamox; ***Canad.:*** Diamox; ***Cz.:*** Diluran; ***Fin.:*** Diamox; Odemin; ***Fr.:*** Defiltran; Diamox; ***Ger.:*** Diamox; Diuramid; Glaupax; ***Gr.:*** Diamox; ***Hong Kong:*** Diamox; ***Hung.:*** Huma-Zolamide; ***India:*** Diamox; ***Indon.:*** Diamox; ***Irl.:*** Diamox; ***Israel:*** Uramox; ***Ital.:*** Diamox; ***Mex.:*** Aceta-Diazol; Akezol; ***Neth.:*** Diamox; ***Norw.:*** Diamox; ***NZ:*** Diamox; ***Philipp.:*** Cetamid; Diamox; ***Pol.:*** Diuramid; ***Port.:*** Carbinib; ***Rus.:*** Diacarb (Диакарб); ***S.Afr.:*** Azomid; Diamox; ***Spain:*** Edemox; ***Switz.:*** Diamox; Glaupax; ***Thai.:*** Diamox; ***Turk.:*** Diazomid; ***UK:*** Diamox; ***USA:*** Diamox.

Adimolol

Other names: Adimololum; Imidolol; MEN-935.

Адимолол

Clinical profile: Adimolol is a long-acting beta blocker.

WADA Status: Banned in and out of competition as specified below

WADA Class: Beta-Blockers

Unless otherwise specified, beta-blockers are prohibited *In-Competition* only in the following sports.

- Aeronautics (FAI)
- Archery (FITA, IPC) (also prohibited *Out-of-Competition*)
- Automobile (FIA)
- Billiards (WCBS)
- Bobsleigh (FIBT)

- Boules (CMSB, IPC bowls)
- Bridge (FMB)
- Curling (WCF)
- Gymnastics (FIG)
- Motorcycling (FIM)
- Modern Pentathlon (UIPM) for disciplines involving shooting
- Nine-pin bowling (FIQ)
- Powerboating (UIM)
- Sailing (ISAF) for match race helms only
- Shooting (ISSF, IPC) (also prohibited *Out-of-Competition*)
- Skiing/Snowboarding (FIS) in ski jumping, freestyle aerials/halfpipe and snowboard halfpipe/big air
- Wrestling (FILA)

WADA Class: Specified Substances

Also listed as a specified substance.

"The prohibited List may identify specified substances which are particularly susceptible to unintentional anti-doping rule violations because of their general availability in medicinal products or which are less likely to be successfully abused as doping agents."

A doping violation involving such substances may result in a reduced sanction provided that the "*...Athlete can establish that the Use of such a specfied substance was not intended to enhance sport performance...*"

Adrafinil

Other names: Adrafinilo; Adrafinilum; CRL-40028.

Адрафинил

Clinical profile: Adrafinil is a central stimulant and alpha$_1$-adrenergic agonist used for mental function impairment in the elderly.

WADA Status: Banned in competition

WADA Class: Stimulants

Includes adrafinil and any optical isomers.

Preparations
Single ingredient: ***Fr.:*** Olmifon.

Adrenaline

Other names: Epinephrine; Adrenaliini; Adrenalin; Adrenalina; Adrénaline; Adrenalinum; Epinefriini; Epinefrin; Epinefrina; Epinefryna; Épinéphrine; Epinephrinum; Epirenamine; Levorenin; Suprarenin.

Эпинефрин

Adrenaline Acid Tartrate

Other names: Epinephrine Bitartrate; Adrenaliinitartraatti; Adrenaline Bitartrate; Adrenaline Tartrate; Adrénaline, Tartrate d'; Adrenalini Bitartras; Adrenalini tartras; Adrenalinii Tartras; Adrenalinium Hydrogentartaricum; Adrenalino tartratas; Adrenalin-tartarát; Adrenalintartrat; Bitartrato de epinefrina; Epinefrin-tartarát; Epinefryny wodorowinian; Epinephrine Acid Tartrate; Épinéphrine, Bitartrate d'; Epinephrine Hydrogen Tartrate; Epinephrini Bitartras; Epinephrini Tartras; Epirenamine Bitartrate.

Эпинефрина Битартрат

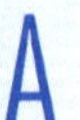

Adrenaline Hydrochloride

Other names: Epinephrine Hydrochloride; Adrenalin Hidroklorür; Épinéphrine, Chlorhydrate d'; Epinephrini Hydrochloridum; Hidrocloruro de epinefrina.

Эпинефрина Гидрохлорид

Clinical profile: Adrenaline is a direct-acting sympathomimetic with a potent effect on alpha and beta adrenoceptors. Major clinical applications of adrenaline include the emergency management of anaphylaxis and anaphylactic shock and use in advanced cardiac life support. It has been given in the treatment of acute asthma. Adrenaline is also used as an adjunct for its vasoconstrictor properties in local anaesthetics for dental use, and as a haemostatic. In ophthalmology adrenaline is used in the treatment of open-angle glaucoma.

WADA Status: Banned in competition

WADA Class: Stimulants

Adrenaline associated with local anaesthetic agents or by local administration (e.g. nasal, ophthalmologic) is not prohibited.

Preparations

Single ingredient: ***Arg.:*** EpiPen; ***Austral.:*** EpiPen; ***Austria:*** EpiPen; Suprarenin; ***Belg.:*** EpiPen; ***Braz.:*** Drenalin; Nefrin; ***Canad.:*** EpiPen; Twinject; Vaponefrin; ***Cz.:*** EpiPen; Glaucon; ***Denm.:*** EpiPen; ***Fin.:*** EpiPen; ***Fr.:*** Anahelp; Anapen; ***Ger.:*** Anapen; Fastjekt; InfectoKrupp; Suprarenin; ***Gr.:*** Anapen; EpiPen; ***Hung.:*** Anapen; EpiPen; Tonogen; ***Irl.:*** Anapen; ***Israel:*** EpiPen; ***Ital.:*** Fastjekt; ***Mex.:*** Pinadrina; ***Neth.:*** EpiPen; ***Norw.:*** EpiPen; ***NZ:*** EpiPen; ***Philipp.:*** Adrenin; ***Pol.:*** Anapen; EpiPen; Fastjekt; ***S.Afr.:*** Adrenotone; Ana-Guard; EpiPen; Eppy; Simplene; ***Spain:*** Adreject; ***Swed.:*** Anapen; EpiPen; ***Switz.:*** EpiPen; ***UK:*** Anapen; EpiPen; ***USA:*** AsthmaHaler Mist; AsthmaNefrin; Epinal; EpiPen; microNefrin; Nephron; Primatene Mist Suspension; Primatene Mist; S-2.

Multi-ingredient: ***Arg.:*** Yanal; ***Austral.:*** Rectinol; ***Hung.:*** Hemorid; ***India:*** Brovon; ***Irl.:*** Ganda; ***Port.:*** Adrinex; ***Spain:*** Coliriocilina Adren Astr; Epistaxol; ***Switz.:*** Haemocortin; ***UK:*** Brovon; ***USA:*** Ana-Kit; Emergent-Ez.

Adjunct-ingredient: ***Arg.:*** Caina G; Duracaine; Gobbicaina; Larjancaina; Xylocaina; ***Austral.:*** Citanest Dental; Marcain; Nurocain; Xylocaine; ***Austria:*** Neo-Xylestesin forte; Neo-Xylestesin; Scandonest; Septanest; Ubistesin; Ultracain Dental; Xylanaest; Xylocain; ***Belg.:*** Citanest; Marcaine; Xylocaine; ***Braz.:*** Bupiabbott Plus; Lidocabbott; Lidogeyer; Marcaina; Neocaina; Novabupi; Xylestesin; Xylocaina; ***Canad.:*** Marcaine; Sensorcaine; Xylocaine; ***Cz.:*** Marcaine; Scandonest; Supracain; Ubistesin; Ultracain D-S; Xylestesin-A; ***Denm.:*** Carbocain; Marcain; Scandonest; Septanest; Septocaine; Ubistesin; Xylocain; Xyloplyin; ***Fin.:*** Marcain; Septocaine; Ubistesin; Ultracain D-Suprarenin; Xylocain; ***Fr.:*** Alphacaine; Ubistesin Adrenalinee; Xylocaine; ***Ger.:*** Ubistesin; Ultracain D-S; Ultracain Suprarenin; Xylocain; Xylocitin; Xylonest; ***Gr.:*** Marcaine; Xylocaine; ***Hong Kong:*** Marcain; Ubistesin; Xylestesin-A; Xylocaine; ***Hung.:*** Ubistesin; Ultracain D-S; ***India:*** Gesicain; Xylocaine; ***Indon.:*** Extracaine; Pehacain; ***Irl.:*** Marcain; Xylocaine; ***Israel:*** Kamacaine; Marcaine; ***Ital.:*** Alfacaina; Bupicain; Bupiforan; Bupisen; Bupisolver; Bupixamol; Carbocaina; Carbosen; Cartidont; Citocartin; Ecocain; Marcaina; Mepi-Mynol; Mepicain; Mepident; Mepiforan; Mepisolver; Mepivamol; Optocain; Sarticain; Scandonest; Septanest; Ubistesin; Xilo-Mynol; Xylonor; Xyloplyina; ***Malaysia:*** Marcain; ***Mex.:*** Buvacaina; Pisacaina; Unicaine; Xylocaina; ***Neth.:*** Bupiforan; Citanest; Lignospan; Marcaine; Scandicaine; Septanest; Ubistesin; Ultracain D-S; Xylocaine; ***Norw.:*** Marcain; Septocaine; Xylocain; ***NZ:*** Marcain; Septanest; Topicaine; Xylestesin-A; Xylocaine; ***Philipp.:*** Dentocaine; ***Pol.:*** Marcaine; ***Port.:*** Artinostrum; Bupinostrum; Lidonostrum; Lincaina; Scandinibsa; Xilonibsa; ***Rus.:*** Ultracain (Ультракаин); ***S.Afr.:*** Macaine; Xylotox; ***Singapore:*** Xylocaine; ***Spain:*** Anestesia Topi Braun C/A; Articaina C/E; Meganest; Octocaine; Scandinibsa; Ultracain; Xilonibsa; Xylonor Especial; ***Swed.:*** Carbocain; Marcain; Xylocain; ***Switz.:*** Alphacaine; Carbostesin; Rapidocaine; Rudocaine; Scandonest; Septanest; Ubistesin; Ultracaine D-S; Xylocain; Xylonest; ***Thai.:*** Lidocation; Xylocaine; ***Turk.:*** Jetokain; Jetosel; Ultracain; ***UAE:*** Ecocain; ***UK:*** Marcain; Septanest; Xylocaine; ***USA:*** Citanest; Marcaine; Octocaine; Sensorcaine; Septocaine; Xylocaine.

Adrenalone

Other names: Adrenalon; Adrenalona; Adrénalone; Adrenaloni; Adrenalonum.

Адреналон

Adrenalone Hydrochloride

Other names: Adrénalone, Chlorhydrate d'; Adrenaloni Hydrochloridum; Adrenalonu chlorowodorek; Hidrocloruro de adrenalona.

Адреналона Гидрохлорид

Clinical profile: Adrenalone is used as a local haemostatic and vasoconstrictor. It has also been used with adrenaline in eye drops for glaucoma.

WADA Status: Banned in competition

WADA Class: Stimulants

Includes stimulants or substances with a similar chemical structure or similar biological effect(s).

WADA Class: Specified Substances

Also listed as a specified substance.

"The prohibited List may identify specified substances which are particularly susceptible to unintentional anti-doping rule violations because of their general availability in medicinal products or which are less likely to be successfully abused as doping agents."

A doping violation involving such substances may result in a reduced sanction provided that the "*...Athlete can establish that the Use of such a specfied substance was not intended to enhance sport performance...*"

Albumin

Other names: Albümin; Albúmina; Albumine; Albuminum.

Clinical profile: Albumin is the major protein involved in maintaining colloid osmotic pressure in the blood. Albumin solutions are used for plasma volume replacement and to restore colloid osmotic pressure. They have been used in acute hypovolaemic shock, burns, and severe acute albumin loss. Albumin is also used in neonatal hyperbilirubinaemia and as an exchange fluid in therapeutic plasmapheresis.

WADA Status: Banned in and out of competition

WADA Class: Diuretics and Other Masking Agents

Masking agents including alpha-reductase inhibitors or plasma expanders or substances with similar biological effect(s).

Preparations

Single ingredient: ***Arg.:*** Buminate; ***Austral.:*** Albumex; ***Austria:*** Albuminativ; ***Braz.:*** Albuminar; Beribumin; Blaubimax; ***Canad.:*** Plasbumin; ***Chile:*** Plasbumin; ***Denm.:*** Octalbin; ***Fin.:*** Albuminativ; Octalbin; ***Fr.:*** Octalbine; Vialebex; ***Ger.:*** Humanalbin; ***Gr.:*** Zenalb; ***Hong Kong:*** Albuminar; Albutein; Biseko; Buminate; Kamapharm; Plasbumin; ***Indon.:*** Albapure; Alburaas; Albutein; Farmin; Fimalbumin; Octalbin; Plasbumin; ***Israel:*** Albuminar; Egg Plus; ***Ital.:*** Albital; Alburex; Albutein; Plasbumin; ***Malaysia:*** Albutein; Buminate; Zenalb; ***Mex.:*** Octalbin; Vanderbumin; ***Neth.:*** Cealb; Octalbine; ***NZ:*** Albumex; ***Philipp.:*** Albumax; Albuminar; Albutein; Plasbumin; ***Pol.:*** Biseko; ***Rus.:*** Plasbumin (Плазбумин); ***S.Afr.:*** Albusol; ***Singapore:*** Albutein; Zenalb; ***Spain:*** Octalbin; Plasbumin; ***Swed.:*** Albuminativ; ***Switz.:*** Albuman; ***Thai.:*** Alburaas; Albutein; Buminate; Zenalb; ***Turk.:*** Alba; Albuman; Albuminar; Cealb; Plasbumin; Zenalb; ***UK:*** Albutein; Zenalb; ***USA:*** Albumarc; Albuminar; Albutein; Buminate; Plasbumin.

Multi-ingredient: ***Denm.:*** Pharmalgen Albumin; ***Swed.:*** Tisseel Duo Quick.

Alclometasone Dipropionate

Other names: Alclométasone, Dipropionate d'; Alclometasoni Dipropionas; Alklometasondipropionat; Alklometasonidipropionaatti; Dipropionato de alclometaso-

A

na; Sch-22219.

Алькламетазона Дипропионат

Clinical profile: Alclometasone dipropionate is a corticosteroid used topically in the treatment of various skin disorders.

WADA Status: Banned in competition

WADA Class: Glucocorticosteroids

All glucocorticosteroids are prohibited when administered orally, rectally, intravenously or intramuscularly. Their use requires a Therapeutic Use Exemption approval. Other routes of administration (intraarticular / periarticular / peritendinous / epidural / intradermal injections and inhalation) require an Abbreviated Therapeutic Use Exemption except as noted below.

Topical preparations when used for dermatological (including iontophoresis / phonophoresis), auricular, nasal, ophthalmic, buccal, gingival and perianal disorders are not prohibited and do not require any form of Therapeutic Use Exemption.

WADA Class: Specified Substances

Also listed as a specified substance.

"The prohibited List may identify specified substances which are particularly susceptible to unintentional anti-doping rule violations because of their general availability in medicinal products or which are less likely to be successfully abused as doping agents."

A doping violation involving such substances may result in a reduced sanction provided that the "*...Athlete can establish that the Use of such a specfied substance was not intended to enhance sport performance...*"

Preparations

Single ingredient: ***Cz.:*** Afloderm; ***Ger.:*** Delonal; ***Gr.:*** Lomesone; ***Hong Kong:*** Perderm; ***Indon.:*** Cloderm; Perderm; ***Irl.:*** Modrasone; ***Ital.:*** Legederm; ***Malaysia:*** Perderm; ***Mex.:*** Logoderm; ***Neth.:*** Aclosone; ***Port.:*** Miloderme; ***Rus.:*** Afloderm (Афлодерм); ***UK:*** Modrasone; ***USA:*** Aclovate; ***Venez.:*** Demiderm.

Alcohol

Other names: Aethanolum; Alcool; Alkol; Etanol; Etanol (96%); Etanol bezwodny; Etanoli; Etanolis; Éthanol; Ethanol; Ethanolum; Ethyl Alcohol.

Clinical profile: Alcohol is a bactericidal antiseptic and disinfectant with little activity against bacterial spores. It is used as a disinfectant for skin and hard surfaces, as a solvent, and as a pharmaceutical preservative. Additional indications include sclerotherapy, severe and chronic pain, and spasticity. Alcoholic beverages are widely used and abused for their effects on the CNS.

WADA Status: Banned in competition as specified below

WADA Class: Alcohol

Prohibited *In-Competition* only, in the following sports. Detection will be conducted by analysis of breath and/or blood. The doping violation threshold (haematological values) for each Federation is reported in parenthesis.

- Aeronautics (FAI) (0.20 g/L)
- Archery (FITA, IPC) (0.10 g/L)
- Automobile (FIA) (0.10 g/L)
- Boules (IPC bowls) (0.10 g/L)
- Karate (WKF) (0.10 g/L)
- Modern Pentathlon (UIPM) for disciplines involving shooting (0.10 g/L)
- Motorcycling (FIM) (0.10 g/L)
- Powerboating (UIM) (0.30 g/L)

WADA Class: Specified Substances

Also listed as a specified substance.

"The prohibited List may identify specified substances which are particularly susceptible to

A

unintentional anti-doping rule violations because of their general availability in medicinal products or which are less likely to be successfully abused as doping agents."

A doping violation involving such substances may result in a reduced sanction provided that the "...*Athlete can establish that the Use of such a specfied substance was not intended to enhance sport performance...*"

Preparations

Single ingredient: ***Austral.:*** Microshield Antimicrobial Hand Gel; ***Canad.:*** Avagard D; Biobase; Duonalc-E Mild; Instant Hand Sanitizer; One Step Hand Sanitizer; President's Choice Hand Sanitizer; Purell; ***Fr.:*** Curethyl; Optrex; Pharmadose alcool; ***Ger.:*** AHD 2000; Amphisept E; Fugaten; Klosterfrau Franzbranntwein Menthol; Sterillium Virugard; ***Indon.:*** Handy Clean; ***Malaysia:*** QuicKlean; ***Philipp.:*** AHD 2000; ***USA:*** Alcare; Bodi Line Action; Gel-Stat.

Multi-ingredient: ***Austral.:*** Dermatech Liquid; Johnsons Clean & Clear Invisible Blemish Treatment; Johnsons Clean & Clear Oil Controlling Toner; Microshield Handrub; Microshield Tincture; ***Austria:*** Dodesept Gefarbt; Dodesept N; Dodesept; Skinsept mucosa; Skinsept; ***Canad.:*** Avagard CHG; Biobase-G; Chase Kolik Gripe Water; Duonalc-E; Green Antiseptic Mouthwash & Gargle; ***Chile:*** Acnoxyl Locion Tonica; Alcolex; Listerine; Listermint Con Fluor; Oralfresh Citrus; Oralfresh Clasico; Oralfresh Menta; ***Cz.:*** Promanum N; Skinsept mucosa; Softa-Man; ***Fin.:*** Otiborin; Somanol + Ethanol; ***Fr.:*** Alco-Aloe; Aniospray 29; ***Ger.:*** Aerodesin; Autoderm Extra; Bacillol AF; Bacillol; Betaseptic; Freka-Derm; Freka-Nol; Freka-Sept 80; Hospidermin; Hospisept; Incidin Spezial; Incidin; Klosterfrau Franzbranntwein Latschenkiefer; Klosterfrau Franzbranntwein Latschenkiefer; Klosterfrau Franzbranntwein; Mucasept-A; Promanum N; Riwa Franzbranntwein; Skinsept G; Skinsept mucosa; Softa Man; Softasept N; Spitacid; ***Gr.:*** Faragel-Forte; ***Hong Kong:*** Listerine Tartar Control; Listerine; ***India:*** Daslin; Dettolin; ***Indon.:*** Allerin; Benadryl CM; Berlifed; Chlorphemin; Coricidin; Dactylen; Domeryl; Eksedryl Expectorant; Inadryl Plus; Inadryl; Koffex; Listerine Coolmint; Listerine; Neo Novapon; Nichodryl; OBH; Paradryl; ***Israel:*** Alcosept; Oxy Clean Medicated; Salisol; Septadine; Spirit Salicyl; V-Tabur; ***Ital.:*** Bemonalcool; Citroclorex; Citromed 80 and 85; Citromed Chirurgico; Citrosil Alcolico Azzuro; Citrosil Alcolico Bruno; Citrosil Alcolico Incolore; Citrosteril Strumenti; Clorexan Ferri; Eso Ferri Alcolico; Esoalcolico Incolore; Esoform Alcolico; Forbrand; Formedico; Incidin Spezial; Incidur Spray; Jodieci; Melsept Spray; Neomedil; Panseptil; Sekumatic; Simpottantacinque; Softa Man; ***Neth.:*** Softa-Man; ***Philipp.:*** BSI Medicated Spray; Dermablend Clarifying; Listerine Coolmint; Listerine Original; Zilactin; Ziladent; ***Port.:*** Promanum; ***S.Afr.:*** Clearasil Medicated Facial Cleanser; Dry & Clear Medicated Skin Cleanser; Listerine Antiseptic; Oxipor VHC; Specific Nerve Pain Remedy; ***Singapore:*** Hexodane Handrub; Listerine Cool Mint; Listerine Fresh Burst; Listerine Tartar Control; Listerine; ***Spain:*** Alcohocel; Alcohol Benzalconio; Alcohol CL Benz; Alcohol Poten; Alcohol Potenciado; Beta Alcanforado; Beta Romero; Embrocacion Gras; Farmalcohol; Linimento Naion; Menalcol; Mercrotona; ***Switz.:*** Betaseptic; Promanum N; Sclerovein; Softasept N; ***Thai.:*** Hand Joy; ***UK:*** Brushtox; Clearasil Pore Cleansing Lotion; Medi-Wipe; Oxy Cleanser; Oxy Cleanser; Oxy Duo Pads; Oxy Duo Pads; Spectrum; ***USA:*** Banadyne-3; Clearasil Double Clear; Clearasil Double Textured Pads; Lipmagik; Massengill Disposable; Massengill; Maximum Strength Anbesol; Orasol; Stri-Dex Pads; ***Venez.:*** Frixonil.

Alfatradiol

Other names: Alfatradiolum; Alpha-estradiol; Epiestradiol; 17α-Estradiol; NSC-20293.

Альфатрадиол

Clinical profile: Alfatradiol is the 17-alpha isomer of estradiol but has much weaker oestrogenic actions. It is a 5α-reductase inhibitor and is used topically for alopecia androgenetica.

WADA Status: Banned in and out of competition

WADA Class: Diuretics and Other Masking Agents

Masking agents including alpha-reductase inhibitors or plasma expanders or substances with similar biological effect(s).

WADA Class: Specified Substances

Also listed as a specified substance.

"The prohibited List may identify specified substances which are particularly susceptible to unintentional anti-doping rule violations because of their general availability in medicinal products or which are less likely to be successfully abused as doping agents."

A doping violation involving such substances may result in a reduced sanction pro-

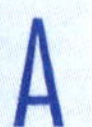

vided that the "...*Athlete can establish that the Use of such a specfied substance was not intended to enhance sport performance...*"

Preparations
Single ingredient: ***Arg.:*** Avixis; ***Ger.:*** Ell-Cranell alpha; Pantostin; ***Mex.:*** Avixis.
Multi-ingredient: ***Ger.:*** Ell-Cranell dexa.

Alfentanil Hydrochloride

Other names: Alfentaniilihydrokloridi; Alfentanil, chlorhydrate d'; Alfentanil Hidroklorür; Alfentanil-hidroklorid; Alfentanil-hydrochlorid; Alfentanilhydroklorid; Alfentanili hydrochloridum; Alfentanilio hidrochloridas; Hidrocloruro de alfentanilo; R-39209.

Альфентанила Гидрохлорид

Clinical profile: Alfentanil is a short-acting opioid analgesic related to fentanyl. It is used in surgical procedures as an analgesic and adjunct to general anaesthetics or as a primary anaesthetic. Alfentanil is also used as an analgesic and respiratory depressant in the management of mechanically ventilated patients under intensive care.

WADA Status: Banned in competition

WADA Class: Narcotics

Includes specified narcotics.

Preparations
Single ingredient: ***Arg.:*** Brevafen; ***Austral.:*** Rapifen; ***Austria:*** Rapifen; ***Belg.:*** Rapifen; ***Braz.:*** Alfast; Rapifen; ***Canad.:*** Alfenta; ***Chile:*** Rapifen; ***Cz.:*** Rapifen; ***Denm.:*** Rapifen; ***Fin.:*** Rapifen; ***Fr.:*** Rapifen; ***Ger.:*** Rapifen; ***Gr.:*** Rapifen; ***Hong Kong:*** Rapifen; ***Hung.:*** Rapifen; ***Irl.:*** Rapifen; ***Israel:*** Rapifen; ***Ital.:*** Fentalim; ***Mex.:*** Rapifen; ***Neth.:*** Rapifen; ***Norw.:*** Rapifen; ***NZ:*** Rapifen; ***S.Afr.:*** Rapifen; ***Spain:*** Fanaxal; Limifen; ***Swed.:*** Rapifen; ***Switz.:*** Rapifen; ***Turk.:*** Rapifen; ***UK:*** Rapifen; ***USA:*** Alfenta; ***Venez.:*** Rapifen.

Alprenolol

Other names: Alprénolol; Alprenololi; Alprenololum.

Альпренолол

Alprenolol Benzoate

Other names: Alprénolol, benzoate d'; Alprenololi benzoas; Benzoato de alprenolol.

Альпренолола Бензоат

Alprenolol Hydrochloride

Other names: Alprénolol, chlorhydrate d'; Alprenolol-hidroklorid; Alprenolol-hydrochlorid; Alprenololhydroklorid; Alprenololi hydrochloridum; Alprenololihydrokloridi; Alprenololio hidrochloridas; H56/28; Hidrocloruro de alprenolol.

Альпренолола Гидрохлорид

Clinical profile: Alprenolol is a non-cardioselective beta blocker that has been used in the management of hypertension, angina pectoris, and cardiac arrhythmias.

WADA Status: Banned in and out of competition as specified below

WADA Class: Beta-Blockers

Unless otherwise specified, beta-blockers are prohibited *In-Competition* only in the following sports.

- Aeronautics (FAI)

- Archery (FITA, IPC) (also prohibited *Out-of-Competition*)
- Automobile (FIA)
- Billiards (WCBS)
- Bobsleigh (FIBT)
- Boules (CMSB, IPC bowls)
- Bridge (FMB)
- Curling (WCF)
- Gymnastics (FIG)
- Motorcycling (FIM)
- Modern Pentathlon (UIPM) for disciplines involving shooting
- Nine-pin bowling (FIQ)
- Powerboating (UIM)
- Sailing (ISAF) for match race helms only
- Shooting (ISSF, IPC) (also prohibited *Out-of-Competition*)
- Skiing/Snowboarding (FIS) in ski jumping, freestyle aerials/halfpipe and snowboard halfpipe/big air
- Wrestling (FILA)

WADA Class: Specified Substances

Also listed as a specified substance.

"The prohibited List may identify specified substances which are particularly susceptible to unintentional anti-doping rule violations because of their general availability in medicinal products or which are less likely to be successfully abused as doping agents."

A doping violation involving such substances may result in a reduced sanction provided that the "*...Athlete can establish that the Use of such a specfied substance was not intended to enhance sport performance...*"

Alsactide

Other names: Alsactida; Alsactidum.

Альсактид

Clinical profile: Alsactide is a synthetic polypeptide structurally related to corticotropin. It has been used diagnostically in the investigation of adrenocortical insufficiency, and has also been used therapeutically for conditions in which corticotropin treatment is indicated.

WADA Status: Banned in and out of competition

WADA Class: Hormones and Related Substances: Corticotrophins

Includes corticotrophin or substances with a similar chemical structure or similar biological effect(s), or one of their releasing factors.

Altizide

Other names: Althiazide; Altizida; Altizidum; P-1779.

Альтизид

Clinical profile: Altizide is a thiazide diuretic used in the treatment of oedema and hypertension.

WADA Status: Banned in and out of competition

WADA Class: Diuretics and Other Masking Agents

Includes diuretics or substances with a similar chemical structure or similar biological effect(s).

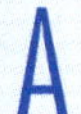

Preparations
Multi-ingredient: ***Belg.:*** Aldactazine; ***Fr.:*** Aldactazine; Practazin; Spiroctazine; ***Port.:*** Aldactazine; ***Spain:*** Aldactacine.

Amcinonide

Other names: Amcinónida; Amcinonidum; Amcinopol; CL-34699.

Амцинонид

Clinical profile: Amcinonide is a corticosteroid used topically in the treatment of various skin disorders.

WADA Status: Banned in competition

WADA Class: Glucocorticosteroids

All glucocorticosteroids are prohibited when administered orally, rectally, intravenously or intramuscularly. Their use requires a Therapeutic Use Exemption approval. Other routes of administration (intraarticular / periarticular / peritendinous / epidural / intradermal injections and inhalation) require an Abbreviated Therapeutic Use Exemption except as noted below.

Topical preparations when used for dermatological (including iontophoresis / phonophoresis), auricular, nasal, ophthalmic, buccal, gingival and perianal disorders are not prohibited and do not require any form of Therapeutic Use Exemption.

WADA Class: Specified Substances

Also listed as a specified substance.

"The prohibited List may identify specified substances which are particularly susceptible to unintentional anti-doping rule violations because of their general availability in medicinal products or which are less likely to be successfully abused as doping agents."

A doping violation involving such substances may result in a reduced sanction provided that the "*...Athlete can establish that the Use of such a specfied substance was not intended to enhance sport performance...*"

Preparations
Single ingredient: ***Belg.:*** Amicla; ***Canad.:*** Amcort; Cyclocort; ***Ger.:*** Amciderm; ***Mex.:*** Visderm H; ***Thai.:*** Amciderm.

Amezinium Metilsulfate

Other names: Ametsiniummetilsulfaatti; Amezinii Metilsulfas; Amezinium Methylsulphate; Amézinium, Métilsulfate d'; Ameziniummetilsulfat; Metilsulfato de amezinio.

Амезиния Метилсульфат

Clinical profile: Amezinium metilsulfate is a sympathomimetic used in the treatment of hypotensive states.

WADA Status: Banned in competition

WADA Class: Stimulants

Includes stimulants or substances with a similar chemical structure or similar biological effect(s).

WADA Class: Specified Substances

Also listed as a specified substance.

"The prohibited List may identify specified substances which are particularly susceptible to unintentional anti-doping rule violations because of their general availability in medicinal products or which are less likely to be successfully abused as doping agents."

A doping violation involving such substances may result in a reduced sanction pro-

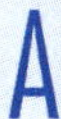

vided that the "...Athlete can establish that the Use of such a specfied substance was not intended to enhance sport performance..."

Preparations
Single ingredient: ***Belg.:*** Regulton; ***Ger.:*** Regulton; Supratonin.

Amfetamine

Other names: Amfetamiini; Amfetamin; Amfétamine; Amfetaminum; Amphetamine; Amphetaminum; Anfetamina; Racemic Desoxynorephedrine.

Амфетамин

Amfetamine Sulfate

Other names: Amfetamiinisulfaatti; Amfétamine, sulfate d'; Amfetamine Sulphate; Amfetamini sulfas; Amfetamino sulfatas; Amfetaminsulfat; Amfetamin-sulfát; Amfetamin-szulfát; Amphetamine Sulfate; Amphetamine Sulphate; Amphetamini Sulfas; Phenaminum; Phenylaminopropanum Racemicum Sulfuricum; Sulfato de anfetamina.

Амфетамина Сульфат

Clinical profile: Amfetamine is an indirect-acting sympathomimetic used as a central stimulant.

WADA Status: Banned in competition

WADA Class: Stimulants

Includes amfetamine and any optical isomers.

Preparations
Multi-ingredient: ***Belg.:*** Epipropane; ***Canad.:*** Adderall; ***USA:*** Adderall.

Amfetaminil

Other names: Amfétaminil; Amfetaminilum; Amphetaminil; Anfetaminilo.

Амфетаминил

Clinical profile: Amfetaminil has been used in the treatment of narcolepsy.

WADA Status: Banned in competition

WADA Class: Stimulants

Includes amfetaminil and any optical isomers.

Amidefrine Mesilate

Other names: 5190; Amidéfrine, Mésilate d'; Amidefrini Mesilas; Amidephrine Mesylate; Mesilato de amidefrina; MJ-5190.

Амидефрина Мезилат

Clinical profile: Amidefrine is a sympathomimetic with alpha-adrenergic activity. It is used as a nasal decongestant.

WADA Status: Banned in competition

A

WADA Class: Stimulants

Includes stimulants or substances with a similar chemical structure or similar biological effect(s).

WADA Class: Specified Substances

Also listed as a specified substance.

"The prohibited List may identify specified substances which are particularly susceptible to unintentional anti-doping rule violations because of their general availability in medicinal products or which are less likely to be successfully abused as doping agents."

A doping violation involving such substances may result in a reduced sanction provided that the "*...Athlete can establish that the Use of such a specfied substance was not intended to enhance sport performance...*"

Preparations
Single ingredient: ***Austria:*** Fentrinol.

Amiloride Hydrochloride

Other names: Amilorid Hidroklorür; Amilorid hydrochlorid dihydrát; Amiloride, chlorhydrate d'; Amilorid-hidroklorid; Amiloridhydroklorid; Amiloridi hydrochloridum; Amiloridi Hydrochloridum Dihydricum; Amiloridihydrokloridi; Amilorido hidrochloridas; Amilorydu chlorowodorek; Amipramizide; Cloridrato de Amilorida; Hidrocloruro de amilorida; MK-870.

Амилорида Гидрохлорид

Clinical profile: Amiloride hydrochloride is a weak diuretic with potassium-sparing properties. It is used mainly as an adjunct to thiazide and loop diuretics in the treatment of oedema and hypertension.

WADA Status: Banned in and out of competition

WADA Class: Diuretics and Other Masking Agents

Includes diuretics or substances with a similar chemical structure or similar biological effect(s).

Preparations
Single ingredient: ***Austral.:*** Kaluril; Midamor; ***Austria:*** Midamor; ***Canad.:*** Midamor; ***Cz.:*** Amiclaran; ***Denm.:*** Nirulid; ***Fr.:*** Modamide; ***NZ:*** Midamor; ***UK:*** Amilamont; ***USA:*** Midamor.

Multi-ingredient: ***Arg.:*** Diflux; Diur Pot; Diurex A; Errolon A; Hidrenox A; Lasiride; Moduretic; Nuriban A; Plenacor D; Ren-Ur; Vericordin Compuesto; ***Austral.:*** Amizide; Moduretic; ***Austria:*** Aldoretic; Amiloral/HCT; Amiloretik; Amilorid comp; Amilostad HCT; Lanuretic; Loradur; Moducrin; Moduretic; ***Belg.:*** Co-Amiloride; Frusamil; Moduretic; ***Braz.:*** Amiretic; Diupress; Diurisa; Moduretic; ***Canad.:*** Apo-Amilzide; Gen-Amilazide; Moduret; Novamilor; Nu-Amilzide; ***Chile:*** Furdiuren; Hidrium; Hidropid; ***Cz.:*** Amicloton; Amilorid/HCT; Apo-Amilzide; Limorid; Loradur; Moduretic; Rhefluin; ***Denm.:*** Amilco; Buram; Frusamil; Sparkal; ***Fin.:*** Amitrid; Diuramin; Diurex; Miloride; Moduretic; Sparkal; ***Fr.:*** Logirene; Moducren; Moduretic; ***Ger.:*** Amilocomp beta; Amiloretik; Amilorid comp; Amilorid/HCT; Diaphal; Diursan; Moducrin; Moduretik; Tensoflux; ***Gr.:*** Frumil; Ividol; Moduretic; Tiaden; ***Hong Kong:*** Amithiazide; Apo-Amilzide; Moducren; Moduretic; Navispare; Sefaretic; ***Hung.:*** Amilorid Comp; Amilozid-B; ***India:*** Biduret; Frumil; Hipres-D; ***Indon.:*** Lorinid; ***Irl.:*** Buram; Fru-Co; Frumil; Moducren; Moduret; ***Israel:*** Kaluril; ***Ital.:*** Moduretic; ***Malaysia:*** Ami-Hydrotride; Amizide; Apo-Amilzide; ***Mex.:*** Moduretic; ***Neth.:*** Moduretic; ***Norw.:*** Moduretic; Normorix; ***NZ:*** Amizide; Frumil; ***Pol.:*** Tialorid; ***Port.:*** Aldoretic; Amiloride Composto; Diurene; Moducren; Moduretic; ***S.Afr.:*** Adco-Retic; Amiloretic; Betaretic; Hexaretic; Moducren; Moduretic; Servatrin; ***Singapore:*** Apo-Amilzide; ***Spain:*** Ameride; Diuzine; Kalten; ***Swed.:*** Amiloferm; Moduretic; Normorix; Sparkal; ***Switz.:*** Amiloride/HCTZ; Comilorid; Ecodurex; Escoretic; Grodurex; Kalten; Moducren; Moduretic; Rhefluin; ***Thai.:*** Bilduretic; Hydrozide Plus; Hyperretic; Miretic; Moduretic; Moure-M; Poli-Uretic; Renase; Sefaretic; ***Turk.:*** Moduretic;

UK: Amil-Co; Aridil; Burinex A; Fru-Co; Frumil; Kalten; Komil; Moducren; Moduret; Moduretic; Navispare; *USA:* Moduretic; *Venez.:* Furdiuren; Moduretic.

Aminoglutethimide

Other names: Aminoglutethimid; Aminoglutéthimide; Aminoglutethimidum; Aminoglutetimid; Aminoglutetimida; Aminoglutetimidas; Aminoglutetimidi; Ba-16038.

Аминоглутетимид

Clinical profile: Aminoglutethimide is an aromatase inhibitor related to glutethimide which has been used in the treatment of advanced breast and prostate cancer and in Cushing's syndrome.

WADA Status: Banned in and out of competition

WADA Class: Hormone Antagonists and Modulators
Includes aromatase inhibitors.

Preparations
Single ingredient: *Austral.:* Cytadren; *Hong Kong:* Orimetene; *Rus.:* Mamomit (Мамомит).

Amiphenazole Hydrochloride

Other names: Amiphénazol, Chlorhydrate d'; Amiphenazole Chloride; Amiphenazoli Hydrochloridum; Hidrocloruro de amifenazol.

Амифеназола Гидрохлорид

Clinical profile: Amiphenazole has been used as a respiratory stimulant.

WADA Status: Banned in competition

WADA Class: Stimulants
Includes amiphenazole and any optical isomers.

Ammonium Phosphate

Other names: 545 (ammonium polyphosphates); Amonowy wodorofosforan; Diammonium Hydrogen Phosphate; Dibasic Ammonium Phosphate; Fosfato de amonio.

Clinical profile: Ammonium phosphate was formerly used as a diuretic. It may be used as a buffering agent in pharmaceutical preparations. Ammonium biphosphate (monobasic ammonium phosphate) has been used to acidify urine and as a phosphate supplement.

WADA Status: Banned in and out of competition

WADA Class: Diuretics and Other Masking Agents
Includes diuretics or substances with a similar chemical structure or similar biological effect(s).

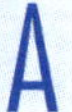

Preparations
Multi-ingredient: ***Fr.:*** Phosphore Medifa; ***Pol.:*** Phosphor.

Amosulalol Hydrochloride

Other names: Amosulalol, Chlorhydrate d'; Amosulaloli Hydrochloridum; Hidrocloruro de amosulalol; YM-09538.

Амосулалола Гидрохлорид

Clinical profile: Amosulalol is a beta blocker that also has alpha-blocking activity. It has been used in the management of hypertension.

WADA Status: Banned in and out of competition as specified below

WADA Class: Beta-Blockers

Unless otherwise specified, beta-blockers are prohibited *In-Competition* only in the following sports.

- Aeronautics (FAI)
- Archery (FITA, IPC) (also prohibited *Out-of-Competition*)
- Automobile (FIA)
- Billiards (WCBS)
- Bobsleigh (FIBT)
- Boules (CMSB, IPC bowls)
- Bridge (FMB)
- Curling (WCF)
- Gymnastics (FIG)
- Motorcycling (FIM)
- Modern Pentathlon (UIPM) for disciplines involving shooting
- Nine-pin bowling (FIQ)
- Powerboating (UIM)
- Sailing (ISAF) for match race helms only
- Shooting (ISSF, IPC) (also prohibited *Out-of-Competition*)
- Skiing/Snowboarding (FIS) in ski jumping, freestyle aerials/halfpipe and snowboard halfpipe/big air
- Wrestling (FILA)

WADA Class: Specified Substances

Also listed as a specified substance.

"The prohibited List may identify specified substances which are particularly susceptible to unintentional anti-doping rule violations because of their general availability in medicinal products or which are less likely to be successfully abused as doping agents."

A doping violation involving such substances may result in a reduced sanction provided that the "*...Athlete can establish that the Use of such a specfied substance was not intended to enhance sport performance...*"

Anastrozole

Other names: Anastrotsoli; Anastrozol; Anastrozolum; ICI-D1033; ZD-1033.

Анастрозол

Clinical profile: Anastrozole is a selective nonsteroidal aromatase inhibitor that is used in the treatment of breast cancer.

WADA Status: Banned in and out of competition

WADA Class: Hormone Antagonists and Modulators

Includes aromatase inhibitors.

Preparations
Single ingredient: ***Arg.:*** Anaskebir; Anastraze; Anebol; Arimidex; Aromenal; Distalene; Gon-

donar; Leprofen; Pantestone; Puricap; Trozolite; ***Austral.:*** Arimidex; ***Austria:*** Arimidex; ***Belg.:*** Arimidex; ***Braz.:*** Arimidex; ***Canad.:*** Arimidex; ***Chile:*** Arimidex; Trozolet; ***Cz.:*** Arimidex; ***Denm.:*** Arimidex; ***Fin.:*** Arimidex; ***Fr.:*** Arimidex; ***Ger.:*** Arimidex; ***Gr.:*** Arimidex; ***Hong Kong:*** Arimidex; ***Hung.:*** Arimidex; ***India:*** Altraz; Armotraz; ***Indon.:*** Arimidex; ***Irl.:*** Arimidex; ***Israel:*** Arimidex; ***Ital.:*** Arimidex; ***Malaysia:*** Arimidex; ***Mex.:*** Arimidex; ***Neth.:*** Arimidex; ***Norw.:*** Arimidex; ***NZ:*** Arimidex; ***Philipp.:*** Arimidex; ***Pol.:*** Arimidex; Atrozol; ***Port.:*** Arimidex; ***Rus.:*** Arimidex (Аримидекс); ***S.Afr.:*** Arimidex; ***Singapore:*** Arimidex; ***Spain:*** Arimidex; ***Swed.:*** Arimidex; ***Switz.:*** Arimidex; ***Thai.:*** Arimidex; ***Turk.:*** Arimidex; ***UK:*** Arimidex; ***USA:*** Arimidex; ***Venez.:*** Arimidex; Trozolet.

Androstanolone

Other names: Androstanolo; Androstanolon; Androstanolona; Androstanoloni; Androstanolonum; Dihidrotestosterona; Dihydrotestosterone; Estanolona; Stanolon; Stanolone.

Андростанолон

Clinical profile: Androstanolone has anabolic and androgenic properties. It is applied topically for male hypogonadism and gynaecomastia, and for lichen sclerosus in both men and women.

WADA Status: Banned in and out of competition

WADA Class: Anabolic; Androgenic Steroids (endogenous)

Includes endogenous anabolic androgenic steroids or specified metabolites or isomers.

Preparations
Single ingredient: ***Belg.:*** Andractim; ***Fr.:*** Andractim.

Androstenedione

Other names: Androstenodiona.

Clinical profile: Androstenedione is a naturally occurring precursor of androgens and oestrogens. It has been employed as hormone replacement for men.

WADA Status: Banned in and out of competition

WADA Class: Anabolic; Androgenic Steroids (endogenous)

Includes endogenous anabolic androgenic steroids or specified metabolites or isomers.

Preparations
Multi-ingredient: ***Thai.:*** Metharmon-F.

Aniracetam

Other names: Aniracétam; Aniracetamum; Ro-13-5057.

Анирацетам

Clinical profile: Aniracetam is a nootropic drug that has been tried in senile dementia.

WADA Status: Banned in competition

WADA Class: Stimulants

Includes stimulants or substances with a similar chemical structure or similar biological effect(s).

A

WADA Class: Specified Substances

Also listed as a specified substance.

"The prohibited List may identify specified substances which are particularly susceptible to unintentional anti-doping rule violations because of their general availability in medicinal products or which are less likely to be successfully abused as doping agents."

A doping violation involving such substances may result in a reduced sanction provided that the "*...Athlete can establish that the Use of such a specfied substance was not intended to enhance sport performance...*"

Preparations
Single ingredient: ***Arg.:*** Aniran; Pergamid; ***Gr.:*** Memodrin; Referan; ***Ital.:*** Ampamet.

Arbutamine Hydrochloride

Other names: Arbutamine, Chlorhydrate d'; Arbutamini Hydrochloridum; GP-2-121-3 (arbutamine or arbutamine hydrochloride); Hidrocloruro de arbutamina.
Арбутамина Гидрохлорид

Clinical profile: Arbutamine is a sympathomimetic with beta-agonist properties and has been used for cardiac stress testing.

WADA Status: Banned in competition

WADA Class: Stimulants

Includes stimulants or substances with a similar chemical structure or similar biological effect(s).

WADA Class: Specified Substances

Also listed as a specified substance.

"The prohibited List may identify specified substances which are particularly susceptible to unintentional anti-doping rule violations because of their general availability in medicinal products or which are less likely to be successfully abused as doping agents."

A doping violation involving such substances may result in a reduced sanction provided that the "*...Athlete can establish that the Use of such a specfied substance was not intended to enhance sport performance...*"

Arformoterol Tartrate

Other names: Arformotérol, Tartrate d'; Arformoteroli Tartras; *R,R*-Formoterol Tartrate; Tartrato de arformoterol.
Арформотерола Тартрат

Clinical profile: Arformoterol tartrate is a long-acting selective beta$_2$-adrenoceptor agonist used for its bronchodilator properties in chronic obstructive pulmonary disease. Arformoterol is the *R,R*-enantiomer of the beta$_2$ agonist formoterol.

WADA Status: Banned in and out of competition

WADA Class: Beta-2 Agonists

Includes beta-2 agonists or their isomers.

WADA Class: Specified Substances

Also listed as a specified substance.

"The prohibited List may identify specified substances which are particularly susceptible to unintentional anti-doping rule violations because of their general availability in medicinal products or which are less likely to be successfully abused as doping agents."

A doping violation involving such substances may result in a reduced sanction pro-

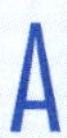

vided that the "*...Athlete can establish that the Use of such a specfied substance was not intended to enhance sport performance...*"

Preparations
Single ingredient: ***USA:*** Brovana.

Arginine

Other names: Arg; Arginiini; Arginin; Arginina; Argininas; L-Arginine; Argininum; R. Аргинин

Arginine Aspartate

Other names: Arginiiniaspartaatti; Arginina, aspartato de; Argininaspartat; Arginin-aspartát; Arginine, aspartate d'; Arginini aspartas; Arginino aspartatas; Aspargininum.

Arginine Glutamate

Other names: Arginine, Glutamate d'; Arginini Glutamas; Glutamato de arginina. Аргинина Глутамат

Arginine Hydrochloride

Other names: Arginiinihydrokloridi; Arginine, chlorhydrate d'; L-Arginine Monohydrochloride; Arginin-hidroklorid; Arginin-hydrochlorid; Argininhydroklorid; Arginini hydrochloridum; Arginino hidrochloridas; Hidrocloruro de arginina. Аргинина Гидрохлорид

Clinical profile: Arginine is a basic amino acid which is essential for infant growth. It is used as a dietary supplement. Arginine stimulates the release of growth hormone by the pituitary gland and may be used for the evaluation of growth disorders. It is also used in certain conditions accompanied by hyperammonaemia, and as an acidifying agent in severe metabolic alkalosis. It has been used in forced acid diuresis to hasten drug elimination after overdose.

WADA Status: Banned in and out of competition

WADA Class: Hormones and Related Substances: Growth Hormone, Insulin-like Growth Factors, Mechano Growth Factors
Includes growth hormone or insulin-like growth factors or mechano growth factor or substances with a similar chemical structure or similar biological effect(s), or one of their releasing factors.

Preparations
Single ingredient: ***Arg.:*** Laclorene; ***Austria:*** Sangenor; ***Braz.:*** Reforgan; Targifor; ***Fr.:*** Dynamisan; Eucol; Pargine; Sargenor; Tiadilon; ***Ital.:*** Bioarginina; Dynamisan; Sargenor; ***Port.:*** Asparten; Bio-Energol Plus; Sargenor; ***Spain:*** Potenciator; Sargenor; Sargisthene; Sorbenor; ***Switz.:*** Dynamisan; ***USA:*** R-Gene.
Multi-ingredient: ***Arg.:*** Acrea; Holomagnesio Vital; ***Austria:*** Leberinfusion; Rocmaline; ***Braz.:*** Dinavital C; Ornihepat; Ornitargin; Targifor C; ***Chile:*** Ureadin 30; ***Cz.:*** Citrargine; ***Fr.:*** Arginotri-B; Fastenyl; Hepagrume; Hepargitol; Rocmaline; Sargenor a la Vitamine C; ***Hung.:*** Glutarsin E; ***Indon.:*** Sirec; ***Ital.:*** Calciofix; Ipoazotal Complex; Isoram; Linfoiodine; Sargenor Plus; Somatron; ***Spain:*** Dynamogen; ***Switz.:*** Activital Forte; Arginotri-B; Vitasprint Complex.

Armodafinil

Other names: Armodafinilo; Armodafinilum; CEP-10953; CRL-40982. Армодафинил

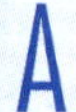

Clinical profile: Armodafinil is a central stimulant used in the treatment of excessive daytime sleepiness associated with the narcoleptic syndrome, obstructive sleep apnoea, and shift-work sleep disorder.

WADA Status: Banned in competition

WADA Class: Stimulants

Includes stimulants or substances with a similar chemical structure or similar biological effect(s).

WADA Class: Specified Substances

Also listed as a specified substance.

"The prohibited List may identify specified substances which are particularly susceptible to unintentional anti-doping rule violations because of their general availability in medicinal products or which are less likely to be successfully abused as doping agents."

A doping violation involving such substances may result in a reduced sanction provided that the "*...Athlete can establish that the Use of such a specfied substance was not intended to enhance sport performance...*"

Preparations
Single ingredient: ***USA:*** Nuvigil.

Arotinolol Hydrochloride

Other names: Arotinolol, Chlorhydrate d'; Arotinololi Hydrochloridum; Hidrocloruro de arotinolol; S-596.

Аротинолола Гидрохлорид

Clinical profile: Arotinolol is a non-cardioselective beta blocker that also has alpha$_1$-blocking activity. It is used in the management of hypertension, angina pectoris, cardiac arhythmias, and essential tremor.

WADA Status: Banned in and out of competition as specified below

WADA Class: Beta-Blockers

Unless otherwise specified, beta-blockers are prohibited *In-Competition* only in the following sports.

- Aeronautics (FAI)
- Archery (FITA, IPC) (also prohibited *Out-of-Competition*)
- Automobile (FIA)
- Billiards (WCBS)
- Bobsleigh (FIBT)
- Boules (CMSB, IPC bowls)
- Bridge (FMB)
- Curling (WCF)
- Gymnastics (FIG)
- Motorcycling (FIM)
- Modern Pentathlon (UIPM) for disciplines involving shooting
- Nine-pin bowling (FIQ)
- Powerboating (UIM)
- Sailing (ISAF) for match race helms only
- Shooting (ISSF, IPC) (also prohibited *Out-of-Competition*)
- Skiing/Snowboarding (FIS) in ski jumping, freestyle aerials/halfpipe and snowboard halfpipe/big air
- Wrestling (FILA)

WADA Class: Specified Substances

Also listed as a specified substance.

"The prohibited List may identify specified substances which are particularly susceptible to unintentional anti-doping rule violations because of their general availability in medicinal products or which are less likely to be successfully abused as doping agents."

A doping violation involving such substances may result in a reduced sanction pro-

vided that the "*...Athlete can establish that the Use of such a specfied substance was not intended to enhance sport performance...*"

Preparations
Single ingredient: ***Jpn:*** Almarl.

A

Atenolol

Other names: Aténolol; Atenololi; Atenololis; Atenololum; ICI-66082.
Атенолол

Clinical profile: Atenolol is a cardioselective beta blocker used in the management of hypertension, angina pectoris, cardiac arrhythmias, and myocardial infarction. It may also be used in the prophylactic treatment of migraine.

WADA Status: Banned in and out of competition as specified below

WADA Class: Beta-Blockers

Unless otherwise specified, beta-blockers are prohibited *In-Competition* only in the following sports.

- Aeronautics (FAI)
- Archery (FITA, IPC) (also prohibited *Out-of-Competition*)
- Automobile (FIA)
- Billiards (WCBS)
- Bobsleigh (FIBT)
- Boules (CMSB, IPC bowls)
- Bridge (FMB)
- Curling (WCF)
- Gymnastics (FIG)
- Motorcycling (FIM)
- Modern Pentathlon (UIPM) for disciplines involving shooting
- Nine-pin bowling (FIQ)
- Powerboating (UIM)
- Sailing (ISAF) for match race helms only
- Shooting (ISSF, IPC) (also prohibited *Out-of-Competition*)
- Skiing/Snowboarding (FIS) in ski jumping, freestyle aerials/halfpipe and snowboard halfpipe/big air
- Wrestling (FILA)

WADA Class: Specified Substances

Also listed as a specified substance.

"*The prohibited List may identify specified substances which are particularly susceptible to unintentional anti-doping rule violations because of their general availability in medicinal products or which are less likely to be successfully abused as doping agents.*"

A doping violation involving such substances may result in a reduced sanction provided that the "*...Athlete can establish that the Use of such a specfied substance was not intended to enhance sport performance...*"

Preparations
Single ingredient: ***Arg.:*** Atel; Atenoblock; Atenovit; Cardioblock; Corpaz; Fabotenol; Felobits; Ilaten; Myocord; Plenacor; Prenormine; Telvodin; Tensilol; Tozolden; Vericordin; ***Austral.:*** Anselol; Atehexal; Noten; Tenormin; Tensig; ***Austria:*** Arcablock; Atehexal; Atenolan; Betasyn; Tenormin; ***Belg.:*** Atenotop; Docateno; Tenormin; ***Braz.:*** Ablok; Angipress; Atecard; Ateneo; Atenobal; Atenol; Atenolab; Atenopress; Atenorm; Atenuol; Atepress; Biotenor; Ditenol; Neotenol; Plenacor; Sifnolol; ***Canad.:*** Apo-Atenol; Novo-Atenol; Nu-Atenol; Tenormin; ***Chile:*** Betacar; Grifotenol; Labotensil; ***Cz.:*** Apo-Atenol; Ateblocor; Atehexal; Atenobene; Catenol; Corotenol; Tenormin; ***Denm.:*** Atenet; Atenodan; Atenor; Tenormin; Uniloc; ***Fin.:*** Atenblock; Atenol; Tenoblock; Tenoprin; ***Fr.:*** Betatop; Tenormine; ***Ger.:*** Ate Lich; Atebeta; Atehexal; Ateno; Atenogamma; Cuxanorm; Jenatenol; Juvental; Tenormin; ***Gr.:*** Adenamin; Azectol; Blocotenol; Fealin; Mesonex; Neocardon; Synarome; Tenormin; Umoder; ***Hong Kong:*** Adoll; Antipressan; Apo-Atenol; CP-Atenol; Hypernol; Lo-Ten; Martenol; Normaten; Nortelol; Oraday; Tenormin; Ternolol; Tredol; Vascoten; Velorin; ***Hung.:*** Atenobene; Atenomel; Blokium; Prinorm; ***India:*** Aten; Beta; Beten; Cadpres; Hipres; Lonol; Teno; Tenolol; Tenormin; ***Indon.:*** Betablok; Farnormin; Hiblok; Internolol; Tenblok; Tenormin; Tensinorm; Zumablok; ***Irl.:*** Amolin; Atecor; Ateni; Atenogen; Atenomel; Tenormin; Trantalol; ***Israel:*** Normalol; Normiten; ***Ital.:*** Atenol; Atermin; Seles Beta;

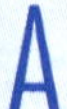

Tenomax; Tenormin; ***Malaysia:*** Apo-Atenol; Loten; Normaten; Noten; Oraday; Ranlol; Tenormin; Ternolol; Urosin; Vascoten; ***Mex.:*** Atenol; Atoken; Biofilen; Blotex; Min-T; Nosbal; Tenormin; Trebanol; ***Neth.:*** Tenormin; ***Norw.:*** Tenormin; Uniloc; ***NZ:*** Lo-Ten; ***Philipp.:*** Atestad; Cardioten; Durabeta; Tenor-Bloc; Tenormin; Tenostat; Tensimin; Therabloc; Velorin; ***Pol.:*** Normocard; ***Port.:*** Ancoren; Blokium; Tenormin; Tessifol; ***Rus.:*** Atenolan (Атенолан); Betacard (Бетакард); Catenol (Катенол); Hypoten (Хайпотен); Tenolol (Тенолол); ***S.Afr.:*** Atenoblok; Hexa-Blok; Ten-Bloka; Tenormin; Venapulse; ***Singapore:*** Apo-Atenol; Hypernol; Normaten; Noten; Prenolol; Tenolol; Tenormin; Vascoten; ***Spain:*** Blokium; Neatenol; Tanser; Tenormin; ***Swed.:*** Tenormin; ***Switz.:*** Atenil; Cardaxen; Selobloc; Tenormin; ***Thai.:*** Atcard; Atenol; Coratol; Nolol; Nortelol; Oraday; Preloc; Prenolol; Tenocor; Tenol; Tenolol; Tenormin; Tetalin; Vascoten; Velorin; ***Turk.:*** Nortan; Tensidif; Tensinor; ***UAE:*** Tensotin; ***UK:*** Antipressan; Atenix; Tenormin; ***USA:*** Tenormin; ***Venez.:*** Beloc; Blokium; Ritmilan; Tenormin.

Multi-ingredient: ***Arg.:*** Plenacor D; Prenoretic; Vericordin Compuesto; ***Austria:*** Arcablock comp; Atenolan comp; Atenolol comp; Beta-Adalat; Nif-Ten; Polinorm; Tenoretic; ***Belg.:*** Tenif; Tenoretic; ***Braz.:*** Ablok Plus; Angipress CD; Atenoclor; Atenoric; Atenuol CRT; Nifelat; Tenoretic; ***Canad.:*** Apo-Atenidone; Tenoretic; ***Cz.:*** Atedon; Atenolol Compositum; Tenoretic; ***Denm.:*** Tenidon; Tenoretic; ***Fin.:*** Nif-Ten; ***Fr.:*** Beta-Adalate; Tenordate; Tenoretic; ***Ger.:*** Ate Lich comp; Atehexal comp; Atel; AteNif beta; Ateno comp; Atenogamma comp; Atenolol AL comp; Atenolol comp; Bresben; Diu-Atenolol; Nif-Ten; Nifatenol; Teneretic; TRI-Normin; ***Gr.:*** Chlotenor; Obosan; Tenoretic; Typofen; ***Hong Kong:*** Nif-Ten; Target; Tenoret; Tenoretic; ***Hung.:*** Blokium Diu; ***India:*** Amdepin-AT; Amlopres AT; Amlostat-AT; Cardif Beta; Cardules Plus; Depten; Hipres-D; Nifetolol; Presolar; Tenochek; Tenoclor; Tenofed; Tenolol-AM; Tenoric; ***Indon.:*** Nif-Ten; Tenoret; Tenoretic; ***Irl.:*** Atecor CT; Atenetic; Beta-Adalat; Nif-Ten; Tenoret; Tenoretic; ***Ital.:*** Atenigron; Atinorm; Carmian; Clortanol; Diube; Eupres; Igroseles; Mixer; Nif-Ten; Nor-Pa; Normopress; Target; Tenoretic; ***Malaysia:*** Tenoret; Tenoretic; ***Mex.:*** Plenacor; Tenoretic; ***Neth.:*** Tenoretic; ***Philipp.:*** Nif-Ten; Tenoretic; ***Port.:*** Blokium Diu; Tenoretic; ***Rus.:*** Atehexal Compositum (Атегексал Композитум); Tenochek (Теночек); Tenoric (Тенорик); Tenorox (Тенорокс); ***S.Afr.:*** Adco-Loten; Tenchlor; Tenoretic; ***Singapore:*** Beta Nicardia; Nif-Ten; Nifetex; Tenoret; Tenoretic; ***Spain:*** Blokium Diu; Kalten; Neatenol Diu; Neatenol Diuvas; Normopresil; Tenoretic; ***Switz.:*** Atedurex; Beta-Adalat; Cardaxen plus; Cotenolol-Neo; Kalten; Nif-Atenil; Nif-Ten; Tenoretic; ***Turk.:*** Tenoretic; ***UK:*** AtenixCo; Beta-Adalat; Kalten; Tenchlor; Tenif; Tenoret; Tenoretic; Totaretic; ***USA:*** Tenoretic; ***Venez.:*** Blokiuret; Tenoretic.

Azosemide

Other names: Azosemida; Azosémide; Azosemidum; BM-02001; Ple-1053.
Азосемид

Clinical profile: Azosemide is a loop diuretic that has been used in the management of oedema.

WADA Status: Banned in and out of competition

WADA Class: Diuretics and Other Masking Agents

Includes diuretics or substances with a similar chemical structure or similar biological effect(s).

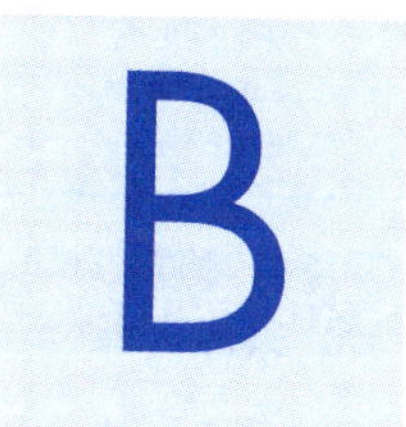

Bambuterol Hydrochloride

Other names: Bambutérol, chlorhydrate de; Bambuterol-hidroklorid; Bambuterol-hydrochlorid; Bambuterolhydroklorid; Bambuteroli hydrochloridum; Bambuterolihydrokloridi; Bambuterolio hidrochloridas; Hidrocloruro de bambuterol; KWD-2183.

Бамбутерола Гидрохлорид

Clinical profile: Bambuterol is a sympathomimetic with bronchodilator activity. It is a prodrug of terbutaline and is used in the management of diseases with persistent reversible airways obstruction such as chronic asthma or chronic obstructive pulmonary disease.

WADA Status: Banned in and out of competition

WADA Class: Beta-2 Agonists

Includes beta-2 agonists or their isomers.

WADA Class: Specified Substances

Also listed as a specified substance.

"The prohibited List may identify specified substances which are particularly susceptible to unintentional anti-doping rule violations because of their general availability in medicinal products or which are less likely to be successfully abused as doping agents."

A doping violation involving such substances may result in a reduced sanction provided that the "*...Athlete can establish that the Use of such a specfied substance was not intended to enhance sport performance...*"

Preparations

Single ingredient: ***Austria:*** Bambec; ***Braz.:*** Bambec; ***Cz.:*** Bambec; ***Denm.:*** Bambec; ***Fr.:*** Oxeol; ***Ger.:*** Bambec; ***India:*** Bambudil; ***Malaysia:*** Bambec; ***Norw.:*** Bambec; ***NZ:*** Bambec; ***Philipp.:*** Bambec; ***Singapore:*** Bambec; ***Spain:*** Bambec; ***Swed.:*** Bambec; ***Thai.:*** Bambec; ***UK:*** Bambec.

Multi-ingredient: ***India:*** Montair Plus.

Bazedoxifene Acetate

Other names: Acetato de bazedoxifeno; Bazédoxifène, Acétate de; Bazedoxifeni Acetas; WAY-140424; WAY-TSE-424.

Базедоксифена Ацетат

Clinical profile: Bazedoxifene acetate is a selective oestrogen receptor modulator under investigation with conjugated oestrogens in the management of menopausal vasomotor symptoms and osteoporosis.

Beclometasone Dipropionate

WADA Status: Banned in and out of competition

WADA Class: Hormone Antagonists and Modulators

Includes selective estrogen receptor modulators.

B

Beclometasone Dipropionate

Other names: Béclométasone, dipropionate de; Beclometasoni dipropionas; Beclometasoni Diproprionas; Beclomethasone Dipropionate; Beklometasondipropionat; Beklometason-dipropionát; Beklometasonidipropionaatti; Beklometazon Dipropiyonat; Beklometazon-diproprionát; Beklometazono dipropionatas; Beklometazonu dipropionian; 9α-Chloro-16β-methylprednisolone Dipropionate; Dipropionato de beclometasona; Sch-18020W.

Беклометазона Дипропионат

Clinical profile: Beclometasone dipropionate is a glucocorticoid corticosteroid used by inhalation in the management of asthma. It is also used as a nasal spray in the prophylaxis and treatment of allergic rhinitis, and applied topically in the treatment of various skin disorders.

WADA Status: Banned in competition

WADA Class: Glucocorticosteroids

All glucocorticosteroids are prohibited when administered orally, rectally, intravenously or intramuscularly. Their use requires a Therapeutic Use Exemption approval. Other routes of administration (intraarticular / periarticular / peritendinous / epidural / intradermal injections and inhalation) require an Abbreviated Therapeutic Use Exemption except as noted below.

Topical preparations when used for dermatological (including iontophoresis / phonophoresis), auricular, nasal, ophthalmic, buccal, gingival and perianal disorders are not prohibited and do not require any form of Therapeutic Use Exemption.

WADA Class: Specified Substances

Also listed as a specified substance.

"The prohibited List may identify specified substances which are particularly susceptible to unintentional anti-doping rule violations because of their general availability in medicinal products or which are less likely to be successfully abused as doping agents."

A doping violation involving such substances may result in a reduced sanction provided that the "*...Athlete can establish that the Use of such a specfied substance was not intended to enhance sport performance...*"

Preparations

Single ingredient: ***Arg.:*** Airbeclosona; Menaderm Simple; Propavent; Rectomenaderm; Rinosol; ***Austral.:*** Aldecin; Beconase; Becotide; Qvar; ***Austria:*** Aerocortin; Beclomet; Beconase; Becotide; Clenil; ***Belg.:*** Beclometatop; Beclophar; Beconase; Qvar; ***Braz.:*** Beclosol; Clenil; Miflasona; ***Canad.:*** Gen-Beclo; Propaderm; Qvar; Rivanase; ***Chile:*** Beclosema; Destap; Filair; Flumates; ***Cz.:*** Aldecin; Beclazone; Becloforte; Beclomet; Becodisks; Beconase; Becotide; Clenil; Ecobec; Miflason; Nasobec; ***Denm.:*** AeroBec; Beclomet; Beconase; ***Fin.:*** AeroBec; Beclomet; Beclonasal; Beconase; ***Fr.:*** Asmabec; Beclo-Rhino; Beclojet; Beclone; Beclospin; Beconase; Becotide; Bemedrex; Ecobec; Humex Rhume des Foins; Miflasone; Nexxair; Prolair; Qvar; ***Ger.:*** AeroBec; Beclo; Beclobreathe; Beclohexal; Beclomet; Beclorhinol; Beclotumant; Beconase Aquosum; Bronchocort; Junik; ratioAllerg; Rhinivict; Sanasthmax; Sanasthmyl; Ventolair; ***Gr.:*** Becolex; Bidiclin; Clenil Forte Jet; Clenil Rino; Qvar; Respocort; Rinosol; ***Hong Kong:*** Beclate; Beclazone; Becodisks; Beconase; Becotide; Cycloson; Nasobec; Qvar; ***Hung.:*** Beclonasal; ***India:*** Beclate; ***Indon.:*** Beclomet; Beconase; Becotide; Cleniderm; ***Irl.:*** Asmabec; Beclazone; Beclo-Rhino; Beconase; Becotide; Nasobec; Qvar; ***Israel:*** Becloforte; Rhinocort; Viarex; ***Ital.:*** Becotide; Clenil; Clenilexx; Clipper; Klostenal; Menaderm Simplex; Prontinal; Rino Clenil; Topster; Turbinal; ***Jpn:*** Propaderm; Rhinocort; Salcoat; ***Malaysia:*** Atomase; Beclomet; Beconase; Qvar; ***Mex.:*** Beclazone; Beconase; Becotide; Dobipro; Riferina; ***Neth.:*** Aldecin; Beclodin; Becloforte; Beconase; Becotide; Clenil; Qvar; Viarin; ***Norw.:*** AeroBec; Beclomet; Becotide; ***NZ:*** Alanase; Atomase; Beclazone; Beconase Hayfever; Qvar; Respocort; ***Philipp.:*** Qvar; ***Pol.:*** Becodisk; Cortare; Nasobec; ***Port.:*** Aldecina; Beclotaide; ***Rus.:*** Aldecin (Альдецин); Beclazone (Беклазон); Becloforte

(Беклофорте); Beclojet (Беклоджет); Becodisk (Бекодиск); Becotide (Бекотид); Clenil (Кленил); Nasobec (Насобек); ***S.Afr.:*** Beclate; Becloforte; Beconase; Becotide; Qvar; Ventnaze; ***Singapore:*** Beclo Asma; Beclomet; Decomit; ***Spain:*** Beclo Asma; Beclo Rino; Becloenema; Becloforte; Beclomet; Beclosona; Beconase; Becotide; Dereme; Menaderm Simple; Recto Menaderm NF; ***Swed.:*** AeroBec; Beclomet; Becotide; ***Switz.:*** BECeco; Beclonarin; Becodisk; Beconase; Beconasol; ***Thai.:*** Atomase; Beclomet; Beconase; Bemase; Clenil; Rino Clenil; ***Turk.:*** Becloforte; Becodisks; Becotide; Beklamet; Beklazon; Filair; ***UAE:*** Beclohale; ***UK:*** AeroBec; Asmabec; Beceze; Beclazone; Beclogen; Becodisks; Beconase; Clenil; Clipper; Filair; Hayfever Relief; Nasobec; Pollenase Nasal; Pulvinal Beclometasone Dipropionate; Qvar; Vivabec; ***USA:*** Beclovent; Beconase; Qvar; ***Venez.:*** Beclofortil; Beclorino; Beclosil; Beconase; Biobeclasona; Biobeclod; Genbeclo; Nasair.

Multi-ingredient: ***Arg.:*** Beclasma; Biotaer Nebulizable; Butocort; Butosol; Menaderm N; Salbutol Beclo; Ventide; ***Austria:*** Ventide; ***Braz.:*** Aerotide; Clenil Compositum; ***Chile:*** Aero-Plus; Aerosoma; Asmavent-B; Belomet; Butotal B; Herolan Aerosol; Ventide; ***Cz.:*** Clenigen; ***Hong Kong:*** Ventide; ***India:*** Aerocort; Anovate; Beclate-C; Beclate-N; Candibiotic; Candid B; Candiderma +; Cloben-G; Clocip B; Clocip NB; NC-Derm; Otek-AC+; Pilovate; Sigmaderm; Stecort-NM; Translipo-Triple; ***Indon.:*** Ventide; ***Ital.:*** Clenil Compositum; Menaderm; ***Mex.:*** Ventide; ***Philipp.:*** Candibec; ***Rus.:*** Candibiotic (Кандибиотик); Candid B (Кандид Б); ***Spain:*** Butosol; Menaderm Clio; Menaderm Neomicina; Menaderm Otologico; ***Thai.:*** Clenil Compositum; ***Turk.:*** Ventide; ***UK:*** Fostair; ***Venez.:*** Aerocort; Beclosal; Butosol; Venticort; Ventide.

Befunolol Hydrochloride

Other names: Béfunolol, Chlorhydrate de; Befunololi Hydrochloridum; BFE-60; Hidrocloruro de befunolol.

Бефунолола Гидрохлорид

Clinical profile: Befunolol hydrochloride is a beta blocker used in the management of ocular hypertension and open-angle glaucoma.

WADA Status: Banned in and out of competition as specified below

WADA Class: Beta-Blockers

Unless otherwise specified, beta-blockers are prohibited *In-Competition* only in the following sports.

- Aeronautics (FAI)
- Archery (FITA, IPC) (also prohibited *Out-of-Competition*)
- Automobile (FIA)
- Billiards (WCBS)
- Bobsleigh (FIBT)
- Boules (CMSB, IPC bowls)
- Bridge (FMB)
- Curling (WCF)
- Gymnastics (FIG)
- Motorcycling (FIM)
- Modern Pentathlon (UIPM) for disciplines involving shooting
- Nine-pin bowling (FIQ)
- Powerboating (UIM)
- Sailing (ISAF) for match race helms only
- Shooting (ISSF, IPC) (also prohibited *Out-of-Competition*)
- Skiing/Snowboarding (FIS) in ski jumping, freestyle aerials/halfpipe and snowboard halfpipe/big air
- Wrestling (FILA)

WADA Class: Specified Substances

Also listed as a specified substance.

"The prohibited List may identify specified substances which are particularly susceptible to unintentional anti-doping rule violations because of their general availability in medicinal products or which are less likely to be successfully abused as doping agents."

A doping violation involving such substances may result in a reduced sanction provided that the "*...Athlete can establish that the Use of such a specfied substance was not intended to enhance sport performance...*"

Preparations
Single ingredient: ***Ital.:*** Betaclar; ***Jpn:*** Bentos; ***Mon.:*** Bentos.

Bemetizide

Other names: Bemetizida; Bémétizide; Bemetizidum; Diu-60.

Беметизид

Clinical profile: Bemetizide is a thiazide diuretic used in the treatment of oedema and hypertension.

WADA Status: Banned in and out of competition

WADA Class: Diuretics and Other Masking Agents

Includes diuretics or substances with a similar chemical structure or similar biological effect(s).

Preparations
Multi-ingredient: ***Ger.:*** dehydro sanol tri; Diucomb.

Bendacort

Other names: AF-2071; Cortazac; Hydrocortisone Bendazac.

Clinical profile: Bendacort is the 21-ester of the corticosteroid hydrocortisone with bendazac and has been applied topically in the management of various skin disorders.

WADA Status: Banned in competition

WADA Class: Glucocorticosteroids

All glucocorticosteroids are prohibited when administered orally, rectally, intravenously or intramuscularly. Their use requires a Therapeutic Use Exemption approval. Other routes of administration (intraarticular / periarticular / peritendinous / epidural / intradermal injections and inhalation) require an Abbreviated Therapeutic Use Exemption except as noted below.

Topical preparations when used for dermatological (including iontophoresis / phonophoresis), auricular, nasal, ophthalmic, buccal, gingival and perianal disorders are not prohibited and do not require any form of Therapeutic Use Exemption.

WADA Class: Specified Substances

Also listed as a specified substance.

"The prohibited List may identify specified substances which are particularly susceptible to unintentional anti-doping rule violations because of their general availability in medicinal products or which are less likely to be successfully abused as doping agents."

A doping violation involving such substances may result in a reduced sanction provided that the "*...Athlete can establish that the Use of such a specfied substance was not intended to enhance sport performance...*"

Bendroflumethiazide

Other names: Bendrofluaz.; Bendrofluazide; Bendroflumethiazid; Bendrofluméthiazide; Bendroflumethiazidum; Bendroflumetiatsidi; Bendroflumetiazid; Bendroflumetiazida; Bendroflumetiazidas; Benzydroflumethiazide; FT-81.

Бендрофлуметиазид

Clinical profile: Bendroflumethiazide is a thiazide diuretic used for hypertension, and for oedema, including that associated with heart failure.

WADA Status: Banned in and out of competition

WADA Class: Diuretics and Other Masking Agents

Includes diuretics or substances with a similar chemical structure or similar biological effect(s).

Preparations
Single ingredient: ***Austral.:*** Aprinox; ***Denm.:*** Centyl; ***Irl.:*** Centyl; ***Norw.:*** Centyl; ***NZ:*** Neo-NaClex; ***Swed.:*** Salures; ***UK:*** Aprinox; Neo-NaClex.
Multi-ingredient: ***Arg.:*** Pertenso; Sumal; ***Austria:*** Sali-Aldopur; ***Braz.:*** Diserim; ***Denm.:*** Centyl med Kaliumklorid; ***Fr.:*** Precyclan; Tensionorme; ***Ger.:*** Dociretic; Pertenso N; Sotaziden N; Tensoflux; ***Irl.:*** Centyl K; Low Centyl K; ***Mex.:*** Corgaretic; ***Neth.:*** Inderetic; ***Norw.:*** Centyl med Kaliumklorid; ***S.Afr.:*** Corgaretic; ***Spain:*** Neatenol Diu; Neatenol Diuvas; Spirometon; ***Swed.:*** Centyl K; Salures-K; ***UK:*** Centyl K; Neo-NaClex-K; Prestim; ***USA:*** Corzide.

Benzfetamine Hydrochloride

Other names: Benzfétamine, Chlorhydrate de; Benzfetamini Hydrochloridum; Benzphetamine Hydrochloride; Hidrocloruro de benzfetamina.
Бензфетамина Гидрохлорид

Clinical profile: Benzfetamine hydrochloride is an amfetamine derivative and a sympathomimetic. It has been used as an anorectic in the treatment of obesity.

WADA Status: Banned in competition

WADA Class: Stimulants

Includes benzfetamine and any optical isomers.

Preparations
Single ingredient: ***USA:*** Didrex.

Benzthiazide

Other names: Benzthiazidum; Benztiazida; P-1393.
Бензтиазид

Clinical profile: Benzthiazide is a thiazide diuretic used for oedema, including that associated with heart failure, and for hypertension.

WADA Status: Banned in and out of competition

WADA Class: Diuretics and Other Masking Agents

Includes diuretics or substances with a similar chemical structure or similar biological effect(s).

Preparations
Multi-ingredient: ***India:*** Ditide; ***Switz.:*** Dyrenium compositum; ***UK:*** Dytide.

Benzylhydrochlorothiazide

Other names: Su-6227.

Clinical profile: Benzylhydrochlorothiazide is a thiazide diuretic that has been used in the treatment of hypertension.

WADA Status: Banned in and out of competition

WADA Class: Diuretics and Other Masking Agents

Includes diuretics or substances with a similar chemical structure or similar biological effect(s).

B

Beta Blockers

Other names: β-Bloqueantes.

Бета-блокаторы

Clinical profile: Beta blockers are competitive inhibitors at beta-adrenergic receptor sites and are used in the management of cardiovascular disorders such as hypertension, angina pectoris, cardiac arrhythmias, and myocardial infarction. Some beta blockers are used in heart failure. They are also given to control symptoms of sympathetic overactivity in alcohol withdrawal, anxiety states, hyperthyroidism, and tremor, and in the prophylaxis of migraine and of bleeding from oesophageal or gastric varices associated with portal hypertension. They are also used with alpha blockers in the initial management of phaeochromocytoma. Some beta blockers are used as eye drops to reduce raised intra-ocular pressure in glaucoma and ocular hypertension.

WADA Status: Banned in and out of competition as specified below

WADA Class: Beta-Blockers

Unless otherwise specified, beta-blockers are prohibited *In-Competition* only in the following sports.

- Aeronautics (FAI)
- Archery (FITA, IPC) (also prohibited *Out-of-Competition*)
- Automobile (FIA)
- Billiards (WCBS)
- Bobsleigh (FIBT)
- Boules (CMSB, IPC bowls)
- Bridge (FMB)
- Curling (WCF)
- Gymnastics (FIG)
- Motorcycling (FIM)
- Modern Pentathlon (UIPM) for disciplines involving shooting
- Nine-pin bowling (FIQ)
- Powerboating (UIM)
- Sailing (ISAF) for match race helms only
- Shooting (ISSF, IPC) (also prohibited *Out-of-Competition*)
- Skiing/Snowboarding (FIS) in ski jumping, freestyle aerials/halfpipe and snowboard halfpipe/big air
- Wrestling (FILA)

WADA Class: Specified Substances

Also listed as a specified substance.

"The prohibited List may identify specified substances which are particularly susceptible to unintentional anti-doping rule violations because of their general availability in medicinal products or which are less likely to be successfully abused as doping agents."

A doping violation involving such substances may result in a reduced sanction provided that the "*...Athlete can establish that the Use of such a specfied substance was not intended to enhance sport performance...*"

Betamethasone

Other names: Beetametasoni; Betadexamethasone; Betametason; Betametasona; Betametazon; Betametazonas; Betamethason; Bétaméthasone; Betamethasonum;

Flubenisolone; Flubenisolonum; 9α-Fluoro-16β-methylprednisolone; β-Methasone; NSC-39470; Sch-4831.

Бетаметазон

Betamethasone Acetate

Other names: Acetato de betametasona; Beetametasoniasetaatti; Betametason-acetat; Betametazon Asetat; Betametazon-acetát; Betametazono acetatas; Betamethason-acetát; Bétaméthasone, acétate de; Betamethasoni acetas.

Бетаметазона Ацетат

Betamethasone Benzoate

Other names: Benzoato de betametasona; Bétaméthasone, Benzoate de; Betamethasoni Benzoas; W-5975.

Бетаметазона Бензоат

Betamethasone Dipropionate

Other names: Beetametasonidipropionaatti; Betametasondipropionat; Betametazon Dipropiyonat; Betametazon-dipropionát; Betametazono dipropionatas; Betametazonu dipropionian; Betamethason-dipropionát; Bétaméthasone, dipropionate de; Betamethasoni dipropionas; Dipropionato de betametasona; Sch-11460.

Бетаметазона Дипропионат

Betamethasone Sodium Phosphate

Other names: Beetametasoninatriumfosfaatti; Betametasonnatrifosfatum; Betametazon Disodyum Fosfat; Betametazon-nátrium-foszfát; Betametazono natrio fosfatas; Betamethasone Disodium Phosphate; Bétaméthasone, phosphate sodique de; Betamethason-fosfát sodná sůl; Betamethasoni natrii phosphas; Fosfato sódico de betametasona; Natrii Betamethasoni Phosphas.

Натрия Бетаметазона Фосфат

Betamethasone Valerate

Other names: Beetametasonivaleraatti; Betametasonvalerat; Betametazon Valerat; Betametazono valeratas; Betametazonu walerianian; Betametazon-valerát; Bétaméthasone, valérate de; Betamethasoni valeras; Betamethason-valerát; Valerato de betametasona.

Бетаметазона Валерат

Clinical profile: Betamethasone is a glucocorticoid corticosteroid. It has been used, either in the form of the free alcohol or in one of the esterified forms, in the treatment of a wide range of conditions that respond to the anti-inflammatory and immunosuppressant effects of corticosteroid therapy.

WADA Status: Banned in competition

WADA Class: Glucocorticosteroids

All glucocorticosteroids are prohibited when administered orally, rectally, intravenously or intramuscularly. Their use requires a Therapeutic Use Exemption approval. Other routes of administration (intraarticular / periarticular / peritendinous / epidural / intradermal injections and inhalation) require an Abbreviated Therapeutic Use Exemption except as noted below.

Topical preparations when used for dermatological (including iontophoresis / phonophoresis), auricular, nasal, ophthalmic, buccal, gingival and perianal disorders are not prohibited and do not require any form of Therapeutic Use Exemption.

WADA Class: Specified Substances

Also listed as a specified substance.

B

"The prohibited List may identify specified substances which are particularly susceptible to unintentional anti-doping rule violations because of their general availability in medicinal products or which are less likely to be successfully abused as doping agents."

A doping violation involving such substances may result in a reduced sanction provided that the "*...Athlete can establish that the Use of such a specfied substance was not intended to enhance sport performance...*"

Preparations

Single ingredient: ***Arg.:*** Betacort; Betacort; Betacort; Betasone-G 12 Horas; Betasone-G; Betatopic; Betnovate Capilar; Betnovate; Blacor; Butasona RL; Butasona; Celestone Cronodose; Celestone; Cevicort NC; Cevicort; Coid; Corteroid Retard; Corteroid; Cortiderma; Cortimar; Cronocorteroid; Cronolevel; Deltalaf; Dermizol; Difenac Forte; Diprosone; Lazar-Cort; Metamar; Micosep B; Quiacort; Transderma B; Valederm; ***Austral.:*** Antroquoril; Betnovate; Celestone Chronodose; Celestone M; Cortival; Diprosone; Eleuphrat; ***Austria:*** Betnesol; Betnovate; Celestan; Diproderm; Diproforte; Diprophos; Solu-Celestan; ***Belg.:*** Betnelan-V; Celestone Chronodose; Celestone; Diprolene; Diprosone; ***Braz.:*** Alersan; Beclonato; Benevat; Beta Long; Betaderm; Betametagen; Betaprospan; Betaspan; Betnelan; Betnolon; Betnovate; Betrat B; Betsona; Celestan; Celestone Soluspan; Celestone; Dermobet; Dermonil; Dermovat; Dibetam; Diprobeta; Diprocort; Diprosone; Diprospan; Duoflam; Sensitex; Valbet; ***Canad.:*** Betaderm; Betaject; Betnesol; Celestone Soluspan; Diprolene Glycol; Diprosone; Prevex B; ratio-Ectosone; ratio-Topilene; ratio-Topisone; Taro-Sone; Valisone; ***Chile:*** Cidoten Rapilento; Cidoten V; Cidoten; Coritex; Cremirit; Cronolevel; Dacam RL; Dacam; Diprolene; Diprospan; Diprospan; Disopranil; Konicortil; Labosona; Oftasona P; Spel; ***Cz.:*** Beloderm; Beta; Betnovate; Celestoderm-V; Diprophos; Diprosone; Kuterid; ***Denm.:*** Betnovat; Bettamousse; Celeston; Celeston; Diproderm; Diprolen; Diprospan; ***Fin.:*** Bemetson; Betapred; Betnovat; Bettamousse; Celestoderm; Celeston Chronodose; Diproderm; Diprolen; ***Fr.:*** Betesil; Betnesol; Betneval; Celestene Chronodose; Celestene; Celestoderm; Diprolene; Diprosone; ***Ger.:*** Bemon; BetaCreme; Betagalen; BetaSalbe; Betnesalic mono; Betnesol-V; Betnesol; Celestamine N; Celestan Depot; Celestan solubile; Celestan-V; Cordes Beta; Deflatop; Diprosis; Diprosone Depot; Diprosone; Linola Cort Beta; Soderm; ***Gr.:*** Betnesol; Betnovate; Celestene; Celestoderm-V; Celestone Chronodose; Celestone; Flogozyme; Galinocort; Locason-N; Movithiol; Osmoran; Propiochrone; Propioform; Sanorvil; ***Hong Kong:*** Betaderma; Betasone; Betazone; Betnovate; Derzid; Diprocel; Diprosone; Diprospan; Synmethasone; ***Hung.:*** Betesil; Diprophos; ***India:*** Betafoam; Betnecip; Betnecort; Betnederm; Betnelan; Betnesol; Betnovate; Topicasone; Valbet; Walacort; ***Indon.:*** Benoson; Betam-Ophtal; Betason; Betnovate; Betodermin; Betopic; Celestoderm-V; Celestone; Corsaderm; Diprosone-OV; Exabet; Mesonta; Metonate; Molason; Oviskin; Proson; Scanderma; Skizon; Vason; ***Irl.:*** Betacap; Betnelan; Betnesol; Betnovate; Bettamousse; Diprosone; ***Israel:*** Betacorten; Betnesol; Betnovate; Bettamousse; Celestone Chronodose; Diprolene; Diprosone; Diprospan; ***Ital.:*** Beben; Bentelan; Beta 21; Betamesol; Betesil; Bettamousse; Celestone Cronodose; Celestone; Diprosone; Ecoval; ***Malaysia:*** Beavate; Beprogel; Beprosone; Besone; Beta; Betasone; Betnosone; Betnovate; Bufencon; Celestoderm-V; Celestone; Dibetasol; Diprocel; Diprosone; Diprospan; Uniflex; ***Mex.:*** Betnovate; Celestone Soluspan; Celestone; Cronolevel; Dermoval; Diprofast; Dipronova; Diprosone; Diprospan; Disons Dex; Erispan; Reubaxona; ***Neth.:*** Betnelan; Betnesol; Celestoderm; Celestone Chronodose; Celestone; Diprolene; Diprosone; ***Norw.:*** Betnovat; Bettamousse; Celeston; Diproderm; ***NZ:*** Beta; Betnesol; Betnovate; Bivate; Celestone Chronodose; Diprolene; Diprosone; ***Philipp.:*** Beta; Betnelan; Betnovate; Celestone; Diprolene; Diprosone; Diprospan; Steroderm; ***Pol.:*** Celestone; Diprolene; Diprophos; Diprosone; Kuterid; ***Port.:*** Betnasol; Betnovate; Celesdepot; Celestone; Cilestoderme; Diprofos; Diprosone; Soluderme; Vabeta; ***Rus.:*** Akriderm (Акридерм); Beloderm (Белодерм); Betasone (Бетазон); Celestoderm-V (Целестодерм-В); Diprospan (Дипроспан); ***S.Afr.:*** Betanoid; Betnesol; Betnovate; Celestone Soluspan; Celestone; Diprosone; Lenasone; Lenovate; Persivate; Repivate; Topivate; ***Singapore:*** Beprogel; Beprosone; Besone; Betacorten; Betasone; Betnovate; Camnovate; Dermasone; Derzid; Dibetasol; Diprocel; Diprosone; Diprospan; ***Spain:*** Betnovate; Bettamousse; Celestoderm-V; Celestoderm; Celestone Cronodose; Celestone; Diproderm; ***Swed.:*** Betapred; Betnovat; Bettamousse; Celeston bifas; Celeston valerat; Celeston; Diproderm; Diprolen; ***Switz.:*** Betnesol; Betnovate; Celestoderm-V; Celestone Chronodose; Celestone; Diprolene; Diprosone; ***Thai.:*** Beprogel; Bepronate; Beprosone; Besone; Bessasone; Beta; Betameth; Bethasone; Betnovate; Betosone; Bipro; Clinivate; Derzid; Diprosone; Diprospan; Diprotop; Polynovate; Sebo; Valbet; ***Turk.:*** Betnovate; Celestoderm-V; Celestone Chronodose; Diprolene; Diprospan; Seroderm; ***UAE:*** Betasone; Betasone; ***UK:*** Betacap; Betnelan; Betnesol; Betnovate RD (Ready Diluted); Betnovate; Bettamousse; Diprosone; Vista-Methasone; ***USA:*** Beta-Val; Cel-U-Jec; Celestone Soluspan; Celestone; Diprolene; Diprosone; Luxiq; Maxivate; Valisone; ***Venez.:*** Beprospen; Betacort; Betaderm; Betagen Solspen; Betagen; Betnovate; Celestoderm; Celestone Soluspan; Celestone; Diprocel; Diprosone; Diprospan; Itisona.

Multi-ingredient: ***Arg.:*** Adenil; Algio Nervomax Fuerte; Antiflogol; Antihemorroidal; Bacticort Complex; Bacticort; Becortin; Betacort Plus; Betametasona B12; Betasalic; Betasone-G Compuesto; Betnovate-C; Betnovate-N; Blamy; Blokium B12; Calmurid; Celestamine-L; Celestamine; Cevaderm; Ciprocort L; Clarityne Cort; Corteroid Gesic; Cortispec; Cortistamin L; Cuta Crema; Denvercrem; Dermizol G; Dermizol Trio; Dermosona; Diclogesic Plus B12; Dioxaflex B12; Diprogenta; Diprosalic; Doxtran B12; Drum B; Factor Dermico; Fucicort; Fusimed B; Gelbiotic Plus; Gentasol; Hifamonil Crema; Histamino Corteroid L; Ingemet; Lazar-Cort Complex; Lisaler Beta; Lotricomb; Macril; Maxisalic; Mencogrin; Mencogrin; Micomazol B; Miklogen; Monizol Cort Crema; Nularef Cort; Oxa B12; Procto-Metadyne; Quadriderm; Quiacort G Plus; Quiacort G; Rodinac B12; Salicort; Sinaler B; Sirotamicin BG; Sorsis Beta; Toflam; Tribiocort; Triliver; Triplex; Vesalion B12; Virobron B12 NF; Vitacortil; Vixidone LB; Xedenol B12; ***Austral.:*** Daivobet; ***Austria:*** Betnesol-N; Betnovate-C; Betnovate-N; Celestamin; Diprogenta; Diprosalic; Fucicort; Psorcutan Beta; ***Belg.:*** Diprophos; Diprosalic; Dovobet; Fucicort; Lotriderm; ***Braz.:*** Betazol Cort; Betnovate-N; Betnovate-Q; Candicort; Celestamil; Celestamine; Cetobeta; Cetocort; Cetocorten; Cremederme; Dermosalic; Dextamine; Dipro AS; Diprogenta; Diprosalic; Emscort; Garasone; Gentacort; Microbiogen; Novacort; Oto Betnovate; Poliderms; Postec; Quadriderm; Quadrikin; Quadrilon; Quadriplus; Qualiderm; Reumix; Tetraderm; Verutex B; ***Canad.:*** Diprosalic; Dovobet; Garasone; Lotriderm; Pentasone; ratio-Topisalic; Valisone-G; ***Chile:*** B-Laboterol; Cam; Celestamine; Clofexan; Clotrimin-B; Cobefen; Contralmor; Creminem-B; Deucoaler; Diproquin; Diprosalic; Diprospan G; Donomix; Fucicort; Gentasone; Gotalgic; Labosalic; Labosona G; Locrim; Lotriderm; Mixgen; Novadrel; Novarnela; Oftagen Compuesto; Oftasona N; Otandrol; Oticum; Otolisan; Plexus; Prodel B; ***Cz.:*** Belogent; Belosalic; Betabioptal; Diprosalic; Fucicort; Garasone; Lotriderm; ***Denm.:*** Betnovat med Chinoform; Celeston med Chinoform; Clotrason; Daivobet; Diprosalic; Fucicort; ***Fin.:*** Bemetson-K; Betnovat-C; Celestoderm cum Garamycin; Daivobet; Diprosalic; Fucicort; ***Fr.:*** Celestamine; Daivobet; Diprosalic; Diprosone Neomycine; Diprostene; ***Ger.:*** Betadermic; Betagentam; Betamethason comp; Daivobet; Diprogenta; Diprosalic; Fucicort; Lotricomb; Psorcutan Beta; Soderm Plus; Sulmycin mit Celestan-V; Terracortril N; ***Gr.:*** Alpider; Befucil; Betacort; Betafusin; Betasid; Betfu; Betnovate-C; Betnovate-N; Celestoderm-V/GA; Dovobet; Fubecot; Fucicort; Fucicream; Fusibet; Garamat; Propiogenta; Propiosalic; Roseti; Sensibio; Staficort; ***Hong Kong:*** Allersan; Aristobet-N; Bechlomin; Becogem; Betnovate-N; Bonjedex; Celestamine; Celestoderm-V with Garamycin; Clobeta-G; Conazole; Daivobet; Dermafacte; Derzid-C; Dextrosone; Diprogenta; Diprosalic; Fucicort; Garasone; Lozopin; Lycobeta-G; Quadriderm; Synbetamine; Triderm; ***Hung.:*** Daivobet; Diprosalic; Fucicort; Garasone; Gentason; ***India:*** Betamil-GM; Betamil-M; Betasalic; Betnederm C; Betnederm GM; Betnederm N; Betnesol-N Nasal; Betnesol-N; Betnor; Betnovate-C; Betnovate-GM; Betnovate-M; Betnovate-N; Betnovate-S; Fourderm AF; Fourderm; Quiss; Supirocin-B; Surfaz-SN; Topicasone with Neomycin; Valbet; ***Indon.:*** Benoson G; Benoson M; Benoson N; Benoson V; Berloson-N; Betagentam; Betasin; Betason-N; Betnovate-N; Bevalex; Biocort; Celestamine; Celestoderm-V with Garamycin; Colergis; Daivobet; Digenta; Diprogenta; Diprosalic; Diprosta; Exabetin; Fucicort; Garasone; Heltiskin; Isotic Betaracin; Krimbeson; Lotriderm; Mastroson; Metaskin-N; Mytaderm; Nilacelin; Ocuson; Polacel; Proson N; Salgen Plus; Scanderma Plus; Skilone; Skinal; Sonigen; Tuderm-N; Zestam; ***Irl.:*** Betnesol-N; Betnovate-C; Betnovate-N; Diprosalic; Dovobet; Fucibet; Lotriderm; ***Israel:*** Betacorten-G; Betnesol-N; Betnovate-C; Betnovate-N; Clotrisone; Daivobet; Diprogenta; Diprosalic; Fucicort; Triderm; ***Ital.:*** Alfaflor; Batasalgin; Beben Clorossina; Betabioptal; Betacream; Betafloroto; Biorinil; Brumeton Colloidale S; Deltavagin; Dermabiolene; Dermatar; Diproform; Diprosalic; Dovobet; Ecoval con Neomicina; Egerian; Eubetal Antibiotico; Eubetal Antibiotico; Fidagenbeta; Fluororinil; Fucicort; Gentalyn Beta; Kamelyn; Sterozinil; Stranoval; Token; Visublefarite; Visumetazone Antibiotico; ***Malaysia:*** Beavate N; Beprogent; Beprosalic; Besone-N; Betacin; Betagen; Betamethasone Clo; Betamethasone G; Betamethasone N; Betamethasone SA; Betnosone N; Betnovate-N; Celestoderm-V with Garamycin; Diprogenta; Diprosalic; Fobancort; Fucicort; Fusidic B; Garasone; Joysun; Triderm-C; Uniflex-N; ***Mex.:*** Artridol; Barmicil Compuesto; Beclogen; Betrigen; Celestamine NS; Clio-Betnovate; Clotricina; Daivobet; Diprosone G; Diprosone Y; Farmalor; Fucicort; Garamicina-V; Garasone; Gelmicin; Miclobet; Prubagen; Quadriderm NF; Tamex; Triderm; ***Neth.:*** Diprosalic; Dovobet; ***Norw.:*** Betnovat med Chinoform; Daivobet; Diprosalic; ***NZ:*** Betnesol Aqueous; Betnovate-C; Daivobet; Fucicort; ***Philipp.:*** Betneton; Betnovate-C; Betnovate-N; Celestamine; Claricort; Clotrasone; Daivobet; Diproform; Diprogenta; Diprosalic; Fucicort; Garasone; Hoebedic; Ophtasone; Quadriderm; Quadrotopic; Triderm; ***Pol.:*** Bedicort G; Betnovate-C; Betnovate-N; Daivobet; Diprogenta; Diprosalic; Lotriderm; Triderm; ***Port.:*** Beta-Micoter; Betnovate-C; Betnovate-N; Daivobet; Diprogenta; Diprosalic; Epione; Flotiran; Fucicort; Psodermil; Quadriderme; ***Rus.:*** Akriderm Genta (Акридерм Гента); Akriderm GK (Акридерм ГК); Akriderm SK (Акридерм СК); Belogent (Белогент); Belosalic (Белосалик); Betagenot (Бетагенот); Celestoderm-V with Garamycin (Целестодерм-В с Гарамицином); Daivobet (Дайвобет); Diprosalic (Дипросалик); Fucicort (Фуцикорт); Triderm (Тридерм); ***S.Afr.:*** Betnesol-N; Betnovate-C; Betnovate-N; Celestamine; Diprogenta; Diprosalic; Lotriderm; Quadriderm; ***Singapore:*** B-Tasone-G; Beprogent; Beprosalic; Besone-N; Bufencon; Combiderm; Conazole; Daivobet; Dermanol-C; Diprogenta; Diprosalic; Fobancort; Fucicort; Garasone; Gentriderm; Gentrisone; Modaderm; Neoderm; Tri-Micon; Triderm; ***Spain:*** Alergical; Beta Micoter; Bronsal; Celesemine; Celestoderm Gentamicina; Celestone S; Clotrasone; Cuatroderm; Daivobet; Diprogenta; Diprosalic; Fucibet; ***Swed.:*** Betnovat med Chinoform; Betnovat med Neomycin; Celeston valerat med chinoform; Celeston valerat med gentamicin; Daivobet; Diprosalic; ***Switz.:*** Betnesalic; Betnovate-C; Betnovate-N; Celestamine; Daivobet; Diprogenta; Diprophos; Diprosalic; Fucicort; Ophtasone; Quadriderm; Triderm; ***Thai.:*** Bacda-B; Beprogent; Beprogenta; Beprolic; Besone-N; Beta-C; Beta-N; Beta-S; Betameth-N; Bethasone-N; Betnovate-C; Betnovate-N; Betosalic; Betosone-CE; Canazol-BE; Clinivate-N; Daivobet; Derzid-C; Derzid-N; Diprosalic; Fango-B; Fucicort; Fungiderm-B; Gynesten-B; Myda-B; Myrazole-B; Topaben-N; Twina; Valbet-N; ***Turk.:*** Betnovate-C; ***UAE:*** Futasone; Supraproct-S; ***UK:*** Betnesol-N; Betnovate-C; Betnovate-N; Diprosalic; Dovobet; Fucibet; Vipsogal; Vista-Methasone N; ***USA:*** Lotrisone; Taclonex; ***Venez.:*** Betaderm con Gentamicina;

Celestamincort; Celestamine; Celestoderm con Gentalyn; Claricort; Diproformo; Diprogenta; Diprosalic; Garabet; Garasone; Lotricomb; Lotrisone; Quadriderm; Triderm; Tridetarmon.

B

Betaxolol Hydrochloride

Other names: ALO-1401-02; Betaksolol Hidroklorür; Betaksololihydrokloridi; Betaksololio hidrochloridas; Bétaxolol, chlorhydrate de; Betaxolol-hidroklorid; Betaxolol-hydrochlorid; Betaxololhydroklorid; Betaxololi hydrochloridum; Hidrocloruro de betaxolol; SL-75212-10.

Бетаксолола Гидрохлорид

Clinical profile: Betaxolol is a cardioselective beta blocker used in the management of hypertension, angina pectoris, and glaucoma.

WADA Status: Banned in and out of competition as specified below

WADA Class: Beta-Blockers

Unless otherwise specified, beta-blockers are prohibited *In-Competition* only in the following sports.

- Aeronautics (FAI)
- Archery (FITA, IPC) (also prohibited *Out-of-Competition*)
- Automobile (FIA)
- Billiards (WCBS)
- Bobsleigh (FIBT)
- Boules (CMSB, IPC bowls)
- Bridge (FMB)
- Curling (WCF)
- Gymnastics (FIG)
- Motorcycling (FIM)
- Modern Pentathlon (UIPM) for disciplines involving shooting
- Nine-pin bowling (FIQ)
- Powerboating (UIM)
- Sailing (ISAF) for match race helms only
- Shooting (ISSF, IPC) (also prohibited *Out-of-Competition*)
- Skiing/Snowboarding (FIS) in ski jumping, freestyle aerials/halfpipe and snowboard halfpipe/big air
- Wrestling (FILA)

WADA Class: Specified Substances

Also listed as a specified substance.

"The prohibited List may identify specified substances which are particularly susceptible to unintentional anti-doping rule violations because of their general availability in medicinal products or which are less likely to be successfully abused as doping agents."

A doping violation involving such substances may result in a reduced sanction provided that the "...*Athlete can establish that the Use of such a specfied substance was not intended to enhance sport performance...*"

Preparations

Single ingredient: ***Arg.:*** Betasel; Tonobexol; ***Austral.:*** Betoptic; Betoquin; ***Austria:*** Betoptic; Kerlone; ***Belg.:*** Betoptic; Kerlone; ***Braz.:*** Betoptic; Presmin; ***Canad.:*** Betoptic; ***Chile:*** Bemaz; Beof; Betoptic; ***Cz.:*** Betoptic; Lokren; ***Denm.:*** Betoptic; ***Fin.:*** Betoptic; Kerlon; ***Fr.:*** Betoptic; Kerlone; ***Ger.:*** Betoptima; Kerlone; ***Gr.:*** Armament; Betoptic; Eifel; Kerlone; ***Hong Kong:*** Betoptic; ***Hung.:*** Betoptic; Lokren; ***India:*** Optipres; ***Indon.:*** Betoptima; Optibet; ***Irl.:*** Betoptic; ***Israel:*** Betoptic; Kerlone; ***Ital.:*** Betoptic; Kerlon; ***Jpn:*** Kerlong; ***Malaysia:*** Betoptic; Kerlone; ***Mex.:*** Betoptic; BTX-HA Ofteno; ***Neth.:*** Betoptic; Kerlon; ***Norw.:*** Betoptic; ***NZ:*** Betoptic; ***Philipp.:*** Betoptic; Kerlone; ***Pol.:*** Betabion; Betoptic; Lokren; Optibetol; ***Port.:*** Bertocil; Betoptic; Davixolol; ***Rus.:*** Betac (Бетак); Betoptic (Бетоптик); Lokren (Локрен); ***S.Afr.:*** Betoptic;

Singapore: Betac; Betoptic; Kerlone; ***Spain:*** Betoptic; ***Swed.:*** Betoptic; ***Switz.:*** Betoptic; ***Thai.:*** Betoptic; ***Turk.:*** Betoptic; ***UK:*** Betoptic; ***USA:*** Betoptic; Kerlone; ***Venez.:*** Betaxol; Betoptic.

Bevantolol Hydrochloride

Other names: Bévantolol, Chlorhydrate de; Bevantololhydroklorid; Bevantololi Hydrochloridum; Bevantololihydrokloridi; CI-775; Hidrocloruro de bevantolol; NC-1400.

Бевантолола Гидрохлорид

Clinical profile: Bevantolol is a cardioselective beta blocker that has been used in the management of hypertension and angina pectoris.

WADA Status: Banned in and out of competition as specified below

WADA Class: Beta-Blockers

Unless otherwise specified, beta-blockers are prohibited *In-Competition* only in the following sports.

- Aeronautics (FAI)
- Archery (FITA, IPC) (also prohibited *Out-of-Competition*)
- Automobile (FIA)
- Billiards (WCBS)
- Bobsleigh (FIBT)
- Boules (CMSB, IPC bowls)
- Bridge (FMB)
- Curling (WCF)
- Gymnastics (FIG)
- Motorcycling (FIM)
- Modern Pentathlon (UIPM) for disciplines involving shooting
- Nine-pin bowling (FIQ)
- Powerboating (UIM)
- Sailing (ISAF) for match race helms only
- Shooting (ISSF, IPC) (also prohibited *Out-of-Competition*)
- Skiing/Snowboarding (FIS) in ski jumping, freestyle aerials/halfpipe and snowboard halfpipe/big air
- Wrestling (FILA)

WADA Class: Specified Substances

Also listed as a specified substance.

"*The prohibited List may identify specified substances which are particularly susceptible to unintentional anti-doping rule violations because of their general availability in medicinal products or which are less likely to be successfully abused as doping agents.*"

A doping violation involving such substances may result in a reduced sanction provided that the "*...Athlete can establish that the Use of such a specfied substance was not intended to enhance sport performance...*"

Bisoprolol Fumarate

Other names: Bisoprolol Fumarat; Bisoprolol, Fumarate de; Bisoprolol Hemifumarate; Bisoprolol, hémifumarate de; Bisoprololfumarat; Bisoprololi Fumaras; Bisoprololi hemifumaras; Bisoprololifumaraatti; CL-297939; EMD-33512 (bisoprolol or bisoprolol fumarate); Fumarato de bisoprolol.

Бизопролола Фумарат

Clinical profile: Bisoprolol is a cardioselective beta blocker used in the management of hypertension, angina pectoris, and heart failure.

WADA Status: Banned in and out of competition as specified below

B

WADA Class: Beta-Blockers

Unless otherwise specified, beta-blockers are prohibited *In-Competition* only in the following sports.

- Aeronautics (FAI)
- Archery (FITA, IPC) (also prohibited *Out-of-Competition*)
- Automobile (FIA)
- Billiards (WCBS)
- Bobsleigh (FIBT)
- Boules (CMSB, IPC bowls)
- Bridge (FMB)
- Curling (WCF)
- Gymnastics (FIG)
- Motorcycling (FIM)
- Modern Pentathlon (UIPM) for disciplines involving shooting
- Nine-pin bowling (FIQ)
- Powerboating (UIM)
- Sailing (ISAF) for match race helms only
- Shooting (ISSF, IPC) (also prohibited *Out-of-Competition*)
- Skiing/Snowboarding (FIS) in ski jumping, freestyle aerials/halfpipe and snowboard halfpipe/big air
- Wrestling (FILA)

WADA Class: Specified Substances

Also listed as a specified substance.

"The prohibited List may identify specified substances which are particularly susceptible to unintentional anti-doping rule violations because of their general availability in medicinal products or which are less likely to be successfully abused as doping agents."

A doping violation involving such substances may result in a reduced sanction provided that the "...*Athlete can establish that the Use of such a specfied substance was not intended to enhance sport performance...*"

Preparations

Single ingredient: ***Arg.:*** Concor; Corbis; Lostaprolol; ***Austral.:*** Bicor; ***Austria:*** Bisocor; Bisostad; Cardiocor; Concor; Darbalan; Nanalan; Rivacor; ***Belg.:*** Bisoprotop; Docbisopro; Emconcor; Isoten; ***Braz.:*** Concor; ***Canad.:*** Monocor; ***Chile:*** Concor; ***Cz.:*** Concor Cor; Concor; ***Denm.:*** Bisocor; Cardicor; Emconcor; ***Fin.:*** Bisomerck; Bisopral; Emconcor; Orloc; ***Fr.:*** Cardensiel; Cardiocor; Detensiel; ***Ger.:*** Biso Lich; Biso-Puren; Biso; BisoAPS; Bisobeta; Bisogamma; Bisohexal; Bisomerck; Concor; Fondril; Jutabis; ***Gr.:*** Abitrol; Blocatens; Pactens; Speridol; ***Hong Kong:*** Concor; ***Hung.:*** Bisoblock; Bisocard; Bisogamma; Bisogen; Concor Cor; Concor; Coviogal; ***India:*** Concor; ***Indon.:*** B-Beta; Concor; Hapsen; Lodoz; Maintate; ***Irl.:*** Bisocor; Bisopine; Cardicor; Emcolol; Emcor; Soprol; ***Israel:*** Bisolol; Cardiloc; Concor; ***Ital.:*** Cardicor; Concor; Congescor; Pluscor; Sequacor; ***Jpn:*** Maintate; ***Malaysia:*** Concor; ***Mex.:*** Concor; ***Neth.:*** Bisoblock; Emcor; ***Norw.:*** Emconcor; ***Philipp.:*** Concore; ***Pol.:*** Bisocard; Bisohexal; Bisopromerck; Bisoratio; Concor; Corectin; ***Port.:*** Concor; ***Rus.:*** Biprol (Бипрол); Bisocard (Бисокард); Bisogamma (Бисогамма); Concor (Конкор); Corbis (Корбис); ***S.Afr.:*** Adco-Bisocor; Bilocor; Bisohexal; Cardicor; Concor; ***Singapore:*** Concor; ***Spain:*** Emconcor; Euradal; Godal; ***Swed.:*** Bisomerck; Emconcor; ***Switz.:*** Bilol; Concor; ***Thai.:*** Concor; Novacor; ***Turk.:*** Concor; ***UK:*** Cardicor; Emcor; Vivacor; ***USA:*** Zebeta; ***Venez.:*** Concor.

Multi-ingredient: ***Arg.:*** Corbis D; Ziac; ***Austria:*** Bisocombin; Bisoprolol comp; Bisoprolol-HCT; Bisostad plus; Concor Plus; Darbalan Plus; Nanalan Plus; Rivacor Plus; ***Belg.:*** Co-Bisoprolol; Emcoretic; Lodoz; Maxsoten; Merck-Co-Bisoprolol; ***Braz.:*** Biconcor; ***Chile:*** Ziac; ***Cz.:*** Concor Plus; ***Fin.:*** Bisoprolol Comp; Emconcor Comp; Orloc Comp; ***Fr.:*** Lodoz; Wytens; ***Ger.:*** Biso comp; Biso-Puren comp; Bisobeta comp; Bisohexal plus; BisoLich comp; Bisomerck Plus; Bisoplus; Bisoprolol Comp; Bisoprolol HCT; Bisoprolol Plus; Concor Plus; Fondril HCT; ***Hong Kong:*** Lodoz; ***Hung.:*** Concor Plus; Lodoz; ***India:*** Lodoz; ***Ital.:*** Lodoz; ***Mex.:*** Biconcor; ***Neth.:*** Emcoretic; ***Norw.:*** Lodoz; ***Philipp.:*** Ziac; ***Port.:*** Concor Plus; ***S.Afr.:*** Ziak; ***Singapore:*** Lodoz; ***Spain:*** Emcoretic; ***Switz.:*** Concor Plus; Lodoz; ***Thai.:*** Lodoz; ***USA:*** Ziac; ***Venez.:*** Biconcor; Ziac.

Bitolterol Mesilate

Other names: Bitoltérol, Mésilate de; Bitolterol Mesylate; Bitolteroli Mesilas; Mesilato de bitolterol; Win-32784.

Битолтерола Мезилат

Clinical profile: Bitolterol is hydrolysed by esterases in tissue and plasma to colterol, a direct-acting sympathomimetic with a selective action on $beta_2$ adrenoceptors. It has been used as a bronchodilator in the management of respiratory disorders such as asthma or chronic obstructive pulmonary disease.

WADA Status: Banned in and out of competition

WADA Class: Beta-2 Agonists
Includes beta-2 agonists or their isomers.

WADA Class: Specified Substances
Also listed as a specified substance.
"The prohibited List may identify specified substances which are particularly susceptible to unintentional anti-doping rule violations because of their general availability in medicinal products or which are less likely to be successfully abused as doping agents."
A doping violation involving such substances may result in a reduced sanction provided that the "*...Athlete can establish that the Use of such a specfied substance was not intended to enhance sport performance...*"

Preparations
Single ingredient: ***USA:*** Tornalate.

B

Blood

Other names: Sangre.

Clinical profile: Whole blood is used as a source of red cell concentrates, clotting factors, platelets, plasma and plasma fractions, and immunoglobulins, each of which has specific indications for use. Because of the risks involved in transfusing whole blood and the need for economy in its use, the appropriate blood component should be used whenever possible. Whole blood may be used where replacement of plasma proteins as well as red blood cells is needed, for example following acute blood loss during surgery and severe haemorrhage. It may also be used to supplement the circulation during cardiac bypass surgery.

WADA Status: Banned in and out of competition

WADA Class: Enhancement of Oxygen Transfer: Blood Doping
Includes blood or red blood cell products that may be used to enhance the uptake, transport or delivery of oxygen.

Boldenone Undecenoate

Other names: Ba-29038; Boldenone Undecylenate; Boldénone, Undécylénate de; Boldenoni Undecylenas; Undecilenato de boldenona.

Болденона Ундециленат

Clinical profile: Boldenone undecenoate is an anabolic steroid that has been used in veterinary practice.

WADA Status: Banned in and out of competition

WADA Class: Anabolic; Androgenic Steroids (exogenous)

Includes exogenous anabolic androgenic steroids or other substances with a similar chemical structure or similar biological effect(s).

Bopindolol Malonate

Other names: Bopindolol Hydrogen Malonate; Bopindolol, Malonate de; Bopindololi Malonas; LT-31-200; Malonato de bopindolol.

Бопиндолола Малонат

Clinical profile: Bopindolol is a non-cardioselective beta blocker used in the management of hypertension and angina pectoris.

WADA Status: Banned in and out of competition as specified below

WADA Class: Beta-Blockers

Unless otherwise specified, beta-blockers are prohibited *In-Competition* only in the following sports.

- Aeronautics (FAI)
- Archery (FITA, IPC) (also prohibited *Out-of-Competition*)
- Automobile (FIA)
- Billiards (WCBS)
- Bobsleigh (FIBT)
- Boules (CMSB, IPC bowls)
- Bridge (FMB)
- Curling (WCF)
- Gymnastics (FIG)
- Motorcycling (FIM)
- Modern Pentathlon (UIPM) for disciplines involving shooting
- Nine-pin bowling (FIQ)
- Powerboating (UIM)
- Sailing (ISAF) for match race helms only
- Shooting (ISSF, IPC) (also prohibited *Out-of-Competition*)
- Skiing/Snowboarding (FIS) in ski jumping, freestyle aerials/halfpipe and snowboard halfpipe/big air
- Wrestling (FILA)

WADA Class: Specified Substances

Also listed as a specified substance.

"*The prohibited List may identify specified substances which are particularly susceptible to unintentional anti-doping rule violations because of their general availability in medicinal products or which are less likely to be successfully abused as doping agents.*"

A doping violation involving such substances may result in a reduced sanction provided that the "*...Athlete can establish that the Use of such a specfied substance was not intended to enhance sport performance...*"

Preparations
Single ingredient: ***Cz.:*** Sandonorm; ***Hung.:*** Sandonorm; ***Switz.:*** Sandonorm.
Multi-ingredient: ***Switz.:*** Sandoretic.

Brinzolamide

Other names: AL-4862; Brintsolamidi; Brinzolamid; Brinzolamida; Brinzolamidum.

Бринзоламид

Clinical profile: Brinzolamide is a carbonic anhydrase inhibitor used to reduce intra-ocular pressure in glaucoma and ocular hypertension.

WADA Status: Banned in and out of competition

WADA Class: Diuretics and Other Masking Agents

Includes diuretics or substances with a similar chemical structure or similar biological effect(s).

Preparations

Single ingredient: ***Arg.:*** Azopt; ***Austral.:*** Azopt; ***Austria:*** Azopt; ***Belg.:*** Azopt; ***Braz.:*** Azopt; ***Canad.:*** Azopt; ***Chile:*** Azopt; ***Cz.:*** Azopt; ***Denm.:*** Azopt; ***Fin.:*** Azopt; ***Fr.:*** Azopt; ***Ger.:*** Azopt; ***Gr.:*** Azopt; ***Hong Kong:*** Azopt; ***Hung.:*** Azopt; ***Indon.:*** Azopt; ***Irl.:*** Azopt; ***Israel:*** Azopt; ***Ital.:*** Azopt; ***Malaysia:*** Azopt; ***Mex.:*** Azopt; ***Neth.:*** Azopt; ***Norw.:*** Azopt; ***NZ:*** Azopt; ***Philipp.:*** Azopt; ***Pol.:*** Azopt; ***Port.:*** Azopt; ***Rus.:*** Azopt (Азопт); ***S.Afr.:*** Azoptic; ***Singapore:*** Azopt; ***Spain:*** Azopt; ***Swed.:*** Azopt; ***Switz.:*** Azopt; ***Thai.:*** Azopt; ***Turk.:*** Azopt; ***UK:*** Azopt; ***USA:*** Azopt; ***Venez.:*** Azopt.

Broxaterol

Other names: Broxatérol; Broxaterolum; Z-1170.

Броксатерол

Clinical profile: Broxaterol is a selective $beta_2$-adrenoceptor agonist which has been investigated for its bronchodilator properties.

WADA Status: Banned in and out of competition

WADA Class: Beta-2 Agonists

Includes beta-2 agonists or their isomers.

WADA Class: Specified Substances

Also listed as a specified substance.

"The prohibited List may identify specified substances which are particularly susceptible to unintentional anti-doping rule violations because of their general availability in medicinal products or which are less likely to be successfully abused as doping agents."

A doping violation involving such substances may result in a reduced sanction provided that the "*...Athlete can establish that the Use of such a specfied substance was not intended to enhance sport performance...*"

Bucindolol Hydrochloride

Other names: Bucindolol, Chlorhydrate de; Bucindololi Hydrochloridum; Hidrocloruro de bucindolol; MJ-13105-1.

Буциндолола Гидрохлорид

Clinical profile: Bucindolol is a non-cardioselective beta blocker with weak $alpha_1$-blocking activity and direct vasodilating activity. It has been investigated in the management of hypertension, heart failure, and other cardiac disorders.

WADA Status: Banned in and out of competition as specified below

WADA Class: Beta-Blockers

Unless otherwise specified, beta-blockers are prohibited *In-Competition* only in the following sports.

- Aeronautics (FAI)
- Archery (FITA, IPC) (also prohibited *Out-of-Competition*)
- Automobile (FIA)
- Billiards (WCBS)
- Bobsleigh (FIBT)
- Boules (CMSB, IPC bowls)
- Bridge (FMB)
- Curling (WCF)
- Gymnastics (FIG)

- Motorcycling (FIM)
- Modern Pentathlon (UIPM) for disciplines involving shooting
- Nine-pin bowling (FIQ)
- Powerboating (UIM)
- Sailing (ISAF) for match race helms only
- Shooting (ISSF, IPC) (also prohibited *Out-of-Competition*)
- Skiing/Snowboarding (FIS) in ski jumping, freestyle aerials/halfpipe and snowboard halfpipe/big air
- Wrestling (FILA)

WADA Class: Specified Substances

Also listed as a specified substance.

"The prohibited List may identify specified substances which are particularly susceptible to unintentional anti-doping rule violations because of their general availability in medicinal products or which are less likely to be successfully abused as doping agents."

A doping violation involving such substances may result in a reduced sanction provided that the "*...Athlete can establish that the Use of such a specfied substance was not intended to enhance sport performance...*"

Budesonide

Other names: Budesonid; Budesónida; Budésonide; Budesonidi; Budesonidum; Budezonid; Budezonidas; S-1320.

Будезонид

Clinical profile: Budesonide is a glucocorticoid corticosteroid used by inhalation in the management of asthma. It is also used for the prophylaxis and treatment of allergic rhinitis and nasal polyps, for the management of childhood croup, inflammatory bowel disease, and collagenous colitis, and in the treatment of various skin disorders.

WADA Status: Banned in competition

WADA Class: Glucocorticosteroids

All glucocorticosteroids are prohibited when administered orally, rectally, intravenously or intramuscularly. Their use requires a Therapeutic Use Exemption approval. Other routes of administration (intraarticular / periarticular / peritendinous / epidural / intradermal injections and inhalation) require an Abbreviated Therapeutic Use Exemption except as noted below.

Topical preparations when used for dermatological (including iontophoresis / phonophoresis), auricular, nasal, ophthalmic, buccal, gingival and perianal disorders are not prohibited and do not require any form of Therapeutic Use Exemption.

WADA Class: Specified Substances

Also listed as a specified substance.

"The prohibited List may identify specified substances which are particularly susceptible to unintentional anti-doping rule violations because of their general availability in medicinal products or which are less likely to be successfully abused as doping agents."

A doping violation involving such substances may result in a reduced sanction provided that the "*...Athlete can establish that the Use of such a specfied substance was not intended to enhance sport performance...*"

Preparations

Single ingredient: ***Arg.:*** Aerovent; Airbude; Budeson; Cuteral; Entocort; Hypersol B; Inflammide; Infliplus; Nastizol Hidrospray; Neumocort; Neumotex; Proetzonide; Pulmo Lisoflam; Rino-B; Spirocort; ***Austral.:*** Budamax; Entocort; Pulmicort; Rhinocort; ***Austria:*** Budiair; Budo-san; Entocort; Miflonide; Novolizer; Pulmicort; Rhinocort; ***Belg.:*** Budenofalk; Docbudeso; Entocort; Merckrhinobudesonide; Miflonide; Pulmicort; Rhinocort; ***Braz.:*** Budecort; Busonid; Entocort; Miflonide; Novopulmon; Pulmicort; ***Canad.:*** Entocort; Pulmicort; Rhinocort; ***Chile:*** Aero-Bud; Aerovial; Budasmal; Budenofalk; Clebudan; Inflammide; Neumocort; Pulmicort; Rhinocort; ***Cz.:*** Apulein; Budenofalk; Easi-Cort; Entocort; Giona; Inflammide; Miflonid; Pulmicort; Rhinocort; Tafen; ***Denm.:*** Budenofalk; Entocort; Giona; Miflonide; Pulairmax; Rhinocort; Rhinosol; Spirocort; ***Fin.:***

Budenofalk; Entocort; Pulmicort; Rhinocort; ***Fr.:*** Entocort; Miflonil; Novopulmon; Pulmicort; Rafton; Rhinocort; ***Ger.:*** Aquacort; Budecort; Budenofalk; Budes; Budiair; Entocort; Miflonide; Novopulmon; Pulmicort; ***Gr.:*** Arsicort; Astrocast; Aurid; Axelovert; Beysonit; Biosonide; Budecol; Budemar; Budenite; Budenofalk; Budeprol; Buderen; Budesan; Budesoderm; Budesonal; Budiair; Busonal; Butekont; Dedostryl; Dexalocal; Esonide; Etrafonil; Farlidone; Ixor; Lisobron; Miflonide; Minalerg; Nalator; Obecirol; Obusonid; Olfosonide; Olyspal; Pulmicort; Pulmiver; Pulmovance; Resata; Rhinobros; Rhinoside; Ribuspir; Rinoster; Serbo; Sonidal; Talgan; Therasound; Udesogel; Udesospray; Velorium; Vericort; Vinecort; Zefecort; Zymacter; Zyolaif; Zytual; ***Hong Kong:*** Budenase; Budenofalk; Cycortide; Entocort; Pulmicort; Rhinocort; ***Hung.:*** Aerox; Budenofalk; Budesogen; Entocort; Miflonide; Neplit; Pulmax; Pulmicort; Rhinocort; ***India:*** Pulmicort; Rhinocort; ***Indon.:*** Budenofalk; Inflammide; Pulmicort; Rhinocort; ***Irl.:*** Budenofalk; Entocort; Pulmicort; Rhinocort; ***Israel:*** Budeson; Budicort; Entocort; Miflonide; Nasocort; ***Ital.:*** Aircort; Bidien; Desonax; Eltair; Entocir; Kesol; Miflo; Miflonide; Preferid; Pulmaxan; Rhinocort; Spirocort; Xavin; ***Malaysia:*** Butacort; Eltair; Inflammide; Pulmicort; Rhinocort; ***Mex.:*** Aerosial; Budosan; Entocort; Miflonide; Numark; Pulmicort; Rhinocort; ***Neth.:*** Budenofalk; Entocort; Pulmicort; Rhinocort; ***Norw.:*** Entocort; Giona; Pulmicort; Rhinocort; ***NZ:*** Butacort; Eltair; Entocort; Pulmicort; ***Philipp.:*** Asmavent; Budecort; Budenofalk; Primavent; ***Pol.:*** Budenofalk; Buderhin; Entocort; Horacort; Miflonide; Neplit; Pulmicort; Rhinocort; Tafen; ***Port.:*** Budo-san; Entocort; Miflonide; Pulmicort; ***Rus.:*** Benacort (Бенакорт); Benarin (Бенарин); Pulmicort (Пульмикорт); Tafen (Тафен); ***S.Afr.:*** Budeflam; Entocord; Inflammide; Inflanaze; Pulmicort; Rhinocort; ***Singapore:*** Budenofalk; Eltair; Esonide; Giona; Inflammide; Pulmicort; Rhinocort; ***Spain:*** Budenofalk; Demotest; Entocord; Miflonide; Neo Rinactive; Novopulm; Olfex; Pulmicort; Pulmictan; Rhinocort; Ribujet; ***Swed.:*** Budenofalk; Entocort; Giona; Pulmicort; Rhinocort; ***Switz.:*** Budenofalk; Cortinasal; Entocort; Miflonide; Pulmicort; Rhinocort; ***Thai.:*** Budecort; Bunase; Eltair; Giona; Pulmicort; Rhinocort; ***Turk.:*** Budenofalk; Entocort; Inflacort; Miflonid; Pulmicort; Rhinocort; ***UAE:*** Sonidar; ***UK:*** Budenofalk; Entocort; Pulmicort; Rhinocort; ***USA:*** Entocort; Pulmicort; Rhinocort; ***Venez.:*** Biosonida; Bronklast; Budecort; Budenas; Miflonide; Pulmicort; Pulmolet; Rhinocort; Rinolet.

Multi-ingredient: ***Arg.:*** Neumoterol; Symbicort; ***Austral.:*** Symbicort; ***Austria:*** Symbicort; ***Belg.:*** Symbicort; ***Braz.:*** Alenia; Foraseq; Symbicort; ***Canad.:*** Symbicort; ***Chile:*** Symbicort; ***Cz.:*** Symbicort; ***Denm.:*** Symbicort; ***Fin.:*** Symbicort; ***Fr.:*** Symbicort; ***Ger.:*** Symbicort; ***Gr.:*** Symbicort; ***Hong Kong:*** Symbicort; ***Hung.:*** Symbicort; ***India:*** Foracort; ***Indon.:*** Symbicort; ***Irl.:*** Symbicort; ***Israel:*** Symbicort; ***Ital.:*** Assieme; Sinestic; Symbicort; ***Malaysia:*** Symbicort; ***Mex.:*** Symbicort; ***Neth.:*** Assieme; Sinestic; Symbicort; ***Norw.:*** Symbicort; ***NZ:*** Symbicort; ***Philipp.:*** Symbicort; ***Pol.:*** Symbicort; ***Port.:*** Assieme; Symbicort; ***Rus.:*** Biasten (Биастен); Simbicort (Симбикорт); ***S.Afr.:*** Symbicord; ***Singapore:*** Symbicort; ***Spain:*** Rilast; Symbicort; ***Swed.:*** Symbicort; ***Switz.:*** Symbicort; ***Thai.:*** Symbicort; ***Turk.:*** Symbicort; ***UK:*** Symbicort; ***USA:*** Symbicort; ***Venez.:*** Foraseq; Symbicort.

Bufetolol Hydrochloride

Other names: Bufétolol, Chlorhydrate de; Bufetololi Hydrochloridum; Hidrocloruro de bufetolol; Y-6124.

Буфетолола Гидрохлорид

Clinical profile: Bufetolol is a beta blocker that has been used in the management of various cardiovascular disorders.

WADA Status: Banned in and out of competition as specified below

WADA Class: Beta-Blockers

Unless otherwise specified, beta-blockers are prohibited *In-Competition* only in the following sports.

- Aeronautics (FAI)
- Archery (FITA, IPC) (also prohibited *Out-of-Competition*)
- Automobile (FIA)
- Billiards (WCBS)
- Bobsleigh (FIBT)
- Boules (CMSB, IPC bowls)
- Bridge (FMB)
- Curling (WCF)
- Gymnastics (FIG)
- Motorcycling (FIM)
- Modern Pentathlon (UIPM) for disciplines involving shooting
- Nine-pin bowling (FIQ)
- Powerboating (UIM)
- Sailing (ISAF) for match race helms only
- Shooting (ISSF, IPC) (also prohibited *Out-of-Competition*)

- Skiing/Snowboarding (FIS) in ski jumping, freestyle aerials/halfpipe and snowboard halfpipe/big air
- Wrestling (FILA)

WADA Class: Specified Substances

Also listed as a specified substance.

"The prohibited List may identify specified substances which are particularly susceptible to unintentional anti-doping rule violations because of their general availability in medicinal products or which are less likely to be successfully abused as doping agents."

A doping violation involving such substances may result in a reduced sanction provided that the *"...Athlete can establish that the Use of such a specfied substance was not intended to enhance sport performance..."*

Bufuralol Hydrochloride

Other names: Bufuralol, Chlorhydrate de; Bufuraloli Hydrochloridum; Hidrocloruro de bufuralol; Ro-03-4787.

Буфуралола Гидрохлорид

Clinical profile: Bufuralol is a non-cardioselective beta blocker.

WADA Status: Banned in and out of competition as specified below

WADA Class: Beta-Blockers

Unless otherwise specified, beta-blockers are prohibited *In-Competition* only in the following sports.

- Aeronautics (FAI)
- Archery (FITA, IPC) (also prohibited *Out-of-Competition*)
- Automobile (FIA)
- Billiards (WCBS)
- Bobsleigh (FIBT)
- Boules (CMSB, IPC bowls)
- Bridge (FMB)
- Curling (WCF)
- Gymnastics (FIG)
- Motorcycling (FIM)
- Modern Pentathlon (UIPM) for disciplines involving shooting
- Nine-pin bowling (FIQ)
- Powerboating (UIM)
- Sailing (ISAF) for match race helms only
- Shooting (ISSF, IPC) (also prohibited *Out-of-Competition*)
- Skiing/Snowboarding (FIS) in ski jumping, freestyle aerials/halfpipe and snowboard halfpipe/big air
- Wrestling (FILA)

WADA Class: Specified Substances

Also listed as a specified substance.

"The prohibited List may identify specified substances which are particularly susceptible to unintentional anti-doping rule violations because of their general availability in medicinal products or which are less likely to be successfully abused as doping agents."

A doping violation involving such substances may result in a reduced sanction provided that the *"...Athlete can establish that the Use of such a specfied substance was not intended to enhance sport performance..."*

Bumetanide

Other names: Bumetanid; Bumetanida; Bumetanidas; Bumétanide; Bumetanidi;

Bumetanidum; Ro-10-6338.

Буметанид

Clinical profile: Bumetanide is a loop diuretic used in the treatment of oedema associated with heart failure and with renal and hepatic disorders, in oliguria due to renal failure or insufficiency, and in hypertension.

WADA Status: Banned in and out of competition

WADA Class: Diuretics and Other Masking Agents

Includes diuretics or substances with a similar chemical structure or similar biological effect(s).

Preparations

Single ingredient: ***Austral.:*** Burinex; ***Austria:*** Burinex; ***Belg.:*** Burinex; ***Braz.:*** Burinax; ***Canad.:*** Burinex; ***Denm.:*** Burinex; ***Fr.:*** Burinex; ***Ger.:*** Burinex; ***Gr.:*** Burinex; ***Hong Kong:*** Burinex; ***Irl.:*** Burinex; ***Malaysia:*** Burinex; ***Mex.:*** Drenural; Miccil; ***Neth.:*** Burinex; ***Norw.:*** Burinex; ***NZ:*** Burinex; ***Philipp.:*** Burinex; ***S.Afr.:*** Burinex; ***Singapore:*** Burinex; ***Spain:*** Fordiuran; ***Swed.:*** Burinex; ***Switz.:*** Burinex; ***UK:*** Burinex; ***USA:*** Bumex; ***Venez.:*** Bumelex.

Multi-ingredient: ***Denm.:*** Buram; Burinex med kaliumklorid; ***Irl.:*** Buram; ***Norw.:*** Burinex K; ***S.Afr.:*** Burinex K; ***Singapore:*** Burinex K; ***UK:*** Burinex A.

Bunitrolol Hydrochloride

Other names: Bunitrolol, Chlorhydrate de; Bunitrololi Hydrochloridum; Hidrocloruro de bunitrolol; Ko-1366 (bunitrolol).

Бунитролола Гидрохлорид

Clinical profile: Bunitrolol is a beta blocker that has been given in the management of cardiovascular disorders.

WADA Status: Banned in and out of competition as specified below

WADA Class: Beta-Blockers

Unless otherwise specified, beta-blockers are prohibited *In-Competition* only in the following sports.

- Aeronautics (FAI)
- Archery (FITA, IPC) (also prohibited *Out-of-Competition*)
- Automobile (FIA)
- Billiards (WCBS)
- Bobsleigh (FIBT)
- Boules (CMSB, IPC bowls)
- Bridge (FMB)
- Curling (WCF)
- Gymnastics (FIG)
- Motorcycling (FIM)
- Modern Pentathlon (UIPM) for disciplines involving shooting
- Nine-pin bowling (FIQ)
- Powerboating (UIM)
- Sailing (ISAF) for match race helms only
- Shooting (ISSF, IPC) (also prohibited *Out-of-Competition*)
- Skiing/Snowboarding (FIS) in ski jumping, freestyle aerials/halfpipe and snowboard halfpipe/big air
- Wrestling (FILA)

WADA Class: Specified Substances

Also listed as a specified substance.

"The prohibited List may identify specified substances which are particularly susceptible to unintentional anti-doping rule violations because of their general availability in medicinal products or which are less likely to be successfully abused as doping agents."

A doping violation involving such substances may result in a reduced sanction pro-

vided that the "*...Athlete can establish that the Use of such a specfied substance was not intended to enhance sport performance...*"

B

Buphenine Hydrochloride

Other names: Buphénine, Chlorhydrate de; Buphenini Hydrochloridum; Hidrocloruro de bufenina; Nylidrin Hydrochloride; Nylidrinium Chloride.

Буфенина Гидрохлорид

Clinical profile: Buphenine produces peripheral vasodilatation through beta-adrenoceptor stimulation and a direct action on the arteries and arterioles of the skeletal muscles. It has been used in the treatment of peripheral vascular and cerebrovascular disease, in rhinitis and nasal congestion, and in premature labour.

WADA Status: Banned in competition

WADA Class: Stimulants

Includes stimulants or substances with a similar chemical structure or similar biological effect(s).

WADA Class: Specified Substances

Also listed as a specified substance.

"*The prohibited List may identify specified substances which are particularly susceptible to unintentional anti-doping rule violations because of their general availability in medicinal products or which are less likely to be successfully abused as doping agents.*"

A doping violation involving such substances may result in a reduced sanction provided that the "*...Athlete can establish that the Use of such a specfied substance was not intended to enhance sport performance...*"

Preparations

Single ingredient: ***Austria:*** Dilatol; ***Canad.:*** Arlidin; ***India:*** Arlidin; ***Mex.:*** Arlidin; Flumil; Nilken.

Multi-ingredient: ***Austria:*** Arbid; Dilaescol; Dilatol-Chinin; Opino; Opino; Tropoderm; ***Fr.:*** Phlebogel; ***Gr.:*** Opino-jel; ***Indon.:*** Opino; ***Switz.:*** Arbid; Visaline.

Bupranolol Hydrochloride

Other names: B-1312; Bupranolol, Chlorhydrate de; Bupranololi Hydrochloridum; Hidrocloruro de bupranolol; KL-255.

Бупранолола Гидрохлорид

Clinical profile: Bupranolol is a beta blocker used in the management of cardiovascular disorders.

WADA Status: Banned in and out of competition as specified below

WADA Class: Beta-Blockers

Unless otherwise specified, beta-blockers are prohibited *In-Competition* only in the following sports.

- Aeronautics (FAI)
- Archery (FITA, IPC) (also prohibited *Out-of-Competition*)
- Automobile (FIA)
- Billiards (WCBS)
- Bobsleigh (FIBT)
- Boules (CMSB, IPC bowls)
- Bridge (FMB)
- Curling (WCF)
- Gymnastics (FIG)
- Motorcycling (FIM)

- Modern Pentathlon (UIPM) for disciplines involving shooting
- Nine-pin bowling (FIQ)
- Powerboating (UIM)
- Sailing (ISAF) for match race helms only
- Shooting (ISSF, IPC) (also prohibited *Out-of-Competition*)
- Skiing/Snowboarding (FIS) in ski jumping, freestyle aerials/halfpipe and snowboard halfpipe/big air
- Wrestling (FILA)

WADA Class: Specified Substances

Also listed as a specified substance.

"The prohibited List may identify specified substances which are particularly susceptible to unintentional anti-doping rule violations because of their general availability in medicinal products or which are less likely to be successfully abused as doping agents."

A doping violation involving such substances may result in a reduced sanction provided that the "*...Athlete can establish that the Use of such a specfied substance was not intended to enhance sport performance...*"

Preparations
Single ingredient: ***Ger.:*** Betadrenol.

Multi-ingredient: ***Austria:*** Betamed.

Buprenorphine

Other names: Buprenorfiini; Buprenorfin; Buprenorfina; Buprenorfinas; Buprénorphine; Buprenorphinum; RX-6029-M.

Бупренорфин

Buprenorphine Hydrochloride

Other names: Buprenorfiinihydrokloridi; Buprenorfin-hidroklorid; Buprenorfin-hydrochlorid; Buprenorfinhydroklorid; Buprenorfino hidrochloridas; Buprénorphine, chlorhydrate de; Buprenorphini hydrochloridum; CL-112302; Hidrocloruro de buprenorfina; NIH-8805; UM-952.

Бупренорфина Гидрохлорид

Clinical profile: Buprenorphine is an opioid agonist and antagonist and is used for the relief of moderate to severe pain and as an adjunct to anaesthesia. It has also been used in the treatment of opioid dependence.

WADA Status: Banned in competition

WADA Class: Narcotics

Includes specified narcotics.

Preparations
Single ingredient: ***Austral.:*** Norspan; Subutex; Temgesic; ***Austria:*** Subutex; Temgesic; Transtec; Tridol; ***Belg.:*** Subutex; Temgesic; Transtec; ***Braz.:*** Temgesic; ***Chile:*** Transtec; ***Cz.:*** Subutex; Temgesic; ***Denm.:*** Anorfin; Norspan; Subutex; Temgesic; Transtec; ***Fin.:*** Subutex; Temgesic; ***Fr.:*** Suboxone; Subutex; Temgesic; ***Ger.:*** Subutex; Temgesic; Transtec; ***Gr.:*** Subutex; ***Hong Kong:*** Subutex; Temgesic; ***Hung.:*** Bupren; Transtec; ***India:*** Norphin; Pentorel; ***Indon.:*** Subutex; ***Irl.:*** BuTrans; Temgesic; Transtec; ***Israel:*** Nopan; Subutex; ***Ital.:*** Subutex; Temgesic; Transtec; ***Malaysia:*** Subutex; Temgesic; ***Mex.:*** Brospina; Temgesic; Transtec; ***Neth.:*** Temgesic; ***Norw.:*** Subutex; Temgesic; ***NZ:*** Suboxone; Temgesic; ***Pol.:*** Bunondol; Transtec; ***Port.:*** Buprex; Subutex; Transtec; ***Rus.:*** Transtec (Транстек); ***S.Afr.:*** Subutex; Temgesic; ***Spain:*** Buprex; Subutex; Tran-

stec; ***Swed.:*** Norspan; Subutex; Temgesic; ***Switz.:*** Subutex; Temgesic; Transtec; ***Thai.:*** Buprine; ***UK:*** BuTrans; Suboxone; Subutex; Temgesic; Transtec; ***USA:*** Buprenex; Suboxone; Subutex.

Buserelin

Other names: Busereliini; Buserelina; Buserelinas; Buséréline; Buserelinum; Buszerelin; S74-6766.

Бусерелин

Buserelin Acetate

Other names: Acetato de buserelina; Buserelin Asetat; Buséréline, Acétate de; Buserelini Acetas; Hoe-766; D-Ser $(Bu^t)^6$ Pro^9 NEt LHRH acetate.

Бусерелина Ацетат

Clinical profile: Buserelin is a gonadorelin analogue used in the treatment of prostatic cancer and endometriosis. It is also used as an adjunct to ovulation induction with gonadotrophins in infertility.

WADA Status: Banned in and out of competition

WADA Class: Hormones and Related Substances: Gonadotrophins

Includes gonadotrophin or a substance with a similar chemical structure or similar biological effect(s), or one of their releasing factors. Prohibited in males only.

Preparations

Single ingredient: ***Arg.:*** Suprefact; ***Austria:*** Suprecur; Suprefact; ***Belg.:*** Suprefact; ***Braz.:*** Suprefact; ***Canad.:*** Suprefact; ***Cz.:*** Suprecur; Suprefact; ***Denm.:*** Suprecur; Suprefact; ***Fin.:*** Suprecur; Suprefact; ***Fr.:*** Bigonist; Suprefact; ***Ger.:*** Profact; Suprecur; ***Gr.:*** Suprefact; ***Hong Kong:*** Suprecur; ***Hung.:*** Suprefact; ***Irl.:*** Suprecur; Suprefact; ***Israel:*** Suprefact; ***Ital.:*** Suprefact; ***Jpn:*** Suprecur; ***Malaysia:*** Suprefact; ***Mex.:*** Suprefact; ***Neth.:*** Suprefact; ***Norw.:*** Suprecur; Suprefact; ***NZ:*** Suprefact; ***Port.:*** Suprefact; ***S.Afr.:*** Suprefact; ***Singapore:*** Suprefact; ***Spain:*** Suprefact; ***Swed.:*** Suprecur; Suprefact; ***Switz.:*** Suprefact; ***Thai.:*** Suprefact; ***Turk.:*** Suprecur; Suprefact; ***UK:*** Suprecur; Suprefact.

Butizide

Other names: Buthiazide; Butitsidi; Butizid; Butizida; Butizidum; Isobutylhydrochlorothiazide; Thiabutazide.

Бутизид

Clinical profile: Butizide is a thiazide diuretic used for oedema, including that associated with heart failure, and for hypertension.

WADA Status: Banned in and out of competition

WADA Class: Diuretics and Other Masking Agents

Includes diuretics or substances with a similar chemical structure or similar biological effect(s).

Preparations
Multi-ingredient: ***Austria:*** Aldactone Saltucin; Buti-Spirobene; ***Indon.:*** Aldazide; ***Ital.:*** Kadiur; Saludopin; ***Mex.:*** Aldazida; ***Philipp.:*** Aldazide; ***S.Afr.:*** Aldazide; ***Switz.:*** Aldozone.

Butofilolol

Other names: Butofilololum; CM-6805a.

Бутофилолол

Clinical profile: Butofilolol is a beta blocker.

WADA Status: Banned in and out of competition as specified below

WADA Class: Beta-Blockers

Unless otherwise specified, beta-blockers are prohibited *In-Competition* only in the following sports.

- Aeronautics (FAI)
- Archery (FITA, IPC) (also prohibited *Out-of-Competition*)
- Automobile (FIA)
- Billiards (WCBS)
- Bobsleigh (FIBT)
- Boules (CMSB, IPC bowls)
- Bridge (FMB)
- Curling (WCF)
- Gymnastics (FIG)
- Motorcycling (FIM)
- Modern Pentathlon (UIPM) for disciplines involving shooting
- Nine-pin bowling (FIQ)
- Powerboating (UIM)
- Sailing (ISAF) for match race helms only
- Shooting (ISSF, IPC) (also prohibited *Out-of-Competition*)
- Skiing/Snowboarding (FIS) in ski jumping, freestyle aerials/halfpipe and snowboard halfpipe/big air
- Wrestling (FILA)

WADA Class: Specified Substances

Also listed as a specified substance.
"*The prohibited List may identify specified substances which are particularly susceptible to unintentional anti-doping rule violations because of their general availability in medicinal products or which are less likely to be successfully abused as doping agents.*"
A doping violation involving such substances may result in a reduced sanction provided that the "*...Athlete can establish that the Use of such a specfied substance was not intended to enhance sport performance...*"

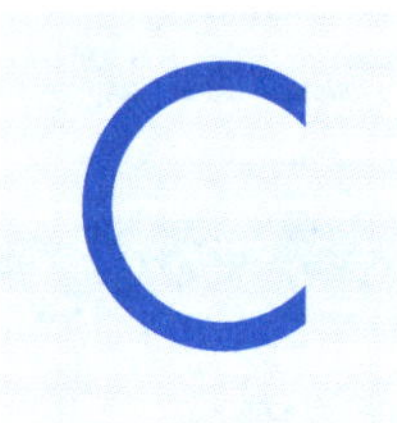

Calusterone

Other names: Calusterona; Calustérone; Calusteronum; 7β,17α-Dimethyltestosterone; NSC-88536; U-22550.

Калустерон

Clinical profile: Calusterone has the properties of androgens and anabolic steroids and has been used in the palliative treatment of breast cancer in postmenopausal women.

WADA Status: Banned in and out of competition

WADA Class: Anabolic; Androgenic Steroids (exogenous)

Includes exogenous anabolic androgenic steroids or other substances with a similar chemical structure or similar biological effect(s).

Cannabidiol

Other names: CBD.

Clinical profile: Cannabidiol is a cannabinoid present in cannabis that is being used or under investigation for a number of potential therapeutic uses, including in combination with 9-tetrahydrocannabinol (dronabinol) in a buccal spray preparation as adjunctive treatment in adults for neuropathic pain in multiple sclerosis and for advanced cancer pain.

WADA Status: Banned in competition

WADA Class: Cannabinoids

E.g. hashish, marijuana

WADA Class: Specified Substances

Also listed as a specified substance.

"The prohibited List may identify specified substances which are particularly susceptible to unintentional anti-doping rule violations because of their general availability in medicinal products or which are less likely to be successfully abused as doping agents."

A doping violation involving such substances may result in a reduced sanction provided that the "*...Athlete can establish that the Use of such a specfied substance was not intended to enhance sport performance...*"

Preparations
Multi-ingredient: ***Canad.:*** Sativex.

Cannabis

Other names: Cáñamo Indiano; Cannab.; Cannabis Indica; Chanvre; Hanfkraut; Indian Hemp.

Clinical profile: Cannabis was formerly employed as a sedative or narcotic. Its main active constituent 9-tetrahydrocannabinol (dronabinol) and a synthetic cannabinol (nabilone) are used as antiemetics in patients receiving cancer chemotherapy; they are also being investigated for a number of other potential therapeutic uses. 9-Tetrahydrocannabinol and cannabidiol, another cannabinoid, are being used in combination in a buccal spray preparation as adjunctive treatment in adults for neuropathic pain in multiple sclerosis and for advanced cancer pain; the combination is also under investigation for other forms of pain and spasticity.

WADA Status: Banned in competition

WADA Class: Cannabinoids

E.g. hashish, marijuana

WADA Class: Specified Substances

Also listed as a specified substance.

"The prohibited List may identify specified substances which are particularly susceptible to unintentional anti-doping rule violations because of their general availability in medicinal products or which are less likely to be successfully abused as doping agents."

A doping violation involving such substances may result in a reduced sanction provided that the "*...Athlete can establish that the Use of such a specfied substance was not intended to enhance sport performance...*"

Canrenone

Other names: Canrenona; Canrénone; Canrenonum; SC-9376.

Канренон

Clinical profile: Canrenone is a potassium-sparing diuretic and an aldosterone antagonist. It is a metabolite of both spironolactone and potassium canrenoate.

WADA Status: Banned in and out of competition

WADA Class: Diuretics and Other Masking Agents

Includes diuretics or substances with a similar chemical structure or similar biological effect(s).

Preparations
Single ingredient: ***Ital.:*** Luvion.

Carazolol

Other names: BM-51052; Carazololum.

Каразолол

Clinical profile: Carazolol is a beta blocker that has been used in the management of various cardiovascular disorders. It is also used in veterinary medicine.

WADA Status: Banned in and out of competition as specified below

WADA Class: Beta-Blockers

Unless otherwise specified, beta-blockers are prohibited *In-Competition* only in the following sports.

- Aeronautics (FAI)
- Archery (FITA, IPC) (also prohibited *Out-of-Competition*)
- Automobile (FIA)
- Billiards (WCBS)
- Bobsleigh (FIBT)
- Boules (CMSB, IPC bowls)
- Bridge (FMB)
- Curling (WCF)
- Gymnastics (FIG)
- Motorcycling (FIM)
- Modern Pentathlon (UIPM) for disciplines involving shooting
- Nine-pin bowling (FIQ)
- Powerboating (UIM)
- Sailing (ISAF) for match race helms only
- Shooting (ISSF, IPC) (also prohibited *Out-of-Competition*)
- Skiing/Snowboarding (FIS) in ski jumping, freestyle aerials/halfpipe and snowboard halfpipe/big air
- Wrestling (FILA)

WADA Class: Specified Substances

Also listed as a specified substance.

"The prohibited List may identify specified substances which are particularly susceptible to unintentional anti-doping rule violations because of their general availability in medicinal products or which are less likely to be successfully abused as doping agents."

A doping violation involving such substances may result in a reduced sanction provided that the "*...Athlete can establish that the Use of such a specfied substance was not intended to enhance sport performance...*"

Carbuterol Hydrochloride

Other names: Carbutérol, Chlorhydrate de; Carbuteroli Hydrochloridum; Hidrocloruro de carbuterol; SKF-40383; SKF-40383-A.

Карбутерола Гидрохлорид

Clinical profile: Carbuterol hydrochloride is a direct-acting sympathomimetic with a selective action on $beta_2$ adrenoceptors. It has been used as a bronchodilator.

WADA Status: Banned in and out of competition

WADA Class: Beta-2 Agonists

Includes beta-2 agonists or their isomers.

WADA Class: Specified Substances

Also listed as a specified substance.

"The prohibited List may identify specified substances which are particularly susceptible to unintentional anti-doping rule violations because of their general availability in medicinal products or which are less likely to be successfully abused as doping agents."

A doping violation involving such substances may result in a reduced sanction pro-

vided that the "...*Athlete can establish that the Use of such a specfied substance was not intended to enhance sport performance...*"

Carfentanil Citrate

Other names: Carfentanil, Citrate de; Carfentanili Citras; Citrato de carfentanilo; R-33799.

Карфентанила Цитрат

Clinical profile: Carfentanil citrate is an opioid analgesic related to fentanyl. It is used in veterinary medicine.

WADA Status: Banned in competition

WADA Class: Narcotics

Includes specified narcotics.

Carperitide

Other names: Carperitida; Carpéritide; Carperitidum; SUN-4936.

Карперитид

Clinical profile: Carperitide is a recombinant atrial natriuretic peptide used in the management of acute heart failure.

WADA Status: Banned in and out of competition

WADA Class: Diuretics and Other Masking Agents

Includes diuretics or substances with a similar chemical structure or similar biological effect(s).

Preparations
Single ingredient: ***Jpn:*** Hanp.

Carteolol Hydrochloride

Other names: Abbott-43326; Cartéolol, chlorhydrate de; Carteololi hydrochloridum; Hidrocloruro de carteolol; Karteolol Hidroklorür; Karteolol-hidroklorid; Karteolol-hydrochlorid; Karteololhydroklorid; Karteololihydrokloridi; Karteololio hidrochloridas; OPC-1085.

Картеолола Гидрохлорид

Clinical profile: Carteolol is a non-cardioselective beta blocker used in the management of glaucoma, hypertension, and some cardiac disorders.

WADA Status: Banned in and out of competition as specified below

WADA Class: Beta-Blockers

Unless otherwise specified, beta-blockers are prohibited *In-Competition* only in the following sports.

- Aeronautics (FAI)
- Archery (FITA, IPC) (also prohibited *Out-of-Competition*)
- Automobile (FIA)
- Billiards (WCBS)
- Bobsleigh (FIBT)
- Boules (CMSB, IPC bowls)

- Bridge (FMB)
- Curling (WCF)
- Gymnastics (FIG)
- Motorcycling (FIM)
- Modern Pentathlon (UIPM) for disciplines involving shooting
- Nine-pin bowling (FIQ)
- Powerboating (UIM)
- Sailing (ISAF) for match race helms only
- Shooting (ISSF, IPC) (also prohibited *Out-of-Competition*)
- Skiing/Snowboarding (FIS) in ski jumping, freestyle aerials/halfpipe and snowboard halfpipe/big air
- Wrestling (FILA)

C

WADA Class: Specified Substances

Also listed as a specified substance.

"The prohibited List may identify specified substances which are particularly susceptible to unintentional anti-doping rule violations because of their general availability in medicinal products or which are less likely to be successfully abused as doping agents."

A doping violation involving such substances may result in a reduced sanction provided that the "*...Athlete can establish that the Use of such a specfied substance was not intended to enhance sport performance...*"

Preparations
Single ingredient: ***Arg.:*** Elebloc; Glacout; Glauteolol; Poenglaucol; Singlauc; ***Austria:*** Arteoptic; Endak; ***Belg.:*** Arteoptic; Carteol; ***Cz.:*** Arteoptic; ***Fr.:*** Carteabak; Carteol; Mikelan; ***Ger.:*** Arteoptic; Endak; ***Gr.:*** Fortinol; Vinitus; ***Hong Kong:*** Arteoptic; ***Irl.:*** Teoptic; ***Ital.:*** Carteol; ***Jpn:*** Mikelan; ***Neth.:*** Arteoptic; Carteabak; Teoptic; ***Philipp.:*** Mikelan; ***Pol.:*** Arteoptic; ***Port.:*** Arteoptic; ***S.Afr.:*** Teoptic; ***Spain:*** Arteolol; Elebloc; Mikelan; ***Switz.:*** Arteoptic; ***Thai.:*** Arteoptic; ***Turk.:*** Carteol; ***UK:*** Teoptic; ***USA:*** Cartrol.
Multi-ingredient: ***Belg.:*** Carteopil; ***Fr.:*** Carpilo; ***Switz.:*** Arteopilo.

Carvedilol

Other names: BM-14190; Carvédilol; Carvedilolum; Karvedilol; Karvediloli; Karvedilolis.

Карведилол

Clinical profile: Carvedilol is a non-cardioselective beta blocker with vasodilating properties and is used in the management of hypertension, angina pectoris, heart failure, and left ventricular dysfunction following myocardial infarction.

WADA Status: Banned in and out of competition as specified below

WADA Class: Beta-Blockers

Unless otherwise specified, beta-blockers are prohibited *In-Competition* only in the following sports.

- Aeronautics (FAI)
- Archery (FITA, IPC) (also prohibited *Out-of-Competition*)
- Automobile (FIA)
- Billiards (WCBS)
- Bobsleigh (FIBT)
- Boules (CMSB, IPC bowls)
- Bridge (FMB)
- Curling (WCF)
- Gymnastics (FIG)
- Motorcycling (FIM)
- Modern Pentathlon (UIPM) for disciplines involving shooting
- Nine-pin bowling (FIQ)
- Powerboating (UIM)
- Sailing (ISAF) for match race helms only
- Shooting (ISSF, IPC) (also prohibited *Out-of-Competition*)
- Skiing/Snowboarding (FIS) in ski jumping, freestyle aerials/halfpipe and snowboard halfpipe/big air
- Wrestling (FILA)

WADA Class: Specified Substances

Also listed as a specified substance.

"The prohibited List may identify specified substances which are particularly susceptible to unintentional anti-doping rule violations because of their general availability in medicinal products or which are less likely to be successfully abused as doping agents."

A doping violation involving such substances may result in a reduced sanction provided that the "*...Athlete can establish that the Use of such a specfied substance was not intended to enhance sport performance...*"

Preparations

Single ingredient: ***Arg.:*** Antibloc; Bidecar; Carvedil; Corafen; Coritensil; Corubin; Dilatrend; Duobloc; Filten; Hipoten; Isobloc; Kollosteril; Rodipal; Rudoxil; Veraten; Vicardol; ***Austral.:*** Dilatrend; Kredex; ***Austria:*** Dilatrend; Hybridil; ***Belg.:*** Dimitone; Kredex; ***Braz.:*** Cardilol; Coreg; Divelol; Ictus; ***Canad.:*** Coreg; ***Chile:*** Betaplex; Blocar; Dilatrend; Dualten; Lodipres; Off-Ten; ***Cz.:*** Apo-Carve; Dilatrend; ***Denm.:*** Carvetone; Dimitone; ***Fin.:*** Cardiol; ***Fr.:*** Kredex; ***Ger.:*** CarLich; Carve-Q; Carve; Carvecard; Carvedigamma; Dilatrend; Dimetil; Querto; ***Gr.:*** Carvedilen; Carvepen; Dilatrend; ***Hong Kong:*** Dilatrend; ***Hung.:*** Carvedigamma; Carvol; Coryol; Dilatrend; Talliton; ***India:*** Carloc; Carvil; Cevas; ***Indon.:*** Carbloxal; Dilbloc; V-Bloc; ***Irl.:*** Biocard; Eucardic; ***Israel:*** Carvedexxon; Dimitone; ***Ital.:*** Carvipress; Colver; Dilatrend; Dilocar; ***Mex.:*** Dilatrend; ***Neth.:*** Eucardic; ***Norw.:*** Kredex; ***NZ:*** Dilatrend; ***Philipp.:*** Dilatrend; ***Pol.:*** Atram; Carvedigamma; Carvetrend; Coryol; Dilatrend; Vivacor; ***Port.:*** Dilbloc; ***Rus.:*** Acridilole (Акридилол); Cardivas (Кардивас); Carvetrend (Карветренд); Carvidil (Карвидил); Coryol (Кориол); Talliton (Таллитон); ***S.Afr.:*** Carloc; Carvetrend; Dilatrend; ***Singapore:*** Dilatrend; ***Spain:*** Coropres; ***Swed.:*** Kredex; ***Switz.:*** Dilatrend; ***Thai.:*** Dilatrend; ***Turk.:*** Dilatrend; ***UK:*** Eucardic; ***USA:*** Coreg; ***Venez.:*** Carbatil; Carvedil; Coventrol; Dilatrend.

Multi-ingredient: ***Arg.:*** Carvedil D; ***Austria:*** Co-Dilatrend; Dilaplus.

Catha

Other names: Abyssinian, African, or Arabian Tea; Kat; Kath; Khat; Miraa; Qat; Somali Tea.

Clinical profile: Catha, the leaves of *Catha edulis* (Celastraceae), is used for its stimulant properties among some cultures of Africa and the Middle East, usually by chewing the leaves. Its effects are reported to resemble those of the amfetamines and are thought to be largely due to the content of cathinone. Cathine, another constituent, has been used as an anorectic.

WADA Status: Banned in competition

WADA Class: Stimulants

Cathine, a constituent of catha, is prohibited when its concentration in urine is greater than 5 micrograms per milliliter.

WADA Class: Specified Substances

Also listed as a specified substance.

"The prohibited List may identify specified substances which are particularly susceptible to unintentional anti-doping rule violations because of their general availability in medicinal products or which are less likely to be successfully abused as doping agents."

A doping violation involving such substances may result in a reduced sanction provided that the "*...Athlete can establish that the Use of such a specfied substance was not intended to enhance sport performance...*"

Cathine

Other names: Cathinum; Catina; (+)-Norpseudoephedrine.

Катин

Clinical profile: Cathine, a constituent of catha [the leaves of *Catha edulis* (Celastraceae)], has been used as an anorectic. Catha is used for its stimulant properties among some cultures of Africa and the Middle East, usually by chewing the leaves. Its effects are reported to resemble those of the amfetamines and are thought to be largely due to the content of cathinone.

WADA Status: Banned in competition

WADA Class: Stimulants

Cathine, a constituent of catha, is prohibited when its concentration in urine is greater than 5 micrograms per milliliter.

WADA Class: Specified Substances

Also listed as a specified substance.

"The prohibited List may identify specified substances which are particularly susceptible to unintentional anti-doping rule violations because of their general availability in medicinal products or which are less likely to be successfully abused as doping agents."

A doping violation involving such substances may result in a reduced sanction provided that the "*...Athlete can establish that the Use of such a specfied substance was not intended to enhance sport performance...*"

C

Cathinone

Other names: Cathinonum; Catinona.

Катинон

Clinical profile: Catha [the leaves of *Catha edulis* (Celastraceae)] is used for its stimulant properties among some cultures of Africa and the Middle East, usually by chewing the leaves. Its effects are reported to resemble those of the amfetamines and are thought to be largely due to the content of cathinone. Cathine, another constituent, has been used as an anorectic.

WADA Status: Banned in competition

WADA Class: Stimulants

Includes stimulants or substances with a similar chemical structure or similar biological effect(s).

WADA Class: Specified Substances

Also listed as a specified substance.

"The prohibited List may identify specified substances which are particularly susceptible to unintentional anti-doping rule violations because of their general availability in medicinal products or which are less likely to be successfully abused as doping agents."

A doping violation involving such substances may result in a reduced sanction provided that the "*...Athlete can establish that the Use of such a specfied substance was not intended to enhance sport performance...*"

Preparations
Single ingredient: ***Ger.:*** Antiadipositum X-112 T; ***S.Afr.:*** Dietene; Eetless; Leanor; Nobese No. 1; Slim 'n Trim; Thinz; ***Switz.:*** Antiadipositum X-112.
Multi-ingredient: ***Mex.:*** Redotex NF; Redotex.

Celiprolol Hydrochloride

Other names: Céliprolol, chlorhydrate de; Celiprolol-hydrochlorid; Celiprololhydroklorid; Celiprololi hydrochloridum; Celiprololio hidrochloridas; Celiprololu chlorowodorek; Hidrocloruro de celiprolol; Seliprololihydrokloridi.

Целипролола Гидрохлорид

Clinical profile: Celiprolol is a cardioselective beta blocker with vasodilator activity. It is used in the management of hypertension and angina pectoris.

WADA Status: Banned in and out of competition as specified below

WADA Class: Beta-Blockers

Unless otherwise specified, beta-blockers are prohibited *In-Competition* only in the following sports.

- Aeronautics (FAI)
- Archery (FITA, IPC) (also prohibited *Out-of-Competition*)
- Automobile (FIA)
- Billiards (WCBS)
- Bobsleigh (FIBT)
- Boules (CMSB, IPC bowls)
- Bridge (FMB)
- Curling (WCF)
- Gymnastics (FIG)
- Motorcycling (FIM)
- Modern Pentathlon (UIPM) for disciplines involving shooting
- Nine-pin bowling (FIQ)
- Powerboating (UIM)
- Sailing (ISAF) for match race helms only
- Shooting (ISSF, IPC) (also prohibited *Out-of-Competition*)
- Skiing/Snowboarding (FIS) in ski jumping, freestyle aerials/halfpipe and snowboard halfpipe/big air
- Wrestling (FILA)

WADA Class: Specified Substances

Also listed as a specified substance.

"The prohibited List may identify specified substances which are particularly susceptible to unintentional anti-doping rule violations because of their general availability in medicinal products or which are less likely to be successfully abused as doping agents."

A doping violation involving such substances may result in a reduced sanction provided that the "...*Athlete can establish that the Use of such a specfied substance was not intended to enhance sport performance...*"

Preparations

Single ingredient: ***Austria:*** Selectol; ***Belg.:*** Selectol; ***Chile:*** Selectol; ***Cz.:*** Celectol; Tenoloc; ***Fin.:*** Selectol; ***Fr.:*** Celectol; ***Ger.:*** Celip; Celipro; Celiprogamma; Selectol; ***Gr.:*** Aplonit; Selectol; Versatil; ***Hong Kong:*** Selectol; ***Irl.:*** Selectol; ***Ital.:*** Cordiax; ***Jpn:*** Selectol; ***Neth.:*** Dilanorm; ***NZ:*** Celol; ***Pol.:*** Celipres; ***Spain:*** Cardem; ***Switz.:*** Selectol; ***UK:*** Celectol.
Multi-ingredient: ***Austria:*** Selecturon.

Cetamolol Hydrochloride

Other names: AI-27303; Cétamolol, Chlorhydrate de; Cetamololi Hydrochloridum; Hidrocloruro de cetamolol.

Цетамолола Гидрохлорид

Clinical profile: Cetamolol hydrochloride is a cardioselective beta blocker.

WADA Status: Banned in and out of competition as specified below

WADA Class: Beta-Blockers

Unless otherwise specified, beta-blockers are prohibited *In-Competition* only in the following sports.

- Aeronautics (FAI)
- Archery (FITA, IPC) (also prohibited *Out-of-Competition*)
- Automobile (FIA)
- Billiards (WCBS)
- Bobsleigh (FIBT)
- Boules (CMSB, IPC bowls)
- Bridge (FMB)
- Curling (WCF)
- Gymnastics (FIG)
- Motorcycling (FIM)
- Modern Pentathlon (UIPM) for disciplines involving shooting
- Nine-pin bowling (FIQ)

- Powerboating (UIM)
- Sailing (ISAF) for match race helms only
- Shooting (ISSF, IPC) (also prohibited *Out-of-Competition*)
- Skiing/Snowboarding (FIS) in ski jumping, freestyle aerials/halfpipe and snowboard halfpipe/big air
- Wrestling (FILA)

WADA Class: Specified Substances

Also listed as a specified substance.

"The prohibited List may identify specified substances which are particularly susceptible to unintentional anti-doping rule violations because of their general availability in medicinal products or which are less likely to be successfully abused as doping agents."

A doping violation involving such substances may result in a reduced sanction provided that the "...*Athlete can establish that the Use of such a specfied substance was not intended to enhance sport performance...*"

Chlorazanil Hydrochloride

Other names: ASA-226 (chlorazanil); Chlorazanil, Chlorhydrate de; Chlorazanili Hydrochloridum; Hidrocloruro de clorazanilo.

Хлоразанила Гидрохлорид

Clinical profile: Chlorazanil hydrochloride is a diuretic.

WADA Status: Banned in and out of competition

WADA Class: Diuretics and Other Masking Agents

Includes diuretics or substances with a similar chemical structure or similar biological effect(s).

Chlorothiazide

Other names: Chlorothiazid; Chlorothiazidum; Chlorotiazidas; Chlorotiazyd; Clorotiazida; Klooritiatsidi; Klorotiazid; Klortiazid.

Хлоротиазид

Chlorothiazide Sodium

Other names: Chlorothiazide Sodique; Clorotiazida sódica; Natrii Chlorothiazidum; Sodium Chlorothiazide.

Натрий Хлоротиазид

Clinical profile: Chlorothiazide is a thiazide diuretic used for oedema, including that associated with heart failure, and for hypertension.

WADA Status: Banned in and out of competition

WADA Class: Diuretics and Other Masking Agents

Includes diuretics or substances with a similar chemical structure or similar biological effect(s).

Preparations
Single ingredient: ***USA:*** Diurigen; Diuril.
Multi-ingredient: ***Gr.:*** Neourizine; ***USA:*** Aldoclor; Diupres.

Chlorphentermine Hydrochloride

Other names: Chlorphentermine, Chlorhydrate de; Chlorphentermini Hydrochloridum; Hidrocloruro de clorfentermina; NSC-76098; S-62; W-2426.
Хлорфентермина Гидрохлорид

Clinical profile: Chlorphentermine hydrochloride is a sympathomimetic that was formerly used as an anorectic but has been implicated in lipid storage disorders and pulmonary hypertension.

WADA Status: Banned in competition

WADA Class: Stimulants

Includes stimulants or substances with a similar chemical structure or similar biological effect(s).

WADA Class: Specified Substances

Also listed as a specified substance.
"The prohibited List may identify specified substances which are particularly susceptible to unintentional anti-doping rule violations because of their general availability in medicinal products or which are less likely to be successfully abused as doping agents."
A doping violation involving such substances may result in a reduced sanction provided that the "*...Athlete can establish that the Use of such a specfied substance was not intended to enhance sport performance...*"

Chlortalidone

Other names: Chlorotalidon; Chlortalidon; Chlortalidonas; Chlortalidonum; Chlorthalidone; Clorotalidona; Clortalidona; G-33182; Klooritalidoni; Klórtalidon; Klortalidon; NSC-69200.
Хлорталидон

Clinical profile: Chlortalidone is a diuretic similar to the thiazide diuretics. It is used for hypertension, and for oedema, including that associated with heart failure. Other indications include diabetes insipidus.

WADA Status: Banned in and out of competition

WADA Class: Diuretics and Other Masking Agents

Includes diuretics or substances with a similar chemical structure or similar biological effect(s).

Preparations
Single ingredient: ***Arg.:*** Euretico; Hygroton; ***Austral.:*** Hygroton; ***Austria:*** Hydrosan; Hygroton; ***Belg.:*** Hygroton; ***Braz.:*** Clordilon; Clortalil; Clortil; Clorton; Drenidra; Higroton; Neolidona; Taluron; ***Cz.:*** Urandil; ***Ger.:*** Hygroton; ***Gr.:*** Hygroton; ***Hung.:*** Hygroton; ***India:*** Thalizide; ***Indon.:*** Hygroton; ***Israel:*** Aquadon; ***Ital.:*** Igroton; ***Mex.:*** Anilid; Bioralin; Hidrona; Hidropharm; Higroton; Sinhidron; ***Neth.:*** Hygroton; ***NZ:*** Hygroton; ***Pol.:*** Hygroton; Urandil; ***Port.:*** Hygroton; ***S.Afr.:*** Hygroton; ***Spain:*** Higrotona; ***Switz.:*** Hygroton; ***Turk.:*** Hygroton; ***UK:*** Hygroton; ***USA:*** Hygroton; Thalitone.
Multi-ingredient: ***Arg.:*** Bemplas; Prenoretic; ***Austria:*** Arcablock comp; Atenolan comp; Atenolol comp; Darebon; Polinorm; Selecturon; Tenoretic; Trasitensin; Trepress; ***Belg.:*** Logroton; Tenoretic; ***Braz.:*** Angipress CD; Atenoclor; Atenoric; Atenuol CRT; Diupress; Higroton Reserpina; Tenoretic; ***Canad.:*** Apo-Atenidone; Tenoretic; ***Cz.:*** Amicloton; Atedon; Atenolol Compositum; Neocrystepin; Tenoretic; Trimecryton; ***Denm.:*** Tenidon; Tenoretic; ***Fr.:*** Logroton; Tenoretic; Trasitensine; ***Ger.:*** Ate Lich comp; Atehexal comp; Atel; Ateno comp; Atenogamma

comp; Atenolol AL comp; Atenolol comp; Diu-Atenolol; Prelis comp; Teneretic; Trepress; TRI-Normin; ***Gr.:*** Chlotenor; Hygroton-Reserpine; Obosan; Tenoretic; Trasitensin; Typofen; ***Hong Kong:*** Target; Tenoret; Tenoretic; ***Hung.:*** Blokium Diu; ***India:*** Catapres Diu; Tenoclor; Tenoric; ***Indon.:*** Tenoret; Tenoretic; ***Irl.:*** Atecor CT; Atenetic; Tenoret; Tenoretic; ***Ital.:*** Atenigron; Carmian; Clortanol; Diube; Eupres; Igroseles; Igroton-Lopresor; Igroton-Reserpina; Target; Tenoretic; Trandiur; Trasitensin; ***Malaysia:*** Logroton; Tenoret; Tenoretic; ***Mex.:*** Higroton-Res; Tenoretic; ***Neth.:*** Tenoretic; ***Philipp.:*** Tenoretic; ***Port.:*** Blokium Diu; Tenoretic; ***Rus.:*** Atehexal Compositum (Атегексал Композитум); Tenoric (Тенорик); Tenorox (Тенорокс); ***S.Afr.:*** Adco-Loten; Tenchlor; Tenoretic; ***Singapore:*** Tenoret; Tenoretic; ***Spain:*** Aldoleo; Blokium Diu; Higrotensin; Normopresil; Tenoretic; Trasitensin; ***Switz.:*** Atedurex; Cardaxen plus; Cotenolol-Neo; Hygroton-Reserpine; Logroton; Sandoretic; Slow-Trasitensine; Tenoretic; ***Turk.:*** Regroton; Tenoretic; ***UK:*** AtenixCo; Kalspare; Tenchlor; Tenoret; Tenoretic; Totaretic; ***USA:*** Clorpres; Demi-Regroton; Regroton; Tenoretic; ***Venez.:*** Blokiuret; Tenoretic.

Chorionic Gonadotrophin

Other names: CG; Choriogonadotrophin; Chorionic Gonadotropin; Chorioninis gonadotropinas; Gonadotrofina coriónica; Gonadotrophine Chorionique; Gonadotrophinum Chorionicum; Gonadotropin choriový; Gonadotropine chorionique; Gonadotropinum chorionicum; hCG; Human Chorionic Gonadotrophin; Koriongonadotropiini; Koriongonadotropin; Korion-gonadotropin; Koriyonik Gonadotrofin; Pregnancy-urine Hormone; PU.

Гонадотропин Хорионический

Clinical profile: Chorionic gonadotrophin is a hormone produced by the placenta and obtained from the urine of pregnant women, with actions predominantly of luteinising hormone. It is given to induce ovulation following follicular stimulation in the treatment of female infertility and as an adjunct to *in-vitro* fertilisation procedures. In males it is used for hypogonadotrophic hypogonadism, cryptorchidism, and delayed puberty.

Choriogonadotropin Alfa

Other names: Choriogonadotropine Alfa; Choriogonadotropinum Alfa; Coriogonadotropina alfa.

Хориогонадотропин Альфа

Clinical profile: Choriogonadotropin alfa is a recombinant chorionic gonadotrophin, with actions predominantly of luteinising hormone. It is given to induce ovulation following follicular stimulation in the treatment of female infertility and as an adjunct to *in-vitro* fertilisation procedures.

WADA Status: Banned in and out of competition

WADA Class: Hormones and Related Substances: Gonadotrophins

Includes gonadotrophin or a substance with a similar chemical structure or similar biological effect(s), or one of their releasing factors. Prohibited in males only.

Preparations

Single ingredient: ***Arg.:*** Dinaron; Endocorion; Gonacor; Ovidrel; Pregnyl; ***Austral.:*** Pregnyl; Profasi; ***Austria:*** Pregnyl; Profasi; ***Belg.:*** Choragon; Ovitrelle; Pregnyl; ***Braz.:*** Choragon; Ovidrel; Pregnyl; Profasi HP; ***Canad.:*** Profasi HP; ***Chile:*** Gonacor; Pregnyl; ***Cz.:*** Praedyn; Pregnyl; Profasi; ***Denm.:*** Ovitrelle; Pregnyl; ***Fin.:*** Ovitrelle; Pregnyl; ***Fr.:*** Ovitrelle; ***Ger.:*** Choragon; Ovitrelle; Predalon; ***Gr.:*** Ovitrelle; Pregnyl; ***Hong Kong:*** Choragon; Choriomon; Ovidrel; Pregnyl; Profasi; ***Hung.:*** Choragon; Ovitrelle; Pregnyl; ***India:*** Corion; Profasi; Provigil; Pubergen; ***Indon.:*** Ovidrel; Pregnyl; ***Irl.:*** Ovitrelle; Pregnyl; Profasi; ***Israel:*** Ovitrelle; Pregnyl; ***Ital.:*** Gonasi HP; Ovitrelle; Pregnyl; ***Malaysia:*** Ovidrel; Pregnyl; ***Mex.:*** Choragon; Choriomon; Ovidrel; Pregnyl; ***Neth.:*** Choragon; Ovitrelle; Pregnyl; ***Norw.:*** Ovitrelle; Pregnyl; ***NZ:*** Ovidrel; Profasi; ***Philipp.:*** Ovidrel; Pregnyl; ***Pol.:*** Choragon; Ovitrelle; Pregnyl; ***Port.:*** Ovitrelle; Pregnyl; Profasi HP; ***Rus.:*** Choragon (Хорагон); Ovitrelle (Овитрель); Pregnyl (Прегнил); ***S.Afr.:*** APL; Pregnyl; Profasi; ***Singapore:*** Ovidrel; Pregnyl; ***Spain:*** Ovitrelle; ***Swed.:*** Ovitrelle; Pregnyl; ***Switz.:*** Choriomon; Ovitrelle; Pregnyl; ***Thai.:*** IVF-C; Ovidrel; Pregnyl; ***Turk.:*** Choragon; Ovitrelle; Pregnyl; Profasi; ***UK:*** Chor-

agon; Ovitrelle; Pregnyl; ***USA:*** Choron; Gonic; Novarel; Ovidrel; Pregnyl; Profasi; ***Venez.:*** Ovidrel; Pregnyl.
Multi-ingredient: ***Mex.:*** Gonakor.

Ciclesonide

Other names: BY-9010; Ciclesonida; Ciclésonide; Ciclesonidum; RPR-251526.

Циклезонид

Clinical profile: Ciclesonide is a glucocorticoid corticosteroid used by inhalation for the management of asthma. It is also under investigation for the topical treatment of allergic rhinitis.

WADA Status: Banned in competition

WADA Class: Glucocorticosteroids

All glucocorticosteroids are prohibited when administered orally, rectally, intravenously or intramuscularly. Their use requires a Therapeutic Use Exemption approval. Other routes of administration (intraarticular / periarticular / peritendinous / epidural / intradermal injections and inhalation) require an Abbreviated Therapeutic Use Exemption except as noted below.

Topical preparations when used for dermatological (including iontophoresis / phonophoresis), auricular, nasal, ophthalmic, buccal, gingival and perianal disorders are not prohibited and do not require any form of Therapeutic Use Exemption.

WADA Class: Specified Substances

Also listed as a specified substance.

"*The prohibited List may identify specified substances which are particularly susceptible to unintentional anti-doping rule violations because of their general availability in medicinal products or which are less likely to be successfully abused as doping agents.*"

A doping violation involving such substances may result in a reduced sanction provided that the "*...Athlete can establish that the Use of such a specfied substance was not intended to enhance sport performance...*"

Preparations
Single ingredient: ***Arg.:*** Alvesco; Cicletex; ***Austral.:*** Alvesco; ***Chile:*** Alvesco; ***Gr.:*** Alvesco; Amavio; Freathe; ***Hong Kong:*** Alvesco; ***Hung.:*** Alvesco; ***India:*** Osonide; ***Irl.:*** Alvesco; ***Mex.:*** Alvesco; ***Neth.:*** Alvesco; ***Pol.:*** Alvesco; ***S.Afr.:*** Alvesco; ***UK:*** Alvesco; ***Venez.:*** Alvesco.

Cicletanine

Other names: (±)-BN-1270; Cicletanina; Ciclétanine; Cicletaninum; (±)-Cycletanide; Win-90000.

Циклетанин

Cicletanine Hydrochloride

Other names: Ciclétanine, Chlorhydrate de; Cicletanini Hydrochloridum; Hidrocloruro de cicletanina.

Циклетанина Гидрохлорид

Clinical profile: Cicletanine is a diuretic used as the hydrochloride in the treatment of hypertension.

WADA Status: Banned in and out of competition

WADA Class: Diuretics and Other Masking Agents

Includes diuretics or substances with a similar chemical structure or similar biological effect(s).

Preparations
Single ingredient: ***Cz.:*** Tenstaten; ***Fr.:*** Tenstaten; ***Ger.:*** Justar.

Ciclomethasone

Other names: RIB-222.

Clinical profile: Ciclomethasone is a glucocorticoid corticosteroid that has been applied topically in allergic and inflammatory skin disorders. It has also been given by inhalation in asthmatic conditions.

WADA Status: Banned in competition

WADA Class: Glucocorticosteroids

All glucocorticosteroids are prohibited when administered orally, rectally, intravenously or intramuscularly. Their use requires a Therapeutic Use Exemption approval. Other routes of administration (intraarticular / periarticular / peritendinous / epidural / intradermal injections and inhalation) require an Abbreviated Therapeutic Use Exemption except as noted below.

Topical preparations when used for dermatological (including iontophoresis / phonophoresis), auricular, nasal, ophthalmic, buccal, gingival and perianal disorders are not prohibited and do not require any form of Therapeutic Use Exemption.

WADA Class: Specified Substances

Also listed as a specified substance.

"The prohibited List may identify specified substances which are particularly susceptible to unintentional anti-doping rule violations because of their general availability in medicinal products or which are less likely to be successfully abused as doping agents."

A doping violation involving such substances may result in a reduced sanction provided that the "*...Athlete can establish that the Use of such a specfied substance was not intended to enhance sport performance...*"

Cicloprolol

Other names: Cicloprololum; Cycloprolol; SL-75-177-10 (cicloprolol or cicloprolol hydrochloride).

Циклопролол

Clinical profile: Cicloprolol has been reported to be a cardioselective beta blocker.

WADA Status: Banned in and out of competition as specified below

WADA Class: Beta-Blockers

Unless otherwise specified, beta-blockers are prohibited *In-Competition* only in the following sports.

- Aeronautics (FAI)
- Archery (FITA, IPC) (also prohibited *Out-of-Competition*)
- Automobile (FIA)
- Billiards (WCBS)
- Bobsleigh (FIBT)
- Boules (CMSB, IPC bowls)
- Bridge (FMB)
- Curling (WCF)
- Gymnastics (FIG)

- Motorcycling (FIM)
- Modern Pentathlon (UIPM) for disciplines involving shooting
- Nine-pin bowling (FIQ)
- Powerboating (UIM)
- Sailing (ISAF) for match race helms only
- Shooting (ISSF, IPC) (also prohibited *Out-of-Competition*)
- Skiing/Snowboarding (FIS) in ski jumping, freestyle aerials/halfpipe and snowboard halfpipe/big air
- Wrestling (FILA)

WADA Class: Specified Substances

Also listed as a specified substance.

"*The prohibited List may identify specified substances which are particularly susceptible to unintentional anti-doping rule violations because of their general availability in medicinal products or which are less likely to be successfully abused as doping agents.*"

A doping violation involving such substances may result in a reduced sanction provided that the "*...Athlete can establish that the Use of such a specfied substance was not intended to enhance sport performance...*"

C

Cinnamedrine

Other names: Cinamedrina; Cinnamédrine; Cinnamedrinum; *N*-Cinnamylephedrine.

Циннамедрин

Cinnamedrine Hydrochloride

Other names: Cinnamédrine, Chlorhydrate de; Cinnamedrini Hydrochloridum; *N*-Cinnamylephedrine Hydrochloride; Hidrocloruro de cinamedrina.

Циннамедрина Гидрохлорид

Clinical profile: Cinnamedrine is reported to have sympathomimetic actions resembling those of ephedrine. It has been used in combination with analgesics in the symptomatic relief of dysmenorrhoea.

WADA Status: Banned in competition

WADA Class: Stimulants

Includes stimulants or substances with a similar chemical structure or similar biological effect(s).

WADA Class: Specified Substances

Also listed as a specified substance.

"*The prohibited List may identify specified substances which are particularly susceptible to unintentional anti-doping rule violations because of their general availability in medicinal products or which are less likely to be successfully abused as doping agents.*"

A doping violation involving such substances may result in a reduced sanction provided that the "*...Athlete can establish that the Use of such a specfied substance was not intended to enhance sport performance...*"

Ciprocinonide

Other names: Ciprocinonida; Ciprocinonidum; RS-2386.

Ципроцинонид

Clinical profile: Ciprocinonide is a derivative of the corticosteroid fluocinolone acetonide that has been applied topically with fluocinonide and procinonide in the management of various skin disorders.

WADA Status: Banned in competition

WADA Class: Glucocorticosteroids

All glucocorticosteroids are prohibited when administered orally, rectally, intravenously or intramuscularly. Their use requires a Therapeutic Use Exemption approval. Other routes of administration (intraarticular / periarticular / peritendinous / epidural / intradermal injections and inhalation) require an Abbreviated Therapeutic Use Exemption except as noted below.

Topical preparations when used for dermatological (including iontophoresis / phonophoresis), auricular, nasal, ophthalmic, buccal, gingival and perianal disorders are not prohibited and do not require any form of Therapeutic Use Exemption.

WADA Class: Specified Substances

Also listed as a specified substance.

"*The prohibited List may identify specified substances which are particularly susceptible to unintentional anti-doping rule violations because of their general availability in medicinal products or which are less likely to be successfully abused as doping agents.*"

A doping violation involving such substances may result in a reduced sanction provided that the "...*Athlete can establish that the Use of such a specfied substance was not intended to enhance sport performance*..."

C

Clenbuterol Hydrochloride

Other names: Clenbutérol, chlorhydrate de; Clenbuteroli hydrochloridum; Hidrocloruro de clenbuterol; Klenbuterol hydrochlorid; Klenbuterol-hidroklorid; Klenbuterolhydroklorid; Klenbuterolihydrokloridi; Klenbuterolio hidrochloridas; NAB-365 (clenbuterol).

Кленбутерола Гидрохлорид

Clinical profile: Clenbuterol hydrochloride is a direct-acting sympathomimetic with a selective action on beta$_2$ adrenoceptors. It is used as a bronchodilator in the management of respiratory disorders such as asthma and chronic obstructive pulmonary disease. It has been abused for its anabolic effects.

WADA Status: Banned in and out of competition

WADA Class: Other Anabolic Agents

Includes other anabolic agents not listed elsewhere.

WADA Class: Beta-2 Agonists

Includes beta-2 agonists or their isomers.

Preparations

Single ingredient: ***Arg.:*** Bronq-C; Clembumar; Oxibron; ***Austria:*** Spiropent; ***Chile:*** Airum; Asmeren; ***Cz.:*** Spiropent; ***Ger.:*** Spiropent; ***Gr.:*** Spiropent; ***Hung.:*** Spiropent; ***Indon.:*** Spiropent; ***Ital.:*** Monores; Spiropent; ***Jpn:*** Spiropent; ***Mex.:*** Novegam; Oxyflux; Spiropent; ***Philipp.:*** Spiropent; ***Port.:*** Broncoterol; Cesbron; ***Spain:*** Ventolase; ***Venez.:*** Brodilan; Brodilin; Buclen; Clenbunal; Risopent.

Multi-ingredient: ***Arg.:*** Mucosolvon Compositum; Oxibron NF; ***Austria:*** Mucospas; ***Ger.:*** Spasmo-Mucosolvan; ***Mex.:*** Ambodil-C; Balsibron-C; Brogal Compositum; Bronolban-M; Broxolan C; Broxofar Compuesto; Broxol Plus; Broxolim-C; Ebromin P; Fludexol-CL; Loxorol; Mucosolvan Compositum; Mucovibrol C; Sekretovit Ex; Septacin Ex; Seraxol; Serbol; ***Port.:*** Mucospas;

Ventoliber; ***Venez.:*** Ambromuco Compositum; Arbixil; Clenbuxol; Litusix Compositum; Mucolin; Mucosolvan Compositum.

Clobenzorex Hydrochloride

Other names: Clobenzorex, Chlorhydrate de; Clobenzorexi Hydrochloridum; Hidrocloruro de clobenzorex; SD-271-12.

Клобензорекса Гидрохлорид

Clinical profile: Clobenzorex hydrochloride is a central stimulant and sympathomimetic that has been used as an anorectic in the treatment of obesity.

WADA Status: Banned in competition

WADA Class: Stimulants

Includes clobenzorex and any optical isomers.

Preparations
Single ingredient: ***Mex.:*** Asenlix; Itravil; Redicres.

Clobetasol Propionate

Other names: CCI-4725; Clobétasol, propionate de; Clobetasoli propionas; GR-2/925; Klobetasol-propionát; Klobetazol Propiyonat; Klobetazolu propionian; Propionato de clobetasol.

Клобетазола Пропионат

Clinical profile: Clobetasol propionate is a corticosteroid used topically in the treatment of various skin disorders.

WADA Status: Banned in competition

WADA Class: Glucocorticosteroids

All glucocorticosteroids are prohibited when administered orally, rectally, intravenously or intramuscularly. Their use requires a Therapeutic Use Exemption approval. Other routes of administration (intraarticular / periarticular / peritendinous / epidural / intradermal injections and inhalation) require an Abbreviated Therapeutic Use Exemption except as noted below.

Topical preparations when used for dermatological (including iontophoresis / phonophoresis), auricular, nasal, ophthalmic, buccal, gingival and perianal disorders are not prohibited and do not require any form of Therapeutic Use Exemption.

WADA Class: Specified Substances

Also listed as a specified substance.

"The prohibited List may identify specified substances which are particularly susceptible to unintentional anti-doping rule violations because of their general availability in medicinal products or which are less likely to be successfully abused as doping agents."

A doping violation involving such substances may result in a reduced sanction provided that the "*...Athlete can establish that the Use of such a specfied substance was not intended to enhance sport performance...*"

Preparations
Single ingredient: ***Arg.:*** Clobesol; Clobex; Dermaclob; Dermadex; Dermexane; Perfracort; Ribatra; Salac; ***Austria:*** Dermovate; ***Belg.:*** Dermovate; ***Braz.:*** Clob-X; Clobesol; Cortalen C; Dermacare; Propiosol; Psorex; Psorin; Therapsor; ***Canad.:*** Clobex; Dermovate; ***Chile:*** Alticort; Clob-X; Clodavan; Cortopic; Dermovate; Koniderm; Xinder; ***Cz.:*** Dermovate; ***Denm.:*** Dermovat; ***Fin.:*** Dermovat; ***Fr.:*** Dermoval; ***Ger.:*** Clobegalen; Dermoxin; Dermoxinale; Karison; ***Gr.:*** Butavate; Clarelux; Rubocort; ***Hong Kong:*** Clobasol; Clobesol; Clobex; Dermo; Dermovate; Dhabesol; Eurobetsol; Medodermone; Uniderm; ***Hung.:*** Closanasol; Dermovate; ***India:*** Cloderm; Lobate; Tenovate; Topifort; ***Indon.:*** Bersol; Closol; Dermovate; Elopro; Forderm; Ika

derm; Kloderma; Klonat; Lamodex; Lotasbat; Primaderm; Psoriderm; ***Irl.:*** Dermovate; ***Israel:*** Dermovate; ***Ital.:*** Clobesol; ***Malaysia:*** Clobet; Cloderm; Dermosol; Dermovate; Dhabesol; Lobesol; Univate; ***Mex.:*** Clobesol; Dermatovate; Lobevat; ***Neth.:*** Clarelux; Clobex; Dermovate; ***Norw.:*** Dermovat; ***NZ:*** Dermol; ***Philipp.:*** Clonate; Closderm; Dermovate; Glevate; ***Pol.:*** Clobederm; Dermklobal; Dermovate; Novate; ***Port.:*** Dermovate; ***Rus.:*** Dermovate (Дермовейт); ***S.Afr.:*** Dermovate; Dovate; Xenovate; ***Singapore:*** Cloderm; Dermosol; Dermovate; Dhabesol; Medodermone; Powercort; Uniderm; Univate; ***Spain:*** Clovate; Decloban; ***Swed.:*** Dermovat; ***Switz.:*** Dermovate; ***Thai.:*** Betasol; Clinoderm; Clobasone; Clobet; Clobetate; Cloderm; Clonovate; Cotaso; Dermovate; P-Vate; Stivate; Uniderm; ***Turk.:*** Dermovate; Psoderm; Psovate; ***UAE:*** Gamavate; ***UK:*** Clarelux; Dermovate; ***USA:*** Clobex; Cormax; Olux; Temovate; ***Venez.:*** Dermovate.

C

Multi-ingredient: ***Arg.:*** Clobeplus; Clobesol LA; Dermadex NN; ***India:*** Cloderm GM; Lobate-G; Lobate-GM; Lobate-M; Tenovate G; Tenovate M; ***Philipp.:*** Dermovate-NN; ***Port.:*** Dermovate-NN; ***Switz.:*** Dermovate-NN; ***UK:*** Dermovate-NN.

Clobetasone Butyrate

Other names: Butirato de clobetasona; CCI-5537; Clobétasone, butyrate de; Clobetasoni Butiras; Clobetasoni butyras; GR-2/1214; Klobetasonbutyrat; Klobetason-butyrát; Klobetasonibutyraatti; Klobetazon Bütirat; Klobetazon-butirát; Klobetazono butiratas.

Клобетазона Бутират

Clinical profile: Clobetasone butyrate is a corticosteroid used topically in the treatment of various eye and skin disorders.

WADA Status: Banned in competition

WADA Class: Glucocorticosteroids

All glucocorticosteroids are prohibited when administered orally, rectally, intravenously or intramuscularly. Their use requires a Therapeutic Use Exemption approval. Other routes of administration (intraarticular / periarticular / peritendinous / epidural / intradermal injections and inhalation) require an Abbreviated Therapeutic Use Exemption except as noted below.

Topical preparations when used for dermatological (including iontophoresis / phonophoresis), auricular, nasal, ophthalmic, buccal, gingival and perianal disorders are not prohibited and do not require any form of Therapeutic Use Exemption.

WADA Class: Specified Substances

Also listed as a specified substance.

"The prohibited List may identify specified substances which are particularly susceptible to unintentional anti-doping rule violations because of their general availability in medicinal products or which are less likely to be successfully abused as doping agents."

A doping violation involving such substances may result in a reduced sanction provided that the "*...Athlete can establish that the Use of such a specfied substance was not intended to enhance sport performance...*"

Preparations

Single ingredient: ***Arg.:*** Eumovate; ***Austria:*** Emovate; ***Belg.:*** Eumovate; ***Braz.:*** Eumovate; ***Canad.:*** Eumovate; ***Denm.:*** Emovat; ***Fin.:*** Emovat; ***Ger.:*** Emovate; ***Gr.:*** Rettavate; ***Hong Kong:*** Eumovate; ***India:*** Eumosone; ***Irl.:*** Eumovate; ***Israel:*** Eumovate; ***Ital.:*** Clobet; Eumovate; Visucloben; ***Malaysia:*** Cortoftal; Eumovate; U-Closone; ***Neth.:*** Emovate; ***NZ:*** Eumovate;

Port.: Emovate; **S.Afr.:** Eumovate; **Singapore:** Amisol; Eumovate; **Spain:** Emovate; **Swed.:** Emovat; **Switz.:** Emovate; **Turk.:** Eumovate; **UK:** Eumovate; **Venez.:** Eumovate.
Multi-ingredient: India: Eumosone-G; Eumosone-M; **Israel:** Cicloderm-C; **Ital.:** Visucloben Antibiotico; Visucloben Decongestionante; **UK:** Trimovate.

Clocortolone Pivalate

Other names: CL-68; Clocortolone, Pivalate de; Clocortoloni Pivalas; Pivalato de clocortolona; SH-863.

Клокортолона Пивалат

Clinical profile: Clocortolone pivalate is a corticosteroid used topically in the treatment of various skin disorders.

WADA Status: Banned in competition

WADA Class: Glucocorticosteroids

All glucocorticosteroids are prohibited when administered orally, rectally, intravenously or intramuscularly. Their use requires a Therapeutic Use Exemption approval. Other routes of administration (intraarticular / periarticular / peritendinous / epidural / intradermal injections and inhalation) require an Abbreviated Therapeutic Use Exemption except as noted below.

Topical preparations when used for dermatological (including iontophoresis / phonophoresis), auricular, nasal, ophthalmic, buccal, gingival and perianal disorders are not prohibited and do not require any form of Therapeutic Use Exemption.

WADA Class: Specified Substances

Also listed as a specified substance.

"The prohibited List may identify specified substances which are particularly susceptible to unintentional anti-doping rule violations because of their general availability in medicinal products or which are less likely to be successfully abused as doping agents."

A doping violation involving such substances may result in a reduced sanction provided that the "*...Athlete can establish that the Use of such a specfied substance was not intended to enhance sport performance...*"

Preparations
Single ingredient: Austria: Glimbal; **Ger.:** Kaban; Kabanimat; **USA:** Cloderm.

Clomifene Citrate

Other names: Chloramiphene Citrate; Citrato de clomifeno; Clomifène, citrate de; Clomifeni citras; Clomiphene Citrate; Klomifeenisitraatti; Klomifen Sitrat; Klomifencitrat; Klomifén-citrát; Klomifen-citrát; Klomifeno citratas; MER-41; MRL-41; NSC-35770.

Кломифена Цитрат

Clinical profile: Clomifene citrate is used for its anti-oestrogenic effects in the treatment of anovulatory infertility.

WADA Status: Banned in and out of competition

WADA Class: Hormone Antagonists and Modulators: Other Anti-estrogenic Substances

Includes other anti-estrogenic substances not listed elsewhere.

Preparations
Single ingredient: Arg.: Genozym; Serofene; **Austral.:** Clomhexal; Clomid; Fermil; Serophene; **Austria:** Serophene; **Belg.:** Clomid; Pergotime; **Braz.:** Clomid; Serophene; **Canad.:** Clomid; Serophene; **Chile:** Zimaquin; **Cz.:** Clomhexal; Clostilbegyt; Serophene; **Denm.:** Pergotime; **Fin.:** Clomifen; **Fr.:** Clomid; Pergotime; **Ger.:** Clomhexal; **Gr.:** Serpafar; **Hong Kong:**

Clostilbegyt; Fertilan; Ova-Mit; Serophene; ***Hung.:*** Clostilbegyt; ***India:*** Clofert; Clopreg; Fertomid; Ovipreg; Ovofar; Siphene; ***Indon.:*** Blesifen; Clomifil; Clovertil; Fensipros; Fertilphen; Fertin; Genoclom; Mestrolin; Ofertil; Pinfetil; Profertil; Provula; ***Irl.:*** Clomid; ***Israel:*** Ikaclomin; ***Ital.:*** Clomid; Prolifen; Serofene; ***Malaysia:*** Clomid; Clostilbegyt; Duinum; Ova-Mit; Ovinum; Phenate; ***Mex.:*** Omifin; ***Neth.:*** Clomid; Serophene; ***Norw.:*** Pergotime; ***NZ:*** Phenate; Serophene; ***Philipp.:*** Clomid; Clostil; I-Clom; Ova-Mit; ***Pol.:*** Clostilbegyt; ***Port.:*** Dufine; ***Rus.:*** Clostilbegyt (Клостилбегит); ***S.Afr.:*** Clomid; Clomihexal; Fertomid; ***Singapore:*** Clomid; Clostilbegyt; Duinum; Ova-Mit; Ovinum; Serophene; ***Spain:*** Omifin; ***Swed.:*** Pergotime; ***Switz.:*** Clomid; Serophene; ***Thai.:*** Clomid; Duinum; Ova-Mit; Ovinum; Serophene; ***Turk.:*** Fertilin; Gonaphene; Klomen; Serophene; ***UK:*** Clomid; ***USA:*** Clomid; Serophene; ***Venez.:*** Serophene; Serophene.

C

Clonazoline Hydrochloride

Other names: Clonazoline, Chlorhydrate de; Clonazolini Hydrochloridum; Hidrocloruro de clonazolina.

Клоназолина Гидрохлорид

Clinical profile: Clonazoline hydrochloride is a sympathomimetic used for its vasoconstrictor activity in the local treatment of nasal congestion.

WADA Status: Banned in competition

WADA Class: Stimulants

Includes stimulants or substances with a similar chemical structure or similar biological effect(s). Clonazoline is an imidazole derivative. Imidazole derivatives for topical use are exempt.

Preparations
Multi-ingredient: ***Ital.:*** Localyn.

Clopamide

Other names: Clopamida; Clopamidum; DT-327; Klopamid; Klopamidi.

Клопамид

Clinical profile: Clopamide is a diuretic similar to the thiazide diuretics. It is used for oedema, including that associated with heart failure, and for hypertension.

WADA Status: Banned in and out of competition

WADA Class: Diuretics and Other Masking Agents

Includes diuretics or substances with a similar chemical structure or similar biological effect(s).

Preparations
Single ingredient: ***Denm.:*** Adurix; ***Hung.:*** Brinaldix; ***India:*** Brinaldix.
Multi-ingredient: ***Austria:*** Brinerdin; ***Belg.:*** Viskaldix; ***Braz.:*** Viskaldix; ***Chile:*** Viskaldix; ***Cz.:*** Crystepin; ***Fr.:*** Viskaldix; ***Ger.:*** Briserin N; Viskaldix; ***Gr.:*** Viskaldix; ***Hung.:*** Viskaldix; ***Irl.:*** Viskaldix; ***Ital.:*** Brinerdina; ***Malaysia:*** Viskaldix; ***Neth.:*** Viskaldix; ***Philipp.:*** Viskaldix; ***Pol.:*** Normatens; ***Port.:*** Brinerdine; ***Rus.:*** Crystepin (Кристепин); Viskaldix (Вискалдикс); ***S.Afr.:*** Brinerdin; ***Switz.:*** Brinerdine; Viskaldix; ***Thai.:*** Bedin; Brinerdin; ***UK:*** Viskaldix.

Cloprednol

Other names: Cloprednolum; RS-4691.

Клопреднол

Clinical profile: Cloprednol is a corticosteroid that is used for its glucocorticoid activity.

WADA Status: Banned in competition

WADA Class: Glucocorticosteroids

All glucocorticosteroids are prohibited when administered orally, rectally, intravenously or intramuscularly. Their use requires a Therapeutic Use Exemption approval. Other routes of administration (intraarticular / periarticular / peritendinous / epidural / intradermal injections and inhalation) require an Abbreviated Therapeutic Use Exemption except as noted below.

Topical preparations when used for dermatological (including iontophoresis / phonophoresis), auricular, nasal, ophthalmic, buccal, gingival and perianal disorders are not prohibited and do not require any form of Therapeutic Use Exemption.

WADA Class: Specified Substances

Also listed as a specified substance.

"The prohibited List may identify specified substances which are particularly susceptible to unintentional anti-doping rule violations because of their general availability in medicinal products or which are less likely to be successfully abused as doping agents."

A doping violation involving such substances may result in a reduced sanction provided that the *"...Athlete can establish that the Use of such a specfied substance was not intended to enhance sport performance..."*

Preparations
Single ingredient: ***Ger.:*** Syntestan.

Cloranolol Hydrochloride

Other names: Cloranolol, Chlorhydrate de; Cloranololi Hydrochloridum; GYKI-41099; Hidrocloruro de cloranolol.

Клоранолола Гидрохлорид

Clinical profile: Cloranolol is a beta blocker that has been used in the management of various cardiovascular disorders.

WADA Status: Banned in and out of competition as specified below

WADA Class: Beta-Blockers

Unless otherwise specified, beta-blockers are prohibited *In-Competition* only in the following sports.

- Aeronautics (FAI)
- Archery (FITA, IPC) (also prohibited *Out-of-Competition*)
- Automobile (FIA)
- Billiards (WCBS)
- Bobsleigh (FIBT)
- Boules (CMSB, IPC bowls)
- Bridge (FMB)
- Curling (WCF)
- Gymnastics (FIG)
- Motorcycling (FIM)
- Modern Pentathlon (UIPM) for disciplines involving shooting
- Nine-pin bowling (FIQ)
- Powerboating (UIM)
- Sailing (ISAF) for match race helms only
- Shooting (ISSF, IPC) (also prohibited *Out-of-Competition*)
- Skiing/Snowboarding (FIS) in ski jumping, freestyle aerials/halfpipe and snowboard halfpipe/big air
- Wrestling (FILA)

WADA Class: Specified Substances

Also listed as a specified substance.

"The prohibited List may identify specified substances which are particularly susceptible to unintentional anti-doping rule violations because of their general availability in medicinal

products or which are less likely to be successfully abused as doping agents."
A doping violation involving such substances may result in a reduced sanction provided that the "*...Athlete can establish that the Use of such a specfied substance was not intended to enhance sport performance...*"

Clorexolone

C

Other names: Clorexolona; Clorexolonum; M&B-8430; RP-12833.
Клорексолон

Clinical profile: Clorexolone is a diuretic similar to the thiazide diuretics and was used in the treatment of oedema and hypertension.

WADA Status: Banned in and out of competition

WADA Class: Diuretics and Other Masking Agents
Includes diuretics or substances with a similar chemical structure or similar biological effect(s).

Clorprenaline Hydrochloride

Other names: 20025; Chlorprenaline Hydrochloride; Clorprénaline, Chlorhydrate de; Clorprenalini Hydrochloridum; Hidrocloruro de clorprenalina; Isophenamine Hydrochloride.
Клорпреналина Гидрохлорид

Clinical profile: Clorprenaline hydrochloride is a sympathomimetic agent with bronchodilating properties.

WADA Status: Banned in competition

WADA Class: Stimulants
Includes stimulants or substances with a similar chemical structure or similar biological effect(s).

WADA Class: Specified Substances
Also listed as a specified substance.
"The prohibited List may identify specified substances which are particularly susceptible to unintentional anti-doping rule violations because of their general availability in medicinal products or which are less likely to be successfully abused as doping agents."
A doping violation involving such substances may result in a reduced sanction provided that the "*...Athlete can establish that the Use of such a specfied substance was not intended to enhance sport performance...*"

Clortermine Hydrochloride

Other names: Clortermine, Chlorhydrate de; Clortermini Hydrochloridum; Hidrocloruro de clortermina; Su-10568.
Клортермина Гидрохлорид

Clinical profile: Clortermine hydrochloride, the ortho isomer of chlorphentermine hydrochloride, is a central stimulant and sympathomimetic that has been used as an anorectic.

WADA Status: Banned in competition

WADA Class: Stimulants

Includes stimulants or substances with a similar chemical structure or similar biological effect(s).

WADA Class: Specified Substances

Also listed as a specified substance.

"The prohibited List may identify specified substances which are particularly susceptible to unintentional anti-doping rule violations because of their general availability in medicinal products or which are less likely to be successfully abused as doping agents."

A doping violation involving such substances may result in a reduced sanction provided that the "*...Athlete can establish that the Use of such a specfied substance was not intended to enhance sport performance...*"

C

Clostebol Acetate

Other names: Acetato de clostebol; 4-Chlorotestosterone Acetate; Chlortestosterone Acetate; Clostébol, Acétate de; Closteboli Acetas.

Клостебола Ацетат

Clinical profile: Clostebol acetate has been used for its anabolic properties. It has also been used in dermatological preparations and in ophthalmological preparations.

WADA Status: Banned in and out of competition

WADA Class: Anabolic; Androgenic Steroids (exogenous)

Includes exogenous anabolic androgenic steroids or other substances with a similar chemical structure or similar biological effect(s).

Preparations
Single ingredient: ***Chile:*** Trofodermin.
Multi-ingredient: ***Braz.:*** Novaderm; Trofodermin; ***Chile:*** Trofodermin Neomicina; ***Ital.:*** Trofodermin; ***Mex.:*** Neobol.

Co-amilofruse

Clinical profile: Compounded preparations of amiloride hydrochloride and furosemide in the proportions, by weight, 1 part to 8 parts have the British Approved Name Co-amilofruse.

WADA Status: Banned in and out of competition

WADA Class: Diuretics and Other Masking Agents

Includes diuretics or substances with a similar chemical structure or similar biological effect(s).

Preparations
Single ingredient: ***UK:*** Aridil; Fru-Co; Frumil; Komil.

Co-amilozide

Clinical profile: Compounded preparations of amiloride hydrochloride and hydrochlorothiazide in the proportions, by weight, 1 part to 10 parts have the British Approved Name Co-amilozide.

WADA Status: Banned in and out of competition

WADA Class: Diuretics and Other Masking Agents

Includes diuretics or substances with a similar chemical structure or similar biological effect(s).

Preparations
Single ingredient: ***UK:*** Amil-Co; Moduret; Moduretic.

Coca

Other names: Coca Leaves; Hoja de Coca.

Clinical profile: Coca, the dried leaves of *Erythroxylum coca* or of *E. truxillense* (Erythroxylaceae), was formerly used for its stimulant action and for the relief of gastric pain, nausea, and vomiting, but it has no place in modern medicine. The practice of coca leaf chewing still continues in South America. Coca is a source of cocaine.

WADA Status: Banned in competition

WADA Class: Stimulants

Includes cocaine and any optical isomers.

Cocaine

Other names: Cocaína; Cocainum; Kokaiini; Kokain; Methyl Benzoylecgonine.

Cocaine Hydrochloride

Other names: Chloridrato de Cocaína; Cocaína, hidrocloruro de; Cocaïne, chlorhydrate de; Cocaine Hydrochlor.; Cocaini hydrochloridum; Cocainium Chloratum; Kokaiinihydrokloridi; Kokain-hidroklorid; Kokain-hydrochlorid; Kokainhydroklorid; Kokaino hidrochloridas; Kokainy chlorowodorek.

Clinical profile: Cocaine, a benzoic acid ester, is a surface anaesthetic but, because of systemic adverse effects and its abuse potential, its use is now almost entirely restricted to surgery of the ear, nose, and throat. It has been largely replaced by other drugs in ophthalmology because of its corneal toxicity, although it may still be useful in removal or debridement of the corneal epithelium.

WADA Status: Banned in competition

WADA Class: Stimulants

Includes cocaine and any optical isomers.

Co-flumactone

Clinical profile: Compounded preparations of equal parts by weight of hydroflumethiazide and spironolactone have the British Approved Name Co-flumactone.

WADA Status: Banned in and out of competition

WADA Class: Diuretics and Other Masking Agents

Includes diuretics or substances with a similar chemical structure or similar biological effect(s).

Preparations
Single ingredient: *UK:* Aldactide.

Co-prenozide

Clinical profile: Compounded preparations of oxprenolol hydrochloride and cyclopenthiazide in the proportions, by weight, 640 parts to 1 part have the British Approved Name Co-prenozide.

WADA Status: Banned in and out of competition as specified below

WADA Class: Beta-Blockers

Unless otherwise specified, beta-blockers are prohibited *In-Competition* only in the following sports.

- Aeronautics (FAI)
- Archery (FITA, IPC) (also prohibited *Out-of-Competition*)
- Automobile (FIA)
- Billiards (WCBS)
- Bobsleigh (FIBT)
- Boules (CMSB, IPC bowls)
- Bridge (FMB)
- Curling (WCF)
- Gymnastics (FIG)
- Motorcycling (FIM)
- Modern Pentathlon (UIPM) for disciplines involving shooting
- Nine-pin bowling (FIQ)
- Powerboating (UIM)
- Sailing (ISAF) for match race helms only
- Shooting (ISSF, IPC) (also prohibited *Out-of-Competition*)
- Skiing/Snowboarding (FIS) in ski jumping, freestyle aerials/halfpipe and snowboard halfpipe/big air
- Wrestling (FILA)

WADA Status: Banned in and out of competition

WADA Class: Diuretics and Other Masking Agents

Includes diuretics or substances with a similar chemical structure or similar biological effect(s).

Preparations
Single ingredient: *UK:* Trasidrex.

Corbadrine

Other names: Corbadrina; Corbadrinum; *l*-3,4-Dihydroxynorephedrine; Levonordefrin; *l*-Nordefrin.
Корбадрин

Clinical profile: Corbadrine is a sympathomimetic that has been added to local anaesthetic preparations in dentistry to diminish absorption and to localise the effect.

WADA Status: Banned in competition

WADA Class: Stimulants

Includes stimulants or substances with a similar chemical structure or similar biological effect(s).

WADA Class: Specified Substances

Also listed as a specified substance.

"The prohibited List may identify specified substances which are particularly susceptible to unintentional anti-doping rule violations because of their general availability in medicinal

products or which are less likely to be successfully abused as doping agents."
A doping violation involving such substances may result in a reduced sanction provided that the "*...Athlete can establish that the Use of such a specfied substance was not intended to enhance sport performance...*"

Preparations
Adjnuct-ingredient: ***USA:*** Carbocaine with Neo-Cobefrin; Isocaine; Polocaine.

Corticorelin

Other names: Corticoliberin; Corticorelina; Corticoréline; Corticorelinum; Corticotrophin-releasing Hormone; Corticotropin-releasing Factor; CRF; CRH; HLC; Hormona liberadora de corticotropina.

Кортикорелин

Corticorelin Triflutate

Other names: Corticorelin Trifluoroacetate; Corticoréline, Triflutate de; Corticorelini Triflutas; Triflutato de corticorelina.

Кортикорелина Трифлутат

Clinical profile: Corticorelin is a hypothalamic polypeptide that stimulates the release of corticotropin from the anterior pituitary. It is used in the differential diagnosis of Cushing's syndrome and other adrenal disorders. It is also under investigation in cerebral oedema.

WADA Status: Banned in and out of competition

WADA Class: Hormones and Related Substances: Corticotrophins
Includes corticotrophin or substances with a similar chemical structure or similar biological effect(s), or one of their releasing factors.

Preparations
Single ingredient: ***Austria:*** CRH; ***Fr.:*** Stimu-ACTH; ***Ger.:*** Cortirel; CRH; ***Neth.:*** CRH; ***USA:*** Acthrel.

Corticotropin

Other names: ACTH; Adrenocorticotrophic Hormone; Adrenocorticotrophin; Corticotrophin; Corticotropina; Corticotropine; Corticotropinum; Kortikotropiini; Kortikotropin.

Кортикотропин

Clinical profile: Corticotropin is a naturally occurring hormone secreted by the anterior lobe of the pituitary gland. It stimulates secretion of corticosteroids by the adrenal cortex and is mainly used parenterally in testing adrenal cortex function. It has also been used therapeutically in conditions for which systemic corticosteroid therapy is indicated.

WADA Status: Banned in and out of competition

WADA Class: Hormones and Related Substances: Corticotrophins
Includes corticotrophin or substances with a similar chemical structure or similar biological effect(s), or one of their releasing factors.

Preparations
Single ingredient: ***Arg.:*** Acthelea; ***USA:*** Acthar.

Cortisone Acetate

Other names: Acetato de cortisona; Compound E Acetate; Cortisone, acétate de; Cortisoni acetas; 11-Dehydro-17-hydroxycorticosterone Acetate; Kortisonacetat; Kortison-acetát; Kortisoniasetaatti; Kortizon-acetát; Kortizono acetatas; Kortyzonu octan.

Кортизона Ацетат

Clinical profile: Cortisone is a glucocorticoid corticosteroid secreted by the adrenal cortex; it also has appreciable mineralocorticoid properties.

WADA Status: Banned in competition

WADA Class: Glucocorticosteroids

All glucocorticosteroids are prohibited when administered orally, rectally, intravenously or intramuscularly. Their use requires a Therapeutic Use Exemption approval. Other routes of administration (intraarticular / periarticular / peritendinous / epidural / intradermal injections and inhalation) require an Abbreviated Therapeutic Use Exemption except as noted below.

Topical preparations when used for dermatological (including iontophoresis / phonophoresis), auricular, nasal, ophthalmic, buccal, gingival and perianal disorders are not prohibited and do not require any form of Therapeutic Use Exemption.

WADA Class: Specified Substances

Also listed as a specified substance.

"*The prohibited List may identify specified substances which are particularly susceptible to unintentional anti-doping rule violations because of their general availability in medicinal products or which are less likely to be successfully abused as doping agents.*"

A doping violation involving such substances may result in a reduced sanction provided that the "*...Athlete can establish that the Use of such a specfied substance was not intended to enhance sport performance...*"

Preparations
Single ingredient: ***Austral.:*** Cortate; ***Ital.:*** Cortone; ***UK:*** Cortisyl; ***USA:*** Cortone.
Multi-ingredient: ***Braz.:*** Corciclen; ***Spain:*** Blefarida; Gingilone.

Cortivazol

Other names: Cortivazolum; H-3625; MK-650; NSC-80998.

Кортивазол

Clinical profile: Cortivazol is a glucocorticoid corticosteroid used in the treatment of musculoskeletal and joint disorders.

WADA Status: Banned in competition

WADA Class: Glucocorticosteroids

All glucocorticosteroids are prohibited when administered orally, rectally, intravenously or intramuscularly. Their use requires a Therapeutic Use Exemption approval. Other routes of administration (intraarticular / periarticular / peritendinous / epidural / intradermal injections and inhalation) require an Abbreviated Therapeutic Use Exemption except as noted below.

Topical preparations when used for dermatological (including iontophoresis / pho-

nophoresis), auricular, nasal, ophthalmic, buccal, gingival and perianal disorders are not prohibited and do not require any form of Therapeutic Use Exemption.

WADA Class: Specified Substances

Also listed as a specified substance.

"The prohibited List may identify specified substances which are particularly susceptible to unintentional anti-doping rule violations because of their general availability in medicinal products or which are less likely to be successfully abused as doping agents."

A doping violation involving such substances may result in a reduced sanction provided that the "*...Athlete can establish that the Use of such a specfied substance was not intended to enhance sport performance...*"

Preparations
Single ingredient: ***Fr.:*** Altim.

Co-tenidone

Clinical profile: Compounded preparations of atenolol and chlortalidone in the proportions, by weight, 4 parts to 1 part have the British Approved Name Co-tenidone.

WADA Status: Banned in and out of competition as specified below

WADA Class: Beta-Blockers

Unless otherwise specified, beta-blockers are prohibited *In-Competition* only in the following sports.

- Aeronautics (FAI)
- Archery (FITA, IPC) (also prohibited *Out-of-Competition*)
- Automobile (FIA)
- Billiards (WCBS)
- Bobsleigh (FIBT)
- Boules (CMSB, IPC bowls)
- Bridge (FMB)
- Curling (WCF)
- Gymnastics (FIG)
- Motorcycling (FIM)
- Modern Pentathlon (UIPM) for disciplines involving shooting
- Nine-pin bowling (FIQ)
- Powerboating (UIM)
- Sailing (ISAF) for match race helms only
- Shooting (ISSF, IPC) (also prohibited *Out-of-Competition*)
- Skiing/Snowboarding (FIS) in ski jumping, freestyle aerials/halfpipe and snowboard halfpipe/big air
- Wrestling (FILA)

WADA Status: Banned in and out of competition

WADA Class: Diuretics and Other Masking Agents

Includes diuretics or substances with a similar chemical structure or similar biological effect(s).

Preparations
Single ingredient: ***UK:*** AtenixCo; Tenchlor; Tenoret; Tenoretic; Totaretic.

Co-triamterzide

Clinical profile: Compounded preparations of triamterene and hydrochlorothiazide in the proportions, by weight, 2 parts to 1 part have the British Approved Name Co-triamterzide.

WADA Status: Banned in and out of competition

WADA Class: Diuretics and Other Masking Agents

Includes diuretics or substances with a similar chemical structure or similar biological effect(s).

Preparations
Single ingredient: ***UK:*** Dyazide; Triamco.

Coumazoline Hydrochloride

Other names: Coumazoline, Chlorhydrate de; Coumazolinum Hydrochloridum; Hidrocloruro de cumazolina; L-5818.

Кумазолина Гидрохлорид

Clinical profile: Coumazoline hydrochloride is a sympathomimetic agent which has been used topically as a nasal vasoconstrictor.

WADA Status: Banned in competition

WADA Class: Stimulants

Includes stimulants or substances with a similar chemical structure or similar biological effect(s). Coumazoline is an imidazole derivative. Imidazole derivatives for topical use are exempt.

Co-zidocapt

Clinical profile: Compounded preparations of hydrochlorothiazide and captopril in the proportions, by weight, 1 part to 2 parts have the British Approved Name Co-zidocapt.

WADA Status: Banned in and out of competition

WADA Class: Diuretics and Other Masking Agents

Includes diuretics or substances with a similar chemical structure or similar biological effect(s).

Preparations
Single ingredient: ***UK:*** Acezide; Capozide; Capto-Co.

Cyclofenil

Other names: Ciclofenilo; Cyclofénil; Cyclofenilum; Cyklofenil; F-6066; H-3452; ICI-48213; Siklofenil; Syklofeniili.

Циклофенил

Clinical profile: Cyclofenil is an anti-oestrogen that has been used in the treatment of anovulatory infertility due to hypothalamic-pituitary dysfunction.

WADA Status: Banned in and out of competition

WADA Class: Hormone Antagonists and Modulators: Other Anti-estrogenic Substances

Includes other anti-estrogenic substances not listed elsewhere.

Preparations
Single ingredient: ***Braz.:*** Menopax; ***Ital.:*** Neoclym; ***Turk.:*** Fertodur.

Cyclopentamine Hydrochloride

Other names: Cyclopentadrin Hydrochloride; Cyclopentamine, Chlorhydrate de; Cyclopentamini Hydrochloridum; Hidrocloruro de ciclopentamina.

Циклопентамина Гидрохлорид

Clinical profile: Cyclopentamine hydrochloride is a sympathomimetic agent formerly used as a nasal decongestant.

WADA Status: Banned in competition

WADA Class: Stimulants

Includes stimulants or substances with a similar chemical structure or similar biological effect(s).

WADA Class: Specified Substances

Also listed as a specified substance.
"The prohibited List may identify specified substances which are particularly susceptible to unintentional anti-doping rule violations because of their general availability in medicinal products or which are less likely to be successfully abused as doping agents."
A doping violation involving such substances may result in a reduced sanction provided that the "*...Athlete can establish that the Use of such a specfied substance was not intended to enhance sport performance...*"

Cyclopenthiazide

Other names: Ciclopentiazida; Cyclopenthiaz.; Cyclopenthiazidum; Cyklopentiazid; NSC-107679; Su-8341; Syklopentiatsidi.

Циклопентиазид

Clinical profile: Cyclopenthiazide is a thiazide diuretic used for hypertension, and for oedema, including that associated with heart failure.

WADA Status: Banned in and out of competition

WADA Class: Diuretics and Other Masking Agents

Includes diuretics or substances with a similar chemical structure or similar biological effect(s).

Preparations
Single ingredient: ***UK:*** Navidrex.
Multi-ingredient: ***Hong Kong:*** Navispare; ***S.Afr.:*** Lenurex-K; ***UK:*** Navispare; Trasidrex.

Cyclothiazide

Other names: Ciclotiazida; Compound 35483; Cyclothiazidum; Cyklotiazid; MDi-193; Syklotiatsidi.

Циклотиазид

Clinical profile: Cyclothiazide is a thiazide diuretic that has been used for hypertension and for oedema.

WADA Status: Banned in and out of competition

WADA Class: Diuretics and Other Masking Agents

Includes diuretics or substances with a similar chemical structure or similar biological effect(s).

C

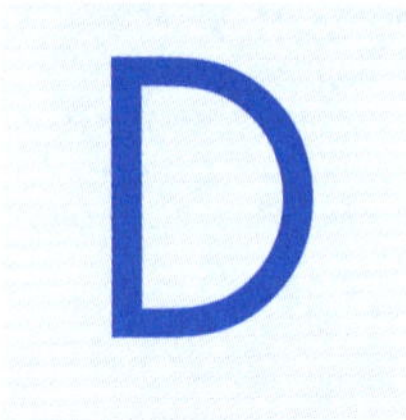

Danazol

Other names: Danatsoli; Danazolum; Win-17757.

Даназол

Clinical profile: Danazol inhibits pituitary gonadotrophin release; it has weak androgenic activity. It is given by mouth in the treatment of endometriosis, benign breast disorders, menorrhagia, and hereditary angioedema. It has also been given in gynaecomastia, pubertal or pre-pubertal breast hypertrophy, and various blood disorders.

WADA Status: Banned in and out of competition

WADA Class: Anabolic; Androgenic Steroids (exogenous)

Includes exogenous anabolic androgenic steroids or other substances with a similar chemical structure or similar biological effect(s).

Preparations

Single ingredient: ***Arg.:*** Ladogal; ***Austral.:*** Azol; Danocrine; ***Austria:*** Danokrin; ***Belg.:*** Danatrol; ***Braz.:*** Ladogal; ***Canad.:*** Cyclomen; ***Cz.:*** Anargil; Danol; ***Fr.:*** Danatrol; ***Gr.:*** Danatrol; ***Hong Kong:*** Anargil; Danocrine; ***Hung.:*** Danoval; ***India:*** Danogen; Gonablok; Zendol; ***Indon.:*** Azol; Danocrine; ***Irl.:*** Danol; ***Israel:*** Danol; ***Ital.:*** Danatrol; ***Malaysia:*** Anargil; Azol; Ladogal; Vabon; ***Mex.:*** Danalem; Ladogal; Novaprin; ***Neth.:*** Danatrol; ***NZ:*** D-Zol; ***Philipp.:*** Ladogal; ***Port.:*** Danatrol; Mastodanatrol; ***Rus.:*** Danoval (Данован); ***S.Afr.:*** Danogen; Ladazol; ***Singapore:*** Azol; Ladogal; ***Spain:*** Danatrol; ***Switz.:*** Danatrol; ***Thai.:*** Anargil; Ectopal; Ladogal; Vabon; ***Turk.:*** Danasin; ***UK:*** Danol; ***Venez.:*** Danogen; Ladogal.

Darbepoetin Alfa

Other names: Darbepoetiinialfa; Darbepoetina alfa; Darbépoétine Alfa; Darbepoetinum Alfa; NESP; Novel Erythropoiesis Stimulating Protein.

Дарбепоэтин Альфа

Clinical profile: Darbepoetin alfa is an analogue of the endogenous protein hormone erythropoietin with similar properties to the epoetins. It is used in the management of anaemia associated with chronic renal failure and for anaemia caused by chemotherapy in non-myeloid malignancies.

WADA Status: Banned in and out of competition

WADA Class: Hormones and Related Substances: Erythropoietin

Includes erythropoietin or a substance with a similar chemical structure or similar biological effect(s), or one of their releasing factors.

Preparations
Single ingredient: ***Austral.:*** Aranesp; ***Austria:*** Aranesp; ***Belg.:*** Aranesp; ***Canad.:*** Aranesp; ***Denm.:*** Aranesp; ***Fin.:*** Aranesp; ***Fr.:*** Aranesp; ***Ger.:*** Aranesp; ***Gr.:*** Aranesp; ***Hong Kong:*** Aranesp; ***Hung.:*** Aranesp; ***Irl.:*** Aranesp; ***Israel:*** Aranesp; ***Ital.:*** Aranesp; Nespo; ***Neth.:*** Aranesp; Nespo; ***Norw.:*** Aranesp; ***Pol.:*** Aranesp; ***Port.:*** Aranesp; ***Spain:*** Aranesp; ***Swed.:*** Aranesp; ***Switz.:*** Aranesp; ***Turk.:*** Aranesp; ***UK:*** Aranesp; ***USA:*** Aranesp.

Deanol

Other names: Démanol.

Clinical profile: Deanol, a precursor of choline, may enhance central acetylcholine formation. It has been employed as a central stimulant and in the treatment of hyperactivity in children but its efficacy has not been substantiated. It has been included in preparations used as tonics and for the management of impaired mental function. Deanol benzilate hydrochloride has been used in antispasmodic preparations.

WADA Status: Banned in competition

WADA Class: Stimulants

Includes stimulants or substances with a similar chemical structure or similar biological effect(s).

WADA Class: Specified Substances

Also listed as a specified substance.
"The prohibited List may identify specified substances which are particularly susceptible to unintentional anti-doping rule violations because of their general availability in medicinal products or which are less likely to be successfully abused as doping agents."
A doping violation involving such substances may result in a reduced sanction provided that the "*...Athlete can establish that the Use of such a specfied substance was not intended to enhance sport performance...*"

Preparations
Single ingredient: ***Arg.:*** DM Active; ***Ger.:*** Risatarun; ***Pol.:*** Bimanol; ***Rus.:*** Nooclerin (Нооклерин).
Multi-ingredient: ***Fr.:*** Acti 5; Debrumyl; ***Port.:*** Actilam; Debrumyl; Forticol; Tonice; Tonice; ***Spain:*** Anti Anorex Triple; Denubil.

Deflazacort

Other names: Azacort; Deflatsakorti; Déflazacort; Deflazacortum; Deflazakort; DL-458-IT; L-5458; MDL-458; Oxazacort.

Дефлазакорт

Clinical profile: Deflazacort is a glucocorticoid corticosteroid that is used in various disorders that respond to its anti-inflammatory and immunosuppressant effects.

WADA Status: Banned in competition

WADA Class: Glucocorticosteroids

All glucocorticosteroids are prohibited when administered orally, rectally, intravenously or intramuscularly. Their use requires a Therapeutic Use Exemption approval. Other routes of administration (intraarticular / periarticular / peritendinous / epidural / intradermal injections and inhalation) require an Abbreviated Therapeutic Use Exemption except as noted below.
Topical preparations when used for dermatological (including iontophoresis / phonophoresis), auricular, nasal, ophthalmic, buccal, gingival and perianal disorders are not prohibited and do not require any form of Therapeutic Use Exemption.

WADA Class: Specified Substances

Also listed as a specified substance.

"*The prohibited List may identify specified substances which are particularly susceptible to unintentional anti-doping rule violations because of their general availability in medicinal products or which are less likely to be successfully abused as doping agents.*"

A doping violation involving such substances may result in a reduced sanction provided that the "*...Athlete can establish that the Use of such a specfied substance was not intended to enhance sport performance...*"

Preparations

Single ingredient: ***Arg.:*** Azacortid; Defas; Flamirex; ***Braz.:*** Calcort; Cortax; Deflanil; Denacen; Flaz-Cort; Flazal; ***Chile:*** Azacortid; Dezartal; ***Ger.:*** Calcort; ***Irl.:*** Calcort; ***Ital.:*** Deflan; Flantadin; ***Mex.:*** Calcort; Setatrep; ***Port.:*** Rosilan; ***Spain:*** Dezacor; Tobolacer; Zamene; ***Switz.:*** Calcort; ***Turk.:*** Flantadin; ***UK:*** Calcort; ***Venez.:*** Calcort.

Deprodone

Other names: Deprodona; Déprodone; Deprodonum; Desolone; RD-20000 (propionate).

Депродон

Clinical profile: Deprodone is a corticosteroid that has been used topically as the propionate.

WADA Status: Banned in competition

WADA Class: Glucocorticosteroids

All glucocorticosteroids are prohibited when administered orally, rectally, intravenously or intramuscularly. Their use requires a Therapeutic Use Exemption approval. Other routes of administration (intraarticular / periarticular / peritendinous / epidural / intradermal injections and inhalation) require an Abbreviated Therapeutic Use Exemption except as noted below.

Topical preparations when used for dermatological (including iontophoresis / phonophoresis), auricular, nasal, ophthalmic, buccal, gingival and perianal disorders are not prohibited and do not require any form of Therapeutic Use Exemption.

WADA Class: Specified Substances

Also listed as a specified substance.

"*The prohibited List may identify specified substances which are particularly susceptible to unintentional anti-doping rule violations because of their general availability in medicinal products or which are less likely to be successfully abused as doping agents.*"

A doping violation involving such substances may result in a reduced sanction provided that the "*...Athlete can establish that the Use of such a specfied substance was not intended to enhance sport performance...*"

Deslorelin

Other names: Deslorelina; Desloréline; Deslorelinum; D-Trp LHRH-PEA.

Дезлорелин

Clinical profile: Deslorelin is a synthetic analogue of gonadorelin investigated in the treatment of precocious puberty, short stature, prostate cancer, and endometriosis.

WADA Status: Banned in and out of competition

WADA Class: Hormones and Related Substances: Gonadotrophins

Includes gonadotrophin or a substance with a similar chemical structure or similar biological effect(s), or one of their releasing factors. Prohibited in males only.

Desonide

Other names: D-2083; Desfluorotriamcinolone Acetonide; Desonid; Desonida; Désonide; Desonidi; Desonidum; 16-Hydroxyprednisolone 16,17-Acetonide; Prednacinolone Acetonide.

Дезонид

Clinical profile: Desonide is a corticosteroid used topically in the treatment of various skin disorders.

WADA Status: Banned in competition

WADA Class: Glucocorticosteroids

All glucocorticosteroids are prohibited when administered orally, rectally, intravenously or intramuscularly. Their use requires a Therapeutic Use Exemption approval. Other routes of administration (intraarticular / periarticular / peritendinous / epidural / intradermal injections and inhalation) require an Abbreviated Therapeutic Use Exemption except as noted below.

Topical preparations when used for dermatological (including iontophoresis / phonophoresis), auricular, nasal, ophthalmic, buccal, gingival and perianal disorders are not prohibited and do not require any form of Therapeutic Use Exemption.

WADA Class: Specified Substances

Also listed as a specified substance.

"The prohibited List may identify specified substances which are particularly susceptible to unintentional anti-doping rule violations because of their general availability in medicinal products or which are less likely to be successfully abused as doping agents."

A doping violation involving such substances may result in a reduced sanction provided that the "*...Athlete can establish that the Use of such a specfied substance was not intended to enhance sport performance...*"

Preparations

Single ingredient: ***Arg.:*** Desoplus; DesOwen; Locatop; ***Austral.:*** DesOwen; ***Braz.:*** Desonol; DesOwen; Steronide; ***Canad.:*** Desocort; ***Chile:*** DesOwen; ***Fin.:*** Apolar; ***Fr.:*** Locapred; Locatop; Tridesonit; ***Hong Kong:*** DesOwen; ***India:*** DesOwen; ***Indon.:*** Apolar; Dermades; Dermanide; Desolex; Nufapolar; ***Israel:*** Locatop; ***Ital.:*** Prenacid; Reticus; Sterades; ***Mex.:*** DesOwen; ***Norw.:*** Apolar; ***Philipp.:*** DesOwen; ***Pol.:*** Locatop; ***Port.:*** Locapred; Zotinar; ***Rus.:*** Prenacid (Пренацид); ***Singapore:*** DesOwen; ***Switz.:*** Locapred; Locatop; ***Turk.:*** Prenacid; ***USA:*** DesOwen; LoKara; Verdeso; ***Venez.:*** Dermosupril; DesOwen; Erilon.

Multi-ingredient: ***Fr.:*** Cirkan a la Prednacinolone; ***Indon.:*** Apolar-N; Desolex-N; ***Norw.:*** Apolar med dekvalin; ***Port.:*** Zotinar-N; ***Venez.:*** Dermosupril C.

Desoximetasone

Other names: A-41-304; Desoksimetasoni; Desoximetason; Desoximetasona; Désoximétasone; Desoximetasonum; Desoxymethasone; Hoe-304; R-2113.

Дезоксиметазон

Clinical profile: Desoximetasone is a corticosteroid used topically in the treatment of various skin disorders.

WADA Status: Banned in competition

WADA Class: Glucocorticosteroids

All glucocorticosteroids are prohibited when administered orally, rectally, intravenously or intramuscularly. Their use requires a Therapeutic Use Exemption approval. Other routes of administration (intraarticular / periarticular / peritendinous / epidural / intradermal injections and inhalation) require an Abbreviated Therapeutic Use Exemption except as noted below.

Topical preparations when used for dermatological (including iontophoresis / phonophoresis), auricular, nasal, ophthalmic, buccal, gingival and perianal disorders are not prohibited and do not require any form of Therapeutic Use Exemption.

WADA Class: Specified Substances

Also listed as a specified substance.

"The prohibited List may identify specified substances which are particularly susceptible to unintentional anti-doping rule violations because of their general availability in medicinal products or which are less likely to be successfully abused as doping agents."

A doping violation involving such substances may result in a reduced sanction provided that the "*...Athlete can establish that the Use of such a specfied substance was not intended to enhance sport performance...*"

D

Preparations

Single ingredient: ***Austria:*** Topisolon; ***Braz.:*** Esperson; ***Canad.:*** Topicort; ***Denm.:*** Ibaril; ***Fin.:*** Ibaril; ***Ger.:*** Topisolon; ***Indon.:*** Dercason; Desomex; Dexocort; Esperson; Inerson; Lerskin; Pyderma; Soderma; Topcort; ***Israel:*** Desicort; ***Ital.:*** Flubason; ***Neth.:*** Ibaril; Topicorte; ***Norw.:*** Ibaril; ***Spain:*** Flubason; ***Switz.:*** Topisolon; ***Thai.:*** Cendexsone; Esperson; Topicorte; ***USA:*** Topicort.

Multi-ingredient: ***Austria:*** Topisolon mit Salicylsaure; ***Braz.:*** Esperson N; ***Indon.:*** Denomix; ***Thai.:*** Topifram.

Dexamethasone

Other names: Deksametasoni; Deksametazon; Deksametazonas; Desamethasone; Dexametason; Dexametasona; Dexametasone; Dexametazon; Dexamethason; Dexaméthasone; Dexamethasonum; 9α-Fluoro-16α-methylprednisolone; Hexadecadrol.

Дексаметазон

Dexamethasone Acetate

Other names: Acetato de dexametasona; Deksametasoniasetaatti; Deksametazono acetatas; Dexametasonacetat; Dexametazon-acetát; Dexamethason-acetát; Dexaméthasone, acétate de; Dexamethasoni acetas.

Дексаметазона Ацетат

Dexamethasone Isonicotinate

Other names: Deksametasoniisonikotinaatti; Deksametazonu izonikotynian; Dexametasonisonikotinat; Dexaméthasone, isonicotinate de; Dexamethasoni isonicotinas; Dexamethason-isonikotinát; Isonicotinato de dexametasona.

Дексаметазона Изоникотинат

Dexamethasone Phosphate

Other names: Dexaméthasone, Phosphate de; Dexamethasoni Phosphas; Fosfato de dexametasona.

Дексаметазона Фосфат

Dexamethasone Sodium Metasulfobenzoate

Other names: Dexaméthasone Métasulfobenzoate Sodique; Dexamethasone

Sodium Metasulphobenzoate; Metasulfobenzoato sódico de dexametasona; Natrii Dexamethasoni Metasulfobenzoas.

Натрий Метасульфобензоат Дексаметазон

Dexamethasone Sodium Phosphate

Other names: Deksametasoninatriumfosfaatti; Deksametazon Sodyum Fosfat; Deksametazono natrio fosfatas; Dexametasonnatriumfosfat; Dexametazon-nátrium-foszfát; Dexaméthasone, phosphate sodique de; Dexamethasone Phosphate Sodium; Dexamethason-fosfát sodná sůl; Dexamethasoni natrii phosphas; Fosfato sódico de dexametasona; Natrii Dexamethasoni Phosphas; Sodium Dexamethasone Phosphate.

Натрия Дексаметазона Фосфат

Clinical profile: Dexamethasone is a glucocorticoid corticosteroid. It has been used, either in the form of the free alcohol or in one of the esterified forms, in the treatment of a wide range of conditions that respond to the anti-inflammatory and immunosuppressant effects of corticosteroid therapy.

WADA Status: Banned in competition

WADA Class: Glucocorticosteroids

All glucocorticosteroids are prohibited when administered orally, rectally, intravenously or intramuscularly. Their use requires a Therapeutic Use Exemption approval. Other routes of administration (intraarticular / periarticular / peritendinous / epidural / intradermal injections and inhalation) require an Abbreviated Therapeutic Use Exemption except as noted below.

Topical preparations when used for dermatological (including iontophoresis / phonophoresis), auricular, nasal, ophthalmic, buccal, gingival and perianal disorders are not prohibited and do not require any form of Therapeutic Use Exemption.

WADA Class: Specified Substances

Also listed as a specified substance.

"The prohibited List may identify specified substances which are particularly susceptible to unintentional anti-doping rule violations because of their general availability in medicinal products or which are less likely to be successfully abused as doping agents."

A doping violation involving such substances may result in a reduced sanction provided that the "*...Athlete can establish that the Use of such a specfied substance was not intended to enhance sport performance...*"

Preparations

Single ingredient: ***Arg.:*** Decadron; Degabina; Dexalaf; Dexalergin; Dexameral; Dexatotal; Duo Decadron; Gotabiotic D; Ingedex; Isopto Maxidex; Lormine; Nexadron; Rupedex; Sedesterol; Trofinan; ***Austral.:*** Dexmethsone; Maxidex; ***Austria:*** Dexabene; Fortecortin; ***Belg.:*** Aacidexam; Dexa-Sine; Maxidex; Oradexon; ***Braz.:*** Cortidex; Cortitop; Decadron; Decadronal; Deflaren; Dexacilin; Dexaden; Dexadermil; Dexaflan; Dexagreen; Dexameson; Dexametax; Dexametonal; Dexametrat; Dexamex; Dexaminor; Dexanil; Dexason; Dexazen; Dexazona; Dexmene; Maxidex; Metaxon; Minidex; Neodex; Netazon; Topidexa; Uni Dexa; ***Canad.:*** Dexasone; Maxidex; ***Chile:*** Maxidex; Oradexon; ***Cz.:*** Baycuten; Dexa; Dexaltin; Dexamed; Dexapos; Dexason; Dexona; Fortecortin; ***Denm.:*** Maxidex; ***Fin.:*** Kaarmepakkaus; Oftan Dexa; Oradexon; ***Fr.:*** Dectancyl; Desocort; Maxidex; ***Ger.:*** afpred-DEXA; Dexa Loscon mono; Dexa-Allvoran; dexa-clinit; Dexa-Effekton; Dexa-ratiopharm; Dexa-Rhinospray Mono; Dexa-sine; Dexa; Dexabene; Dexabeta; DexaEDO; Dexaflam; Dexagalen; Dexagel; Dexahexal; Dexamonozon; Dexapos; Fortecortin; Isopto Dex; Lipotalon; Solupen N; Solutio Cordes Dexa N; Spersadex; Totocortin; Tuttozem N; ***Gr.:*** Decadron; Dexacollyre; Dexaton; Iriniozol; Maxidex; Oradexon; Soldesanil; Thilodexine; ***Hong Kong:*** Dexaltin; Dexamed; Dexasone; Dexmetha; Dexmethsone; Maxidex; ***Hung.:*** Dexa; Maxidex; Oradexon; ***India:*** Decdan; Dexacip; Dexasone; Dexona; Millicortenol; Wymesone; ***Indon.:*** Cetadexon; Cortidex; Danasone; Decilone; Dellamethasone; Dexa-M; Elason; Fortecortin; Indexon; Inthesa-5; Kalmethasone; Lanadexon; Licodexon; Molacort; Nufadex; Oradexon; Prodexon; Pycameth; Pyradexon; Scandexon; ***Irl.:*** Maxidex; ***Israel:*** Dexacort; Maxidex; Sterodex; ***Ital.:*** Decadron; Dermadex; Etacortilen; Luxazone; Megacort; Soldesam; Visumetazone; ***Jpn:*** Limethason; Methaderm; ***Malaysia:*** Decan; Dexalone; Dexaltin; Dexasone; Limethason; Maxidex; ***Mex.:*** Adrecort; Alin; Azona; Baycuten; Beminex; Cortidex; Cryometasona; Decadron; Decadronal; Decorex; Dexafrin; Dexagrin; Dexal; Dexamilan; Dexicar; Dexona; Dibasona; Examsa; Indarzona-N; Lergosin; Maxidex; Metax; Pardex; Reusan; Taprodex; Taxyl; ***Neth.:*** Dexa-POS; Oradexon; ***Norw.:*** Isopto Maxidex; Spersadex; ***NZ:*** Maxidex; ***Philipp.:***

Cordex; Dabrin; Decan; Decilone; Drenex; Isodexam; Maxidex; Midexone; Oradexon; Penodex; Santeson; Scancortin; Vexamet; ***Pol.:*** Dexafree; Dexapolcort; Dexaven; ***Port.:*** Decadron; Dexaval; Ronic; ***Rus.:*** Dexamed (Дексамед); Dexapos (Дексапос); Dexaven (Дексавен); Dexona (Дексона Д); Maxidex (Максидекс); Oftan Dexamethason (Офтан Дексаметазон); ***S.Afr.:*** Decadron; Decasone; Maxidex; Spersadex; ***Singapore:*** Decan; Decordex; Dexaltin; Dexamed; Dexasone; Maxidex; ***Spain:*** Dalamon Inyectable; Fortecortin; Maxidex; ***Swed.:*** Dexacortal; Isopto Maxidex; Opnol; ***Switz.:*** Dexacortin; Dexalocal; Fortecortin; Maxidex; Mephamesone; Spersadex; ***Thai.:*** B Dexol; Decadron; Dexa ANB; Dexaltin; Dexano; Dexasone; Dexion; Dexon; Dexthasol; Dexton; Oradexon; Phenodex; ***Turk.:*** Cebedex; Dekort; Deksalon; Deksamet; Dexa-Sine; Maxidex; Onadron; Spersadex; ***UK:*** Dexsol; Maxidex; ***USA:*** Aeroseb-Dex; Dalalone; Decadron; Decaspray; Dexasone; Dexone; DexPak; Hexadrol; Maxidex; ***Venez.:*** Decalona; Decobel; Dexacort; Dexamin; Maradex.

Multi-ingredient: ***Arg.:*** Alergi; Belbar; Bicrinol; Biocort; Bioptic DX; Ciloxadex; Ciprocort; Decadron con Ciprofloxina; Decadron con Neomicina; Decadron con Tobramicina; Dexa Aminofilin; Dexa Teosona; Dexa-Rhinospray N; Dexabion; Dexalergin; Dexalergin; Dexalergin; Dexamytrex; Dexaprof D; Empecid Cort; Exudrol con Dexametasona; Factioneye; Flexicamin B12; Flexicamin B12; Flogiatrin B12; Fluoropoen; Fotadex; Gotabiotic F; Hongal; Isoptomax; Klonamicin Compuesto; Larsen; Linfol; Melasmax; Naxo TV; Neodexa Plus; Neoftalm Dexa; Neolag; Neosona; Nexadron Compuesto; Nexadron Plus; Paraflex Plus; Polioftal; Polyplex; Proetztotal; Provisual Compuesto; Quidex; Radina Dex; Sincerum Biotic L; Sincerum Biotic; Solocalm Plus; Solocalm Plus; Tacines; Tobrabiotic D; Tobracort; Tobradex; Tobragan D; Toflamixina Plus; Tratomax; Trimepol D; Vixalerg; Vixidone; Xibradex; ***Austral.:*** Otodex; Sofradex; ***Austria:*** Ambene; Dexagenta; Multodrin; Rheumesser; Tobradex; Uromont; ***Belg.:*** De Icol; Dexa-Polyspectran New; Dexa-Rhinospray; Dexagenta-POS; Frakidex; Maxitrol; Percutalgine; Polydexa; Tobradex; ***Braz.:*** Baycuten; Biamotil-D; Cianotrat-Dexa; Cilodex; Cylocort; Decadron Colirio com Neomicina; Decadron Nasal; Dexa-Citoneurin; Dexa-Cronobe; Dexa-Neuriberi; Dexacilin; Dexaclor; Dexacobal; Dexacort; Dexador; Dexadoze; Dexafenicol; Dexagil; Dexalgen; Dexamytrex; Dexaneurin; Dexanevral; Dexanil; Dexavison; Dexazona; Duo-Decadron; Emistin; Fenidex; Gynax-N; Hidrocin; Maxiflox D; Maxitrol; Metcort; Neocortin; Neodex; Nepodex; Otofenicol-D; Rinosbon; Tobracin D; Tobracort; Tobradex; Trivagel N; Vagitrin-N; Vitatonus Dexa; ***Canad.:*** Ciprodex; Maxitrol; Opticort; Sofracort; Tobradex; ***Chile:*** Baycuten; Cilodex; Ciprodex; Dexagin; Grifoftal-D; Maxitrol; Oflono-D; Poentobral Plus; Telugren Plus; Tobradex; Tobragan D; Tobrin-D; Todexona; Tribesona; Xolof D; ***Cz.:*** Dexa-Gentamicin; Doxiproct Plus; Maxitrol; Otobacid N; Sofradex; Spersadex Compositum; Tobradex; ***Denm.:*** Sofradex; Spersadex Comp; ***Fin.:*** Maxitrol; Oftan Dexa-Chlora; Sofradex; ***Fr.:*** Auricularum; Cebedexacol; Chibro-Cadron; Corticetine; Dexagrane; Frakidex; Framyxone; Maxidrol; Percutalgine; Polydexa; Ster-Dex; Tobradex; ***Ger.:*** Corti Biciron N; Cortidexason comp; Dexa Biciron; Dexa Polyspectran; Dexa-Gentamicin; Dexa-Siozwo; Dexamytrex; Dispadex comp; Ell-Cranell dexa; Isopto Max; Lokalison-antimikrobiell Creme N; Nystalocal; Otobacid N; Supertendin; ***Gr.:*** Afacort; Chlorapred; Dexa-Rhinaspray-N; Dexachlor; Dexamycin; Dexamytrex; Dispersadron-C; Gentadex; Isopto Maxitrol; Lofoto; Nezefib; O-Biotic; Otocort; Otomize; Saocin-D; Thilomicine Dex; Tobradex; Urecortin; ***Hong Kong:*** Chloram-D; Dexoph; Dextracin; Eurodron; Frakidex; Maxitrol; Neo-Dex (Improved); Parasone; Polydex-N; Polydexa; Sofradex; Sonexa-C; Spersadex Comp; Tobradex; ***Hung.:*** Dexapolcort N; Doxiproct Plus; Tobradex; ***India:*** Ciplox D; Decdan-N; Dexona Eye/Ear; Dexosyn Plus; Dexosyn-C; Dexosyn-N; Gentacip D; Millicorten-Vioform; Obrasone; Ocupol-D; Ocutob-D; Oflox D; Pyrimon; Sofracort; Sofradex-F; Sofradex; Tobazon DM; ***Indon.:*** Alegi; Alerdex; Baycuten-N; Blecidex; Bralifex Plus; Dexatopic; Dextafen; Dextamine; Inmatrol; Isotic Neolyson; Isotic Tobrizon; Kloramixin D; Lorson; Lotharson; Maxitrol; Oregan; Osatrol; Polidemisin; Pritacort; Sofradex; Soldextam; Spersadex Comp; Tobradex; Trodex; Ximex Optixitrol; ***Irl.:*** Dexa-Rhinaspray Duo; Maxitrol; Otomize; Sofradex; ***Israel:*** Adexone; Auricularum; Desoren; Dethamycin; Dethaphrine; Dex-Otic; Dexamycin; Dexefrin; Maxitrol; Polycutan; Tarocidin D; Tevacutan; ***Ital.:*** Cloradex; Corti-Arscolloid; Desalfa; Desalfa; Desalfa; Desalfa; Desamix Effe; Desamix-Neomicina; Dexoline; Doxiproct; Eta Biocortilen VC; Eta Biocortilen; Luxazone Eparina; Neo Cortofen; Netildex; Tobradex; Visumetazone Antistaminico; Visumetazone Decongestionante; ***Jpn:*** Una A Gel; ***Malaysia:*** Baycuten N; De Icol; Dexa-Gentamicin; Dextracin; Gentadexa; Maxitrol; Neo-Deca; Sofradex; Spersadex Comp; Spersadexoline; Tobradex; ***Mex.:*** Alin Nasal; Alin Oftalmico; Baycuten N; Bexine; Biodexan; Butisel; Cilodex; Cloxona-O; Decadron con Neomicina; Decadron con Nistatina; Dexabion; Dexadutil; Dexamicin; Dexne; Dexne; Dexne; Dexsul; Dextone; Dibutasona; Dinill-D; Doxiproct Plus; Exafenil; Innobion; Lergosin A; Levodexan; Levofenil; Maxitrol; Mildex; Neobacigrin; Neuralin; Nispil; Obrydex; Odexan; Ofodex; Polideltaxin NF; Rinadex Compuesto; Rinidyl DN; Soldrin; Sondex-Of; Tiamidexal; Timpacil; Tobracort; Tobradex; Trazidex; Trineurovita Compuesto; ***Neth.:*** Dexagenta-POS; Dexamytrex; Maxitrol; Sofradex; Tobradex; ***Norw.:*** Maxitrol; Sofradex; Spersadex med kloramfenikol; ***NZ:*** Maxitrol; Sofradex; Tobradex; ***Philipp.:*** Baycuten; Dexamytrex; Dexanicol; Maxirap; Maxitrol; Maxoptic; Postop; Postotic; Spersadex Compound; Syntemax; Tobradex; ***Pol.:*** Dexadent; Dexamytrex; Dexapolcort N; Maxitrol; Tobradex; ***Port.:*** Baycuten; Dexamytrex; Dexaval A; Dexaval N; Dexaval O; Dexaval V; Frakidex; Gentadexa; Polydexa; ***Rus.:*** Ambene (Амбене); Dexa-Gentamicin (Декса-Гентамицин); Dexona (Дексона); Maxitrol (Макситрол); Polydexa (Полидекса); Polydexa with Phenylephrine (Полидекса С Фенилефрином); Tobradex (Тобрадекс); Tobrasone (Тобразон); ***S.Afr.:*** Covomycin-D; Maxitrol; Sofradex; Spersadex Comp; Spersadexoline; Tobradex; ***Singapore:*** Dexamytrex; Dextracin; Maxitrol; Polydexa; Sofradex; Tobradex; ***Spain:*** Amplidermis; Broncoformo Muco Dexa; Cloran Hemidex; Cresophene; Dexa Tavegil; Gentadexa; Hem Anth; Hongosan; Icol; Inzitan; Liquipom Dexa Antib; Maxitrol; Neodexa; Neurodavur Plus; Otix; Phonal; Resorborina; Rino Dexa; Sabanotropico; Sedofarin; Tobradex; Vasodexa; ***Switz.:*** Antikeloides Creme; Chronocorte; Dexalocal-F; Dexasalyl; Dexolan; Doxiproct Plus; Frakidex; Maxitrol; Nystalocal; Pigmanorm; Polydexa; Sebo-Psor; Sofradex; Spersadex Comp; Tobradex; ***Thai.:*** Archidex; Dexacin; Dexamytrex; Dexoph; Dexylin; Eyedex; Maxitrol; Neo-Optal; Neodex; Sofradex; Spersadexoline; Tobradex; Vesoph; ***UK:*** Maxitrol; Otomize; Sofradex; Tobradex; ***USA:*** Ak-Neo-Dex; Ciprodex; Dexasporin; Maxitrol; Neo-Dexameth; NeoDecadron; Neodexasone; Neopolydex; Ocu-Trol; Poly-Dex; Tobradex; ***Venez.:*** Baycuten N; Cyprodex; Decaven; Dexapostafen; Gentidexa; Gentidexa; Maxicort; Maxitrol; Otocort; Poentobral Plus; Poli-Otico; Quinocort; Tobracort; Tobradex; Tobragan D; Todex; Trazidex.

Dexamfetamine Sulfate

Other names: Deksamfetamin Sülfat; Dexamfétamine, Sulfate de; Dexamfetamine Sulphate; Dexamfetamini Sulfas; Dexamphetamine Sulphate; Dexamphetamini Sulfas; Dextro Amphetamine Sulphate; Dextroamphetamine Sulfate; NSC-73713 (dexamfetamine); Sulfato de dexanfetamina.

Дексамфетамина Сульфат

Clinical profile: Dexamfetamine is an optical isomer of amfetamine. It is an indirect-acting sympathomimetic with alpha- and beta-adrenergic agonist activity. It has a marked stimulant effect on the CNS, particularly the cerebral cortex. It is used clinically in the treatment of narcolepsy and attention deficit hyperactivity disorder. It has been used in the treatment of obesity.

WADA Status: Banned in competition

WADA Class: Stimulants

Includes amfetamine and any optical isomers.

Preparations
Single ingredient: ***Canad.:*** Dexedrine; ***UK:*** Dexedrine; ***USA:*** Dexedrine; Dextrostat.
Multi-ingredient: ***Canad.:*** Adderall; ***USA:*** Adderall.

Dexfenfluramine Hydrochloride

Other names: Deksfenfluramiinihydrokloridi; Dexfenfluramine, Chlorhydrate de; Dexfenfluraminhydroklorid; Dexfenfluramini Hydrochloridum; Hidrocloruro de dexfenfluramina; S-5614 (dexfenfluramine).

Дексфенфлурамина Гидрохлорид

Clinical profile: Dexfenfluramine, the *S*-isomer of fenfluramine, is an anorectic. It was formerly used in the treatment of obesity but was withdrawn worldwide following reports of valvular heart defects.

WADA Status: Banned in competition

WADA Class: Stimulants

Includes fenfluramine and any optical isomers.

Dexmethylphenidate Hydrochloride

Other names: Dexméthylphénidate, Chlorhydrate de; Dexmethylphenidati Hydrochloridum; d-Methylphenidate Hydrochloride; d-MPH; Hidrocloruro de dexmetilfenidato; *d-threo*-Methylphenidate.

Дексметилфенидата Гидрохлорид

Clinical profile: Dexmethylphenidate hydrochloride is the *d-threo*-enantiomer of racemic methylphenidate hydrochloride. It is used as a central stimulant in the treatment of hyperactivity disorders in children.

WADA Status: Banned in competition

WADA Class: Stimulants

Includes methylphenidate and any optical isomers.

Preparations
Single ingredient: ***USA:*** Focalin.

Dextran 1

Other names: Dekstraani 1; Dekstranas 1; Dextrán 1; Dextrano 1; Dextranum 1.

Декстран 1

Clinical profile: Dextran 1 consists of dextrans of weight average molecular weight about 1000. It is used to prevent severe anaphylactic reactions to infusions of dextran.

WADA Status: Banned in and out of competition

WADA Class: Diuretics and Other Masking Agents

Masking agents including alpha-reductase inhibitors or plasma expanders or substances with similar biological effect(s).

Preparations
Single ingredient: ***Austral.:*** Promit; ***Austria:*** Praedex; Promit; ***Denm.:*** Promiten; ***Hung.:*** Promit; ***Neth.:*** Promiten; ***Norw.:*** Promiten; ***S.Afr.:*** Promit; ***Swed.:*** Promiten; ***USA:*** Promit.

Multi-ingredient: ***Venez.:*** Optifresh.

Dextran 40

Other names: Dekstraani 40; Dekstran 40; Dekstranas 40; Dextrán 40; Dextrano 40; Dextranum 40; LMD; LMWD; Low-molecular-weight Dextran; LVD.

Декстран 40

Clinical profile: Dextran 40 consists of dextrans of weight average molecular weight about 40 000. It acts as a plasma expander and also reduces blood viscosity and inhibits sludging or aggregation of red blood cells. Dextran 40 is used for short-term plasma expansion, for the prophylaxis and treatment of postoperative thromboembolic disorders, and to improve blood flow and prevent intravascular aggregation in conditions or procedures associated with impaired circulation.

WADA Status: Banned in and out of competition

WADA Class: Diuretics and Other Masking Agents

Masking agents including alpha-reductase inhibitors or plasma expanders or substances with similar biological effect(s).

Preparations
Single ingredient: ***Austria:*** Elorheo; Rheomacrodex; ***Canad.:*** Gentran 40; ***Cz.:*** Rheodextran; ***Denm.:*** Rheomacrodex; ***Hung.:*** Rheomacrodex; ***Israel:*** Rheomacrodex; ***Ital.:*** Eudextran; Plander R; ***Mex.:*** Rheomacrodex; ***Norw.:*** Rheomacrodex; ***Philipp.:*** LM Dextran; ***Rus.:*** Rheomacrodex (Реомакродекс); Rheopolydex (Реополидекс); ***S.Afr.:*** Rheomacrodex; ***Spain:***

Rheomacrodex; ***Swed.:*** Perfadex; Rheomacrodex; ***Thai.:*** Onkovertin; ***Turk.:*** Rheomacrodex; ***UK:*** Gentran 40; ***USA:*** Gentran 40; Rheomacrodex.
Multi-ingredient: ***Indon.:*** Otsutran; ***Port.:*** Bas-Dextrano; ***Rus.:*** Rheogluman (Реоглюман); Rheopolyglukin with Glucose (Реополиглюкин С Глюкозой).

Dextran 60

Other names: Dekstraani 60; Dekstranas 60; Dextrán 60; Dextrano 60; Dextranum 60.

Декстран 60

Clinical profile: Dextran 60 consists of dextrans of weight average molecular weight about 60 000. It is used for short-term plasma expansion and for the prevention of postoperative thromboembolic disorders.

WADA Status: Banned in and out of competition

WADA Class: Diuretics and Other Masking Agents

Masking agents including alpha-reductase inhibitors or plasma expanders or substances with similar biological effect(s).

Preparations
Single ingredient: ***Austria:*** Macrodex; ***Hung.:*** Macrodex; ***Norw.:*** Plasmodex; ***Swed.:*** Plasmodex.

D

Dextran 70

Other names: Dekstraani 70; Dekstran 70; Dekstranas 70; Dextrán 70; Dextrano 70; Dextranum 70; Polyglucin (dextran).

Декстран 70

Clinical profile: Dextran 70 consists of dextrans of weight average molecular weight about 70 000. It is used for short-term plasma expansion and for the prevention of postoperative thromboembolic disorders.

WADA Status: Banned in and out of competition

WADA Class: Diuretics and Other Masking Agents

Masking agents including alpha-reductase inhibitors or plasma expanders or substances with similar biological effect(s).

Preparations
Single ingredient: ***Austral.:*** Hyskon; ***Canad.:*** Gentran 70; ***Cz.:*** Tensiton; ***Denm.:*** Macrodex; RescueFlow; ***Fin.:*** RescueFlow; ***Israel:*** Macrodex; ***Ital.:*** Plander; ***Neth.:*** RescueFlow; ***Norw.:*** Macrodex; RescueFlow; ***S.Afr.:*** Macrodex; RescueFlow; ***Swed.:*** Macrodex; RescueFlow; ***Switz.:*** Dialens; ***Turk.:*** Macrodex; ***UK:*** Gentran 70; RescueFlow; ***USA:*** Gentran 70; Hyskon; Macrodex; ***Venez.:*** Lacridos; Lacrimart; Lagrimas Artificiales.
Multi-ingredient: ***Arg.:*** Alcon Lagrimas; Kalopsis Lagrimas; Phoenix Lagrimas; Tears Naturale; Visine Plus; ***Austral.:*** Bion Tears; Opti-Free Comfort; Poly-Tears; Tears Naturale; Visine Advanced Relief; ***Belg.:*** Alcon Adequad; Lacrystat; Tears Naturale; ***Braz.:*** Lacribell; Lacrima Plus; Trisorb; ***Canad.:*** Artificial Tears; Bion Tears; Tears Naturale Forte; Tears Naturale; Visine Advance Triple Action; ***Chile:*** Lagrimas Artificiales; Naphtears; Nico Drops; Nicotears; Tears Naturale; ***Cz.:*** Tears Naturale; ***Denm.:*** Dacriosol; ***Ger.:*** Isopto Naturale; ***Gr.:*** Tears Naturale; ***Hong Kong:*** Bion Tears; Tears Naturale Forte; ***Hung.:*** Dacrolux; Tears Naturale; ***Indon.:*** Isotic Tearin; Tears Naturale II; Tears; ***Irl.:*** Tears Naturale; ***Israel:*** Tears Naturale; ***Ital.:*** Dacriosol; ***Malaysia:*** Bion Tears; Dacrolux; Tears Naturale; ***Mex.:*** Lacrima Plus; Naphtears; Naturalag; Tears Naturale; Visine Extra; ***Neth.:*** Duratears; ***Norw.:*** Tears Naturale; ***NZ:*** Poly-Tears; Tears Naturale; Visine Advanced Relief; ***Philipp.:*** Gentle Tears; Tears Naturale; ***Pol.:*** Tears Naturale; ***Port.:*** Tears Naturale; ***Rus.:*** Tears Naturale (Слеза Натуральная); ***S.Afr.:*** Tears Naturale; ***Singapore:*** Bion Tears; Tears Naturale; ***Spain:*** Dacrolux; Tears Humectante; ***Swed.:*** Bion Tears; ***Switz.:*** Tears Naturale; ***Thai.:*** Bion Tears; Tears Naturale; ***Turk.:*** Dacrolux; Tears Naturale; ***UK:*** Tears Naturale; ***USA:***

Advanced Relief Visine; Bion Tears; Lacri-Tears; LubriTears; Moisture Drops; Nature's Tears; Ocucoat; Tears Naturale; Tears Renewed.

D

Dextran 75

Other names: Dextrán 75; Dextrano 75; Dextranum 75.

Декстран 75

Clinical profile: Dextran 75 consists of dextrans of weight average molecular weight about 75 000. It is used for short-term plasma expansion.

WADA Status: Banned in and out of competition

WADA Class: Diuretics and Other Masking Agents

Masking agents including alpha-reductase inhibitors or plasma expanders or substances with similar biological effect(s).

Dextran 110

Other names: Dextrán 110; Dextrano 110; Dextranum 110.

Декстран 110

Clinical profile: Dextran 110 consists of dextrans of weight average molecular weight about 110 000. It is used for short-term plasma expansion.

WADA Status: Banned in and out of competition

WADA Class: Diuretics and Other Masking Agents

Masking agents including alpha-reductase inhibitors or plasma expanders or substances with similar biological effect(s).

Dextromoramide

Other names: Dekstromoramidi; Dextrodiphenopyrine; Dextromoramid; Dextromoramida; Dextromoramidum; *d*-Moramid; Pyrrolamidol.

Декстроморамид

Dextromoramide Tartrate

Other names: Bitartrate de Dextromoramide; Dekstromoramiditartraatti; Dekstromoramido tartratas; Dextromoramide Acid Tartrate; Dextromoramide Hydrogen Tartrate; Dextromoramide, tartrate de; Dextromoramidi tartras; Dextromoramid-tartarát; Dextromoramidtartrat; Tartrato de dextromoramida.

Декстроморамида Тартрат

Clinical profile: Dextromoramide is an opioid analgesic structurally related to methadone and used in the treatment of severe pain.

WADA Status: Banned in competition

WADA Class: Narcotics

Includes specified narcotics.

Preparations
Single ingredient: ***Irl.:*** Palfium; ***Neth.:*** Palface; Palfium.

Diamorphine Hydrochloride

Other names: Diacetilmorfina, hidrocloruro de; Diacetylmorphine Hydrochloride; Heroin Hydrochloride.

Clinical profile: Diamorphine hydrochloride is an acetylated morphine derivative which is metabolised to morphine. It is a more potent opioid analgesic than morphine and is used for the relief of severe pain especially in terminal illnesses. Diamorphine is used similarly to morphine for the relief of dyspnoea due to pulmonary oedema resulting from left ventricular failure. It has a powerful cough suppressant effect and has been given to control cough associated with terminal lung cancer.

WADA Status: Banned in competition

WADA Class: Narcotics
Includes specified narcotics.

Preparations
Single ingredient: ***Switz.:*** Diaphin.

Dichlorisone Acetate

Other names: Acetato de diclorisona; Dichlorisone, Acétate de; Dichlorisoni Acetas; Diclorisone Acetate.

Дихлоризона Ацетат

Clinical profile: Dichlorisone acetate is a corticosteroid used topically in the treatment of various skin disorders.

WADA Status: Banned in competition

WADA Class: Glucocorticosteroids
All glucocorticosteroids are prohibited when administered orally, rectally, intravenously or intramuscularly. Their use requires a Therapeutic Use Exemption approval. Other routes of administration (intraarticular / periarticular / peritendinous / epidural / intradermal injections and inhalation) require an Abbreviated Therapeutic Use Exemption except as noted below.
Topical preparations when used for dermatological (including iontophoresis / phonophoresis), auricular, nasal, ophthalmic, buccal, gingival and perianal disorders are not prohibited and do not require any form of Therapeutic Use Exemption.

WADA Class: Specified Substances
Also listed as a specified substance.
"The prohibited List may identify specified substances which are particularly susceptible to unintentional anti-doping rule violations because of their general availability in medicinal products or which are less likely to be successfully abused as doping agents."
A doping violation involving such substances may result in a reduced sanction provided that the *"...Athlete can establish that the Use of such a specfied substance was not intended to enhance sport performance..."*

Diclofenamide

Preparations
Single ingredient: ***Spain:*** Dermaren; Dicloderm Forte.

Diclofenamide

Other names: Dichlorphenamide; Diclofenamida; Diclofénamide; Diclofenamidum; Diklofenamid; Diklofenamidi.

Диклофенамид

Clinical profile: Diclofenamide is an inhibitor of carbonic anhydrase used to reduce intraocular pressure in glaucoma.

WADA Status: Banned in and out of competition

D

WADA Class: Diuretics and Other Masking Agents

Includes diuretics or substances with a similar chemical structure or similar biological effect(s).

Preparations
Single ingredient: ***Cz.:*** Oratrol; ***Ital.:*** Antidrasi; Fenamide; ***Spain:*** Glauconide.

Diethylaminoethanol

Other names: Dietilaminoetanol.

Clinical profile: Diethylaminoethanol is an analogue of deanol and has been used as a central stimulant.

WADA Status: Banned in competition

WADA Class: Stimulants

Includes stimulants or substances with a similar chemical structure or similar biological effect(s).

WADA Class: Specified Substances

Also listed as a specified substance.

"The prohibited List may identify specified substances which are particularly susceptible to unintentional anti-doping rule violations because of their general availability in medicinal products or which are less likely to be successfully abused as doping agents."

A doping violation involving such substances may result in a reduced sanction provided that the "*...Athlete can establish that the Use of such a specfied substance was not intended to enhance sport performance...*"

Preparations
Single ingredient: ***Gr.:*** Durobion.
Multi-ingredient: ***Austria:*** Barokaton.

Diethylpropion Hydrochloride

Other names: Amfepramone Hydrochloride; Amfépramone, Chlorhydrate d'; Amfepramoni Hydrochloridum; Hidrocloruro de anfepramona.

Амфепрамона Гидрохлорид

Clinical profile: Diethylpropion hydrochloride is a central stimulant and indirect-acting sympathomimetic used as an anorectic in the short-term treatment of obesity.

WADA Status: Banned in competition

WADA Class: Stimulants

Includes diethylpropion and any optical isomers.

Preparations
Single ingredient: ***Austral.:*** Tenuate; ***Braz.:*** Dualid S; Inibex S; ***Canad.:*** Tenuate; ***Chile:*** Sacin; ***Denm.:*** Regenon; ***Ger.:*** Regenon; ***Hong Kong:*** Atractil; Prothin; ***Mex.:*** Ifa Norex; Neobes; ***NZ:*** Tenuate Dospan; ***S.Afr.:*** Tenuate Dospan; ***Switz.:*** Regenon; ***Thai.:*** Atractil; Dietil.
Multi-ingredient: ***Arg.:*** Tratobes; ***Indon.:*** Apisate.

Diflorasone Diacetate

Other names: Diacetato de diflorasona; Diflorasone, Diacetate de; Diflorasoni Diacetas; U-34865.

Дифлоразона Диацетат

D

Clinical profile: Diflorasone diacetate is a corticosteroid used topically in the treatment of various skin disorders.

WADA Status: Banned in competition

WADA Class: Glucocorticosteroids

All glucocorticosteroids are prohibited when administered orally, rectally, intravenously or intramuscularly. Their use requires a Therapeutic Use Exemption approval. Other routes of administration (intraarticular / periarticular / peritendinous / epidural / intradermal injections and inhalation) require an Abbreviated Therapeutic Use Exemption except as noted below.

Topical preparations when used for dermatological (including iontophoresis / phonophoresis), auricular, nasal, ophthalmic, buccal, gingival and perianal disorders are not prohibited and do not require any form of Therapeutic Use Exemption.

WADA Class: Specified Substances

Also listed as a specified substance.

"The prohibited List may identify specified substances which are particularly susceptible to unintentional anti-doping rule violations because of their general availability in medicinal products or which are less likely to be successfully abused as doping agents."

A doping violation involving such substances may result in a reduced sanction provided that the "*...Athlete can establish that the Use of such a specfied substance was not intended to enhance sport performance...*"

Preparations
Single ingredient: ***Ger.:*** Florone; ***Mex.:*** Diasorane; ***Spain:*** Murode; ***USA:*** ApexiCon; Florone; Maxiflor; Psorcon.
Multi-ingredient: ***Arg.:*** Filoderma Plus; Filoderma; Griseocrem.

Diflucortolone

Other names: Diflucortolona; Diflucortolonum; Diflukortolon; Diflukortoloni.

Дифлукортолон

Diflucortolone Pivalate

Other names: Diflucortolone, Pivalate de; Diflucortoloni Pivalas; Pivalato de diflucortolona; SH-968.

Дифлукортолона Пивалат

Diflucortolone Valerate

Other names: Diflucortolone, Valérate de; Diflucortoloni Valeras; Diflukortolon

Valerat; Valerato de diflucortolona.

Дифлукортолона Валерат

Clinical profile: Diflucortolone is a corticosteroid used topically, usually as the valerate, in the treatment of various skin disorders.

WADA Status: Banned in competition

WADA Class: Glucocorticosteroids

All glucocorticosteroids are prohibited when administered orally, rectally, intravenously or intramuscularly. Their use requires a Therapeutic Use Exemption approval. Other routes of administration (intraarticular / periarticular / peritendinous / epidural / intradermal injections and inhalation) require an Abbreviated Therapeutic Use Exemption except as noted below.

Topical preparations when used for dermatological (including iontophoresis / phonophoresis), auricular, nasal, ophthalmic, buccal, gingival and perianal disorders are not prohibited and do not require any form of Therapeutic Use Exemption.

WADA Class: Specified Substances

Also listed as a specified substance.

"The prohibited List may identify specified substances which are particularly susceptible to unintentional anti-doping rule violations because of their general availability in medicinal products or which are less likely to be successfully abused as doping agents."

A doping violation involving such substances may result in a reduced sanction provided that the "*...Athlete can establish that the Use of such a specfied substance was not intended to enhance sport performance...*"

Preparations

Single ingredient: ***Arg.:*** Nerisona; ***Austria:*** Neriforte; Nerisona; ***Belg.:*** Nerisona; ***Braz.:*** Nerisona; ***Canad.:*** Nerisone; ***Denm.:*** Nerisona; ***Fr.:*** Nerisone; ***Ger.:*** Nerisona; ***Hong Kong:*** Nerisone; ***Indon.:*** Nerilon; Nerisona; Valeron; ***Israel:*** Neriderm; ***Ital.:*** Cortical; Dermaval; Dervin; Flu-Cortanest; Nerisona; Temetex; ***Malaysia:*** Nerisone; ***Mex.:*** Nerisona; ***Neth.:*** Nerisona; ***NZ:*** Nerisone; ***Philipp.:*** Nerisona; ***Port.:*** Nerisona; ***S.Afr.:*** Nerisone; ***Spain:*** Claral; ***Turk.:*** Temetex; ***UK:*** Nerisone.

Multi-ingredient: ***Arg.:*** Nerisona C; Scheriderm; ***Austria:*** Travocort; ***Belg.:*** Travocort; ***Braz.:*** Bi-Nerisona; ***Canad.:*** Nerisalic; ***Chile:*** Bi-Nerisona; ***Fr.:*** Nerisalic; Nerisone C; ***Ger.:*** Travocort; ***Gr.:*** Travocort; ***Hong Kong:*** Nerisone C; Travocort; ***Indon.:*** Nerisona Combi; Travocort; ***Irl.:*** Travocort; ***Israel:*** Isocort; Multiderm; Tevaderm; ***Ital.:*** Corti-Fluoral; Dermaflogil; Impetex; Nerisalic; Nerisona C; Travocort; ***Malaysia:*** Isoradin; Travocort; ***Mex.:*** Bi-Nerisona; Scheriderm; ***NZ:*** Nerisone C; ***Philipp.:*** Nerisona Combi; Travocort; ***Pol.:*** Travocort; ***Port.:*** Nerisona C; Travocort; ***Rus.:*** Travocort (Травокорт); ***S.Afr.:*** Travocort; ***Singapore:*** Travocort; ***Spain:*** Claral Plus; ***Switz.:*** Travocort; ***Thai.:*** Travocort; ***Turk.:*** Impetex; Nerisona C; Travazol; Travocort; ***Venez.:*** Binerisona.

Difluprednate

Other names: CM-9155; Difluprednato; Difluprednatum; W-6309.

Дифлупреднат

Clinical profile: Difluprednate is a corticosteroid used topically in the treatment of various skin disorders.

WADA Status: Banned in competition

WADA Class: Glucocorticosteroids

All glucocorticosteroids are prohibited when administered orally, rectally, intravenously or intramuscularly. Their use requires a Therapeutic Use Exemption approval. Other routes of administration (intraarticular / periarticular / peritendinous / epidural / intradermal injections and inhalation) require an Abbreviated Therapeutic Use Exemption except as noted below.

Topical preparations when used for dermatological (including iontophoresis / pho-

nophoresis), auricular, nasal, ophthalmic, buccal, gingival and perianal disorders are not prohibited and do not require any form of Therapeutic Use Exemption.

WADA Class: Specified Substances

Also listed as a specified substance.

"The prohibited List may identify specified substances which are particularly susceptible to unintentional anti-doping rule violations because of their general availability in medicinal products or which are less likely to be successfully abused as doping agents."

A doping violation involving such substances may result in a reduced sanction provided that the "*...Athlete can establish that the Use of such a specfied substance was not intended to enhance sport performance...*"

Preparations
Single ingredient: ***Fr.:*** Epitopic.

D

Dilevalol

Other names: Dilévalol; Dilevalolum; *R,R*-Labetalol; Sch-19927 (dilevalol hydrochloride).

Дилевалол

Clinical profile: Dilevalol is a beta blocker with vasodilating activity and was formerly used in the treatment of hypertension. It was withdrawn from the world market in 1990 due to reports of hepatotoxicity.

WADA Status: Banned in and out of competition as specified below

WADA Class: Beta-Blockers

Unless otherwise specified, beta-blockers are prohibited *In-Competition* only in the following sports.

- Aeronautics (FAI)
- Archery (FITA, IPC) (also prohibited *Out-of-Competition*)
- Automobile (FIA)
- Billiards (WCBS)
- Bobsleigh (FIBT)
- Boules (CMSB, IPC bowls)
- Bridge (FMB)
- Curling (WCF)
- Gymnastics (FIG)
- Motorcycling (FIM)
- Modern Pentathlon (UIPM) for disciplines involving shooting
- Nine-pin bowling (FIQ)
- Powerboating (UIM)
- Sailing (ISAF) for match race helms only
- Shooting (ISSF, IPC) (also prohibited *Out-of-Competition*)
- Skiing/Snowboarding (FIS) in ski jumping, freestyle aerials/halfpipe and snowboard halfpipe/big air
- Wrestling (FILA)

WADA Class: Specified Substances

Also listed as a specified substance.

"The prohibited List may identify specified substances which are particularly susceptible to unintentional anti-doping rule violations because of their general availability in medicinal products or which are less likely to be successfully abused as doping agents."

A doping violation involving such substances may result in a reduced sanction pro-

vided that the "*...Athlete can establish that the Use of such a specfied substance was not intended to enhance sport performance...*"

Dimetamfetamine

Other names: Dimétamfétamine; Dimetamfetaminum; Dimetanfetamina; Dimethylamphetamine.

Диметамфетамин

Clinical profile: Dimetamfetamine is an amfetamine derivative and has been used as a central stimulant.

D

WADA Status: Banned in competition

WADA Class: Stimulants

Includes dimetamfetamine and any optical isomers.

Dimetofrine Hydrochloride

Other names: Dimétofrine, Chlorhydrate de; Dimetofrini Hydrochloridum; Dimetophrine Hydrochloride; Hidrocloruro de dimetofrina.

Диметофрина Гидрохлорид

Clinical profile: Dimetofrine hydrochloride is a sympathomimetic that has been used in the treatment of hypotensive states and for cold and influenza symptoms.

WADA Status: Banned in competition

WADA Class: Stimulants

Includes stimulants or substances with a similar chemical structure or similar biological effect(s).

WADA Class: Specified Substances

Also listed as a specified substance.

"*The prohibited List may identify specified substances which are particularly susceptible to unintentional anti-doping rule violations because of their general availability in medicinal products or which are less likely to be successfully abused as doping agents.*"

A doping violation involving such substances may result in a reduced sanction provided that the "*...Athlete can establish that the Use of such a specfied substance was not intended to enhance sport performance...*"

Preparations
Multi-ingredient: ***Ital.:*** Raffreddoremed.

Dioxethedrin Hydrochloride

Other names: Dioxéthédrine, Chlorhydrate de; Dioxethedrine Hydrochloride; Dioxethedrini Hydrochloridum; Hidrocloruro de dioxetedrina.

Диоксетедрина Гидрохлорид

Clinical profile: Dioxethedrin hydrochloride is a sympathomimetic that has been used in preparations intended for the relief of coughs and associated respiratory-tract disorders.

WADA Status: Banned in competition

WADA Class: Stimulants

Includes stimulants or substances with a similar chemical structure or similar biological effect(s).

WADA Class: Specified Substances

Also listed as a specified substance.

"The prohibited List may identify specified substances which are particularly susceptible to unintentional anti-doping rule violations because of their general availability in medicinal products or which are less likely to be successfully abused as doping agents."

A doping violation involving such substances may result in a reduced sanction provided that the "*...Athlete can establish that the Use of such a specfied substance was not intended to enhance sport performance...*"

Dipivefrine

Other names: Dipivalyl Epinephrine; Dipivefriini; Dipivefrin; Dipivefrina; Dipivéfrine; Dipivefrinum; DPE.

Дипивефрин

Dipivefrine Hydrochloride

Other names: Dipivalyl Adrenaline Hydrochloride; Dipivalyl Epinephrine Hydrochloride; Dipivefriinihydrokloridi; Dipivefrin Hydrochloride; Dipivéfrine, chlorhydrate de; Dipivefrin-hydrochlorid; Dipivefrinhydroklorid; Dipivefrini hydrochloridum; Dipivefrino hidrochloridas; Dipiwefryny chlorowodorek; Hidrocloruro de dipivefrina.

Дипивефрина Гидрохлорид

Clinical profile: Dipivefrine is an ester and prodrug of adrenaline used to lower intra-ocular pressure.

WADA Status: Banned in competition

WADA Class: Stimulants

Includes stimulants or substances with a similar chemical structure or similar biological effect(s).

WADA Class: Specified Substances

Also listed as a specified substance.

"The prohibited List may identify specified substances which are particularly susceptible to unintentional anti-doping rule violations because of their general availability in medicinal products or which are less likely to be successfully abused as doping agents."

A doping violation involving such substances may result in a reduced sanction provided that the "*...Athlete can establish that the Use of such a specfied substance was not intended to enhance sport performance...*"

Preparations

Single ingredient: ***Austral.:*** Dipoquin; Propine; ***Belg.:*** Propine; ***Braz.:*** Propine; ***Cz.:*** d Epifrin; Oftanex; ***Denm.:*** Propine; ***Fin.:*** Propine; ***Fr.:*** Propine; ***Ger.:*** d Epifrin; Glaucothil; ***Gr.:*** Glaucodose; Thilodrin; ***Hong Kong:*** Propine; ***Irl.:*** Propine; ***Israel:*** Difrin; ***Ital.:*** Propine; ***Jpn:***

Pivalephrine; ***Malaysia:*** Propine; ***Neth.:*** Diopine; ***Norw.:*** Propine; ***NZ:*** Propine; ***Port.:*** Propine; ***Spain:*** Diopine; ***Swed.:*** Propine; ***UK:*** Propine; ***USA:*** AkPro; Propine.

Multi-ingredient: ***Austria:*** Thiloadren; ***Ger.:*** Thiloadren N; Thilodigon.

Domoprednate

Other names: Domoprednato; Domoprednatum; Ro-12-7024.

Домопреднат

Clinical profile: Domoprednate is a corticosteroid that has been used topically in the treatment of various skin disorders.

D

WADA Status: Banned in competition

WADA Class: Glucocorticosteroids

All glucocorticosteroids are prohibited when administered orally, rectally, intravenously or intramuscularly. Their use requires a Therapeutic Use Exemption approval. Other routes of administration (intraarticular / periarticular / peritendinous / epidural / intradermal injections and inhalation) require an Abbreviated Therapeutic Use Exemption except as noted below.

Topical preparations when used for dermatological (including iontophoresis / phonophoresis), auricular, nasal, ophthalmic, buccal, gingival and perianal disorders are not prohibited and do not require any form of Therapeutic Use Exemption.

WADA Class: Specified Substances

Also listed as a specified substance.

"*The prohibited List may identify specified substances which are particularly susceptible to unintentional anti-doping rule violations because of their general availability in medicinal products or which are less likely to be successfully abused as doping agents.*"

A doping violation involving such substances may result in a reduced sanction provided that the "*...Athlete can establish that the Use of such a specfied substance was not intended to enhance sport performance...*"

Dopexamine Hydrochloride

Other names: Dopeksamiinihydrokloridi; Dopeksamin Hidroklorür; Dopéxamine, Chlorhydrate de; Dopexamine, dichlorhydrate de; Dopexamine dihydrochloride; Dopexaminhydroklorid; Dopexamini dihydrochloridum; Dopexamini Hydrochloridum; FPL-60278 (dopexamine); FPL-60278AR; Hidrocloruro de dopexamina.

Допексамина Гидрохлорид

Clinical profile: Dopexamine hydrochloride is a sympathomimetic with direct and indirect effects. It stimulates beta$_2$ adrenoceptors and peripheral dopamine receptors and also inhibits the neuronal reuptake of noradrenaline. It is used to provide haemodynamic support after cardiac surgery or in exacerbations of chronic heart failure.

WADA Status: Banned in and out of competition

WADA Class: Beta-2 Agonists

Includes beta-2 agonists or their isomers.

Preparations
Single ingredient: ***Cz.:*** Dopacard; ***Denm.:*** Dopacard; ***Fin.:*** Dopacard; ***Fr.:*** Dopacard; ***Ger.:*** Dopacard; ***Irl.:*** Dopacard; ***UK:*** Dopacard.

Dorzolamide Hydrochloride

Other names: Dorzolamid Hidroklorür; Dorzolamide, chlorhydrate de; Dorzolamidi hydrochloridum; Hidrocloruro de dorzolamida; L-671152 (dorzolamide); MK-507; MK-0507.

Дорзоламида Гидрохлорид

Clinical profile: Dorzolamide is a carbonic anhydrase inhibitor used in the management of glaucoma and ocular hypertension.

WADA Status: Banned in and out of competition

WADA Class: Diuretics and Other Masking Agents

Includes diuretics or substances with a similar chemical structure or similar biological effect(s).

Preparations
Single ingredient: ***Arg.:*** Dorlamida; Trusopt; ***Austral.:*** Trusopt; ***Austria:*** Trusopt; ***Belg.:*** Trusopt; ***Braz.:*** Trusopt; ***Canad.:*** Trusopt; ***Chile:*** Glaucotensil; Trusopt; ***Cz.:*** Trusopt; ***Denm.:*** Trusopt; ***Fin.:*** Trusopt; ***Fr.:*** Trusopt; ***Ger.:*** Trusopt; ***Gr.:*** Trusopt; ***Hong Kong:*** Trusopt; ***Hung.:*** Trusopt; ***India:*** Dorzox; ***Irl.:*** Trusopt; ***Israel:*** Trusopt; ***Ital.:*** Trusopt; ***Malaysia:*** Trusopt; ***Mex.:*** Trusopt; ***Neth.:*** Trusopt; ***Norw.:*** Trusopt; ***NZ:*** Trusopt; ***Philipp.:*** Trusopt; ***Pol.:*** Trusopt; ***Port.:*** Trusopt; ***Rus.:*** Trusopt (Трусопт); ***S.Afr.:*** Trusopt; ***Singapore:*** Trusopt; ***Spain:*** Trusopt; ***Swed.:*** Trusopt; ***Switz.:*** Trusopt; ***Thai.:*** Trusopt; ***Turk.:*** Trusopt; ***UK:*** Trusopt; ***USA:*** Trusopt; ***Venez.:*** Dorzol; Glaucotensil D; Trusopt.
Multi-ingredient: ***Arg.:*** Cosopt; Dorlamida T; Glaucotensil TD; Timed D; ***Austral.:*** Cosopt; ***Austria:*** Cosopt; Timsopt; ***Belg.:*** Cosopt; ***Braz.:*** Cosopt; ***Canad.:*** Cosopt; ***Chile:*** Cosopt; Dorsof T; Glaucotensil T; Glausolets Plus; Tiof Plus; ***Cz.:*** Cosopt; ***Denm.:*** Cosopt; ***Fin.:*** Cosopt; ***Fr.:*** Cosopt; ***Ger.:*** Cosopt; ***Gr.:*** Cosopt; ***Hong Kong:*** Cosopt; ***Hung.:*** Cosopt; ***Irl.:*** Cosopt; ***Israel:*** Cosopt; ***Ital.:*** Cosopt; ***Mex.:*** Cosopt; ***Neth.:*** Cosopt; ***Norw.:*** Cosopt; ***NZ:*** Cosopt; ***Philipp.:*** Cosopt; ***Pol.:*** Cosopt; ***Port.:*** Cosopt; ***S.Afr.:*** Cosopt; ***Singapore:*** Cosopt; ***Swed.:*** Cosopt; ***Switz.:*** Cosopt; ***Thai.:*** Cosopt; ***Turk.:*** Cosopt; ***UK:*** Cosopt; ***USA:*** Cosopt; ***Venez.:*** Cosopt; Dobet; Glaucotensil T.

Draquinolol

Other names: Draquinololum; H-I-42-BS.

Драхинолол

Clinical profile: Draquinolol is a cardioselective beta blocker.

WADA Status: Banned in and out of competition as specified below

WADA Class: Beta-Blockers

Unless otherwise specified, beta-blockers are prohibited *In-Competition* only in the following sports.

- Aeronautics (FAI)
- Archery (FITA, IPC) (also prohibited *Out-of-Competition*)
- Automobile (FIA)
- Billiards (WCBS)
- Bobsleigh (FIBT)
- Boules (CMSB, IPC bowls)
- Bridge (FMB)
- Curling (WCF)
- Gymnastics (FIG)
- Motorcycling (FIM)
- Modern Pentathlon (UIPM) for disciplines involving shooting
- Nine-pin bowling (FIQ)

- Powerboating (UIM)
- Sailing (ISAF) for match race helms only
- Shooting (ISSF, IPC) (also prohibited *Out-of-Competition*)
- Skiing/Snowboarding (FIS) in ski jumping, freestyle aerials/halfpipe and snowboard halfpipe/big air
- Wrestling (FILA)

WADA Class: Specified Substances

Also listed as a specified substance.

"*The prohibited List may identify specified substances which are particularly susceptible to unintentional anti-doping rule violations because of their general availability in medicinal products or which are less likely to be successfully abused as doping agents.*"

A doping violation involving such substances may result in a reduced sanction provided that the "*...Athlete can establish that the Use of such a specfied substance was not intended to enhance sport performance...*"

D

Droloxifene

Other names: Droloxifène; Droloxifeno; Droloxifenum; 3-Hydroxytamoxifen; K-21060E.

Дролоксифен

Clinical profile: Droloxifene is a potent anti-oestrogen related to tamoxifen. It has been investigated in the hormonal prophylaxis and treatment of breast cancer and is under study for osteoporosis.

WADA Status: Banned in and out of competition

WADA Class: Hormone Antagonists and Modulators

Includes selective estrogen receptor modulators.

Dronabinol

Other names: Dronabinolum; NSC-134454; Δ^9-Tetrahydrocannabinol; Δ^9-THC.

Дронабинол

Clinical profile: Dronabinol, the major psychoactive constituent of cannabis, has antiemetic properties and is used for the control of nausea and vomiting associated with cancer chemotherapy in patients who have failed to respond adequately to conventional antiemetics. It is also used for its appetite-stimulant effects in the treatment of anorexia associated with weight loss in AIDS patients. Dronabinol is also used with cannabidiol, another cannabinoid, in a buccal spray preparation as adjunctive treatment in adults for neuropathic pain in multiple sclerosis in adults and for advanced cancer pain.

WADA Status: Banned in competition

WADA Class: Cannabinoids

E.g. hashish, marijuana

WADA Class: Specified Substances

Also listed as a specified substance.

"*The prohibited List may identify specified substances which are particularly susceptible to unintentional anti-doping rule violations because of their general availability in medicinal products or which are less likely to be successfully abused as doping agents.*"

A doping violation involving such substances may result in a reduced sanction pro-

vided that the "*...Athlete can establish that the Use of such a specfied substance was not intended to enhance sport performance...*"

Preparations
Single ingredient: ***Canad.:*** Marinol; ***USA:*** Marinol.
Multi-ingredient: ***Canad.:*** Sativex.

Drostanolone Propionate

Other names: Compound 32379; Dromostanolone Propionate; Drostanolone, Propionate de; Drostanoloni Propionas; 2α-Methyldihydrotestosterone Propionate; NSC-12198; Propionato de drostanolona.

Дростанолона Пропионат

Clinical profile: Drostanolone has anabolic and androgenic properties and has been used in the treatment of advanced malignant neoplasms of the breast in postmenopausal women.

WADA Status: Banned in and out of competition

WADA Class: Anabolic; Androgenic Steroids (exogenous)

Includes exogenous anabolic androgenic steroids or other substances with a similar chemical structure or similar biological effect(s).

Dutasteride

Other names: Dutasterid; Dutasterida; Dutastéride; Dutasteridum; GG-745; GI-198745; GI-198745X.

Дутастерид

Clinical profile: Dutasteride is a 5α-reductase inhibitor used in benign prostatic hyperplasia, and under investigation in alopecia and the prevention of prostate cancer.

WADA Status: Banned in and out of competition

WADA Class: Diuretics and Other Masking Agents

Masking agents including alpha-reductase inhibitors or plasma expanders or substances with similar biological effect(s).

WADA Class: Specified Substances

Also listed as a specified substance.

"*The prohibited List may identify specified substances which are particularly susceptible to unintentional anti-doping rule violations because of their general availability in medicinal products or which are less likely to be successfully abused as doping agents.*"

A doping violation involving such substances may result in a reduced sanction provided that the "*...Athlete can establish that the Use of such a specfied substance was not intended to enhance sport performance...*"

Preparations
Single ingredient: ***Arg.:*** Avodart; ***Austria:*** Avodart; Avolve; Zyfetor; ***Belg.:*** Avodart; ***Canad.:*** Avodart; ***Chile:*** Avodart; ***Denm.:*** Avodart; ***Fin.:*** Avodart; ***Fr.:*** Avodart; ***Ger.:*** Avodart; ***Gr.:*** Avodart; Duagen; ***India:*** Duprost; ***Indon.:*** Avodart; ***Irl.:*** Avodart; ***Israel:*** Avodart; ***Ital.:*** Avodart; ***Malaysia:*** Avodart; ***Mex.:*** Avodart; ***Neth.:*** Avodart; Duagen; ***Norw.:*** Avodart; ***Philipp.:*** Avodart; ***Pol.:*** Avodart; ***Port.:*** Avodart; Duagen; ***Rus.:*** Avodart (Аводарт); ***S.Afr.:*** Avodart; ***Singapore:*** Avodart; ***Spain:*** Avidart; Duagen; ***Swed.:*** Avodart; ***Switz.:*** Avodart; ***Turk.:*** Avodart; ***UK:*** Avodart; ***USA:*** Avodart.

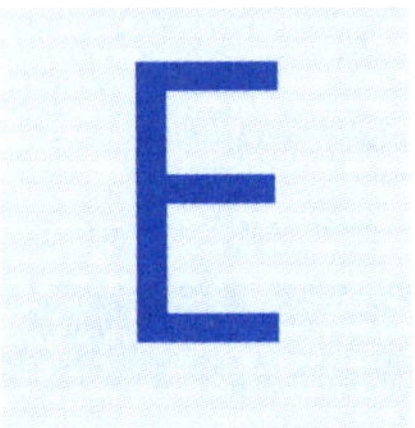

Efaproxiral

Other names: Éfaproxiral; Efaproxiralum; RSR-13.

Эфапроксирал

Efaproxiral Sodium

Other names: Efaproxiral sódico; Éfaproxiral Sodique; Natrii Efaproxiralum.

Натрий Эфапроксирал

Clinical profile: Efaproxiral is an allosteric modifier of haemoglobin that enhances the diffusion of oxygen to hypoxic tumour tissue, making it more sensitive to radiotherapy. It has been investigated in the treatment of brain metastases from solid tumours.

WADA Status: Banned in and out of competition

WADA Class: Enhancement of Oxygen Transfer: Artificial Enhancers

Includes products that may be used to artificially enhance the uptake, transport, or delivery of oxygen.

Endrisone

Other names: Endrisona; Endrisonum; Endrysone.

Эндризон

Clinical profile: Endrisone is a corticosteroid that has been used in eye drops and eye ointments.

WADA Status: Banned in competition

WADA Class: Glucocorticosteroids

All glucocorticosteroids are prohibited when administered orally, rectally, intravenously or intramuscularly. Their use requires a Therapeutic Use Exemption approval. Other routes of administration (intraarticular / periarticular / peritendinous / epidural / intradermal injections and inhalation) require an Abbreviated Therapeutic Use Exemption except as noted below.

Topical preparations when used for dermatological (including iontophoresis / phonophoresis), auricular, nasal, ophthalmic, buccal, gingival and perianal disorders are not prohibited and do not require any form of Therapeutic Use Exemption.

WADA Class: Specified Substances

Also listed as a specified substance.

"The prohibited List may identify specified substances which are particularly susceptible to unintentional anti-doping rule violations because of their general availability in medicinal products or which are less likely to be successfully abused as doping agents."

A doping violation involving such substances may result in a reduced sanction provided that the "*...Athlete can establish that the Use of such a specfied substance was not intended to enhance sport performance...*"

Epanolol

Other names: Epanalol; Épanolol; Epanololi; Epanololum; ICI-141292.

Эпанолол

Clinical profile: Epanolol is reported to be a cardioselective beta blocker.

WADA Status: Banned in and out of competition as specified below

WADA Class: Beta-Blockers

Unless otherwise specified, beta-blockers are prohibited *In-Competition* only in the following sports.

- Aeronautics (FAI)
- Archery (FITA, IPC) (also prohibited *Out-of-Competition*)
- Automobile (FIA)
- Billiards (WCBS)
- Bobsleigh (FIBT)
- Boules (CMSB, IPC bowls)
- Bridge (FMB)
- Curling (WCF)
- Gymnastics (FIG)
- Motorcycling (FIM)
- Modern Pentathlon (UIPM) for disciplines involving shooting
- Nine-pin bowling (FIQ)
- Powerboating (UIM)
- Sailing (ISAF) for match race helms only
- Shooting (ISSF, IPC) (also prohibited *Out-of-Competition*)
- Skiing/Snowboarding (FIS) in ski jumping, freestyle aerials/halfpipe and snowboard halfpipe/big air
- Wrestling (FILA)

WADA Class: Specified Substances

Also listed as a specified substance.

"The prohibited List may identify specified substances which are particularly susceptible to unintentional anti-doping rule violations because of their general availability in medicinal products or which are less likely to be successfully abused as doping agents."

A doping violation involving such substances may result in a reduced sanction provided that the "*...Athlete can establish that the Use of such a specfied substance was not intended to enhance sport performance...*"

Ephedra

Other names: Efedra; Ma-huang.

Хвойник; Эфедра хвощевая (Ephedra equisetina)

Clinical profile: The sympathomimetic action of ephedra (the dried young branches of *Ephedra* species) is due to the presence of ephedrine and pseudoephedrine. It has been used chiefly as a source of these alkaloids. The FDA has banned the sale of ephedra-containing dietary supplements in the USA.

WADA Status: Banned in competition

WADA Class: Stimulants

Ephedrine is prohibited when its concentration in urine is greater than 10 micrograms per milliliter.

WADA Class: Specified Substances

Also listed as a specified substance.

"The prohibited List may identify specified substances which are particularly susceptible to unintentional anti-doping rule violations because of their general availability in medicinal products or which are less likely to be successfully abused as doping agents."

A doping violation involving such substances may result in a reduced sanction provided that the "...*Athlete can establish that the Use of such a specfied substance was not intended to enhance sport performance...*"

Preparations
Multi-ingredient: ***Ger.:*** Cefadrin.

E

Ephedrine

Other names: Efedriini; Efedrin; Efedrina; Efedrinas; Ephedrina; Éphédrine; (−)-Ephedrine; Ephedrinum.

Эфедрин

Ephedrine Hydrochloride

Other names: Efedriinihydrokloridi; Efedrin Hidroklorür; Efedrin hydrochlorid; Efedrina, hidrocloruro de; Efedrin-hidroklorid; Efedrinhydroklorid; Efedrino hidrochloridas; Efedryny chlorowodorek; Ephedrinae Hydrochloridum; Éphédrine, chlorhydrate d'; Ephedrine Chloride; Ephedrini hydrochloridum; Ephedrinium Chloratum; *l*-Ephedrinum Hydrochloricum.

Эфедрина Гидрохлорид

Ephedrine Sulfate

Other names: Efedrina, sulfato de; Ephedrine Sulphate.

Эфедрина Сульфат

Clinical profile: Ephedrine is both a direct- and indirect-acting sympathomimetic; additionally it causes stimulation of the CNS. Its main clinical use is as a nasal decongestant when it may be used alone or in combination preparations. It has also been used as a bronchodilator and in motion sickness. Other uses have included diabetic neuropathy, nocturnal enuresis, and reversal of hypotension induced by spinal or epidural anaesthesia.

Racephedrine Hydrochloride

Other names: Efedriinihydrokloridi, raseeminen; Efedrinhydroklorid, racemisk; Efedrino (raceminio) hidrochloridas; Éphédrine (chlorhydrate d') racémique; *dl*-Ephedrine Hydrochloride; Ephedrini racemici hydrochloridum; *dl*-Ephedrinium Chloride; Hidrocloruro de racefedrina; Racém efedrin-hidroklorid; Racemic Ephedrine Hydrochloride; Racéphédrine, Chlorhydrate de; Racephedrini Hydrochloridum.

Рацефедрина Гидрохлорид

Clinical profile: Racephedrine is a racemic mixture of which ephedrine is the laevo-isomer.

WADA Status: Banned in competition

WADA Class: Stimulants

Ephedrine is prohibited when its concentration in urine is greater than 10 micrograms per milliliter.

WADA Class: Specified Substances

Also listed as a specified substance.

"The prohibited List may identify specified substances which are particularly susceptible to unintentional anti-doping rule violations because of their general availability in medicinal products or which are less likely to be successfully abused as doping agents."

A doping violation involving such substances may result in a reduced sanction provided that the "*...Athlete can establish that the Use of such a specfied substance was not intended to enhance sport performance...*"

Preparations

Single ingredient: ***Arg.:*** Muchan; ***Belg.:*** Ephedronguent; ***Chile:*** Efedrosan; ***Gr.:*** Neo Rhinovit; Rhinolex; ***Hung.:*** Epherit; ***Mex.:*** Tendrin; ***Pol.:*** Efrinol; ***Turk.:*** Rinitalmit; ***UK:*** CAM; ***USA:*** Kondon's Nasal; ***Venez.:*** Colirio Iris.

Multi-ingredient: ***Arg.:*** Amiorel Compuesto; Aqua Lent Colirio; Bisolvon Compositum NF; Clarisoft; Coliria; Exudrol con Dexametasona; Fadatos; Irix; Kalopsis; No-Tos Adultos; Quemicetina Nasal Compuesta; Sintebron; Usualix; Vislus; ***Austria:*** Asthma 23 D; Asthma Efeum; Asthma-Hilfe; Coldargan; Famel cum Ephedrin; Helopyrin; Novipec; Pilka Forte; Piniment; Spirbon; Wick Erkaltungs-Saft fur die Nacht; ***Belg.:*** Argyrophedrine; Endrine Doux; Endrine; ***Braz.:*** Alergotox Efedrina; Asmatiron; Beclase; Canfomenol; Coquevit; Franol; Inhalante Yatropan; Marax; Marsonil; Novotussan; Rinisone; Teutoss; Tonaton; Yatropan; ***Chile:*** Broncodeina; Pulmagol; ***Cz.:*** Ipecarin; Kodynal; Mukoseptonex E; Solutan; Spasmoveralgin Neo; Tussilen; ***Fin.:*** Codesan Comp; Sir. Ephedrin; ***Fr.:*** Osmotol; Rhinamide; Rhino-Sulfuryl; ***Ger.:*** Wick Medinait; ***Gr.:*** Sival-B; ***Hong Kong:*** Antiflu-N-Forte; Bromhexine Compound; Coci-Fedra-C; DEC; Decofam Cough; Dhasedyl; Ephedyl; Fendyl; Marsedyl; Marsedyl; Methor-Co; Methorsedyl; Metoplex; PEC; Phensedyn; Uni-Ramine CE; ***Hung.:*** Coderetta N; Coderit N; Coldargan; Hemorid; Hemorid; ***India:*** Alergin; Asmapax; Cadiphylate; Cofton SF; Dericip Plus; Endrine Mild; Endrine; Gocold; Marax; ***Indon.:*** Asmadex; Asmano; Asmasolon; Asthma Soho; Bronchitin; Cold Cap; Ersylan; Kafsir; Koffex for Children; Mixadin; Neo Napacin; Noscapax; Oskadryl; Phenadex; Poncolin D; Poncolin; Prinasma; Theochodil; Thymcal; ***Israel:*** Pertussol; Proaf; Shiulon; Tussophedrine New Formula; Tussosedan; ***Ital.:*** Argotone; Deltarinolo; Fienamina; Paidorinovit; Pasta Arsenicale; Rinovit; ***Malaysia:*** Asthma; Dexcophan Cough; ***Mex.:*** Alfan; Coderit; Jarabe de Capulin; Paliatil; Piralgina; ***Pol.:*** Rubital Compositum; Syrop Prawoslazowy Zlozony; Tussipect; Tussipect; ***Port.:*** Anti-Asmatico; Ipesandrine; Naso-Prieulina; Prelus; ***Rus.:*** Bronchitussin (Бронхитусен); Bronchocin (Бронхоцин); Broncholytin (Бронхолитин); Solutan (Солутан); ***S.Afr.:*** Brunacod; Codef; Colcleer; Corbar; Coughcod; Dequa-Coff; Docsed; Flusin; Genasma; Grippon; Lenazine Forte; Linctodyl; Natrophylline Compound; Oto-Phen Forte; Phensedyl; Repasma; Vicks Medinite; ***Singapore:*** Beacons Cough; Chlorsedyl; Cophadyl-E; Coughlax; Decofam Cough; Dhasedyl DM; Dhasedyl; Promedyl; Sedilix; ***Spain:*** Bisolvon Compositum; Brota Rectal Balsamico; Cilinafosal Dihidroestreptomicina; Cilinafosal Hidrocortisona; Cilinafosal Neomicina; Cilinafosal; Fludren; Hemoal; Kanafosal Predni; Kanafosal; Medinait; Pazbronquial; Tabletas Quimpe; Voxfor; ***Swed.:*** Lepheton; Lergigan comp; Mollipect; ***Switz.:*** Demo Elixir pectoral N; Euproctol N; Euproctol; Haemolan; Kemeol; Pectocalmine; Pertussex Compositum; Sano Tuss; Vicks Medinait; ***Turk.:*** Antibeksin; Artu; Brodil; Broksin; Defeks; Eupnase; Fenokodin; Hemoralgine; Latusin; Neo Sedeks; Neofedrin; Pedrin; Pektodin; Penikin; Radycodin; Sulfarhin; ***UAE:*** Codaphed Plus; Codaphed; ***UK:*** Do-Do ChestEze; Dolvan; Haymine; Noradran; Paranorm; ***USA:*** Broncholate; Bronkaid Dual Action; Bronkotuss Expectorant; Dynafed Asthma Relief; Hydrophed; KIE; Marax; Pazo; Primatene; Quadrinal; Quelidrine; Rentamine Pediatric; Rynatuss; Tedrigen; Theodrine; Theomax DF; Tri-Tannate Plus Pediatric; Tuss-Tan; ***Venez.:*** Amodion; Pi-Fedrin; Pidrol; Tabonuco.

Epitiostanol

Other names: Épitiostanol; Epitiostanolum; 10275-S.

Эпитиостанол

Clinical profile: Epitiostanol is reported to have anabolic activity and has been used in various breast disorders including neoplasms of the breast.

WADA Status: Banned in and out of competition

WADA Class: Anabolic; Androgenic Steroids (exogenous)

Includes exogenous anabolic androgenic steroids or other substances with a similar chemical structure or similar biological effect(s).

Epitizide

Other names: Epithiazide; Epitizida; Épitizide; Epitizidum; Eptizida; NSC-108164; P-2105.

Эпитизид

Clinical profile: Epitizide is a thiazide diuretic used in the treatment of hypertension and oedema.

WADA Status: Banned in and out of competition

WADA Class: Diuretics and Other Masking Agents

Includes diuretics or substances with a similar chemical structure or similar biological effect(s).

Preparations

Multi-ingredient: ***Belg.:*** Dyta-Urese; ***Neth.:*** Dyta-Urese.

E

Eplerenone

Other names: Eplerenona; Éplérénone; Eplerenonum; SC-66110.

Эплеренон

Clinical profile: Eplerenone is a potassium-sparing diuretic and an aldosterone antagonist that is used in the treatment of hypertension, and in the management of heart failure after myocardial infarction.

WADA Status: Banned in and out of competition

WADA Class: Diuretics and Other Masking Agents

Includes diuretics or substances with a similar chemical structure or similar biological effect(s).

Preparations

Single ingredient: ***Austral.:*** Inspra; ***Austria:*** Inspra; ***Chile:*** Inspra; ***Denm.:*** Inspra; ***Fin.:*** Inspra; ***Fr.:*** Inspra; ***Gr.:*** Inspra; ***Hong Kong:*** Inspra; ***Hung.:*** Inspra; ***Irl.:*** Inspra; ***Mex.:*** Inspra; ***Neth.:*** Inspra; ***Norw.:*** Inspra; ***Spain:*** Elecor; Inspra; ***Swed.:*** Inspra; ***UK:*** Inspra; ***USA:*** Inspra.

Epoetins

Other names: Epoetinas.

Epoetin Alfa

Other names: EPO; Epoetina alfa; Époétine Alfa; Epoetinum Alfa.

Эпоэтин Альфа

Epoetin Beta

Other names: BM-06.019; EPOCH; Epoetina beta; Époétine Bêta; Epoetinum Beta.

Эпоэтин Бета

Epoetin Delta

Other names: Epoetina delta; Époétine Delta; Epoetinum Delta; GA-EPO; HMR-4396.

Эпоетин Дельта

Epoetin Gamma

Other names: BI-71.052; Epoetina gamma; Époétine Gamma; Epoetinum Gamma.

Эпоэтин Гамма

Epoetin Omega

Other names: Epoetina omega; Époétine Oméga; Epoetinum Omega.

Эпоэтин Омега

Clinical profile: Erythropoietin is the main regulator of erythropoiesis in the body. Recombinant human erythropoietin is available as epoetin alfa and epoetin beta, which are used to correct anaemia in chronic renal failure, in patients with non-myeloid malignant disease on chemotherapy, in HIV-positive patients on zidovudine therapy, and in premature neonates. Epoetins may also be used to increase the yield of blood collected for autologous blood transfusion and to reduce the need for allogeneic transfusion.

E

WADA Status: Banned in and out of competition

WADA Class: Hormones and Related Substances: Erythropoietin

Includes erythropoietin or a substance with a similar chemical structure or similar biological effect(s), or one of their releasing factors.

Preparations

Single ingredient: ***Arg.:*** Epogen; Eprex; Eritrogen; Hemax; Hypercrit; Pronivel; Recormon; ***Austral.:*** Eprex; ***Austria:*** Culat; Erypo; NeoRecormon; Recormon; ***Belg.:*** Eprex; NeoRecormon; ***Braz.:*** Eprex; Eritina; Eritromax; Hemax-Eritron; Recormon; Tinax; ***Canad.:*** Eprex; ***Chile:*** Epokine; Eprex; Hypercrit; Recormon; ***Cz.:*** Epomax; Eprex; NeoRecormon; Recormon; ***Denm.:*** Eprex; NeoRecormon; ***Fin.:*** Eprex; NeoRecormon; ***Fr.:*** Eprex; NeoRecormon; ***Ger.:*** Eprex; Erypo; NeoRecormon; ***Gr.:*** Eprex; NeoRecormon; ***Hong Kong:*** Eprex; Recormon; ***Hung.:*** Eprex; NeoRecormon; ***India:*** Wepox; ***Indon.:*** Epotrex-NP; Eprex; Hemapo; Recormon; ***Irl.:*** Eprex; NeoRecormon; ***Israel:*** Eprex; Recormon; ***Ital.:*** Eprex; NeoRecormon; ***Jpn:*** Epogin; Espo; ***Malaysia:*** Eprex; ***Mex.:*** Bioyetin; Epomax; Eprex; Erlan; Exetin-A; Hypercrit; Negortire; Recormon; Yepotin; ***Neth.:*** Dynepo; Eprex; NeoRecormon; ***Norw.:*** Eprex; NeoRecormon; ***NZ:*** Eprex; Recormon; ***Philipp.:*** Epokine; Eposino; Eprex; Recormon; Renogen; ***Pol.:*** Eprex; NeoRecormon; ***Port.:*** NeoRecormon; Recormon; ***Rus.:*** Epocrin (Эпокрин); Eprex (Эпрекс); Erythrostim (Эритростим); Recormon (Рекормон); ***S.Afr.:*** Eprex; Recormon; Repotin; ***Singapore:*** Eprex; Recormon; ***Spain:*** Epopen; Eprex; NeoRecormon; ***Swed.:*** Eprex; NeoRecormon; ***Switz.:*** Eprex; Recormon; ***Thai.:*** Epokine; Eprex; Espogen; Hemax; Recormon; ***Turk.:*** Eprex; NeoRecormon; ***UAE:*** Epotin; ***UK:*** Binocrit; Dynepo; Eprex; NeoRecormon; ***USA:*** Epogen; Procrit; ***Venez.:*** Eprex; Hypercrit; Recormon.

Esatenolol

Other names: (–)-Atenolol; *S*-Atenolol; Ésaténolol; Esatenololum.

Эзатенолол

Clinical profile: Esatenolol, the *S*(–)-isomer of the beta blocker atenolol, has been used similarly to atenolol in the treatment of cardiovascular disorders.

WADA Status: Banned in and out of competition as specified below

WADA Class: Beta-Blockers

Unless otherwise specified, beta-blockers are prohibited *In-Competition* only in the following sports.

- Aeronautics (FAI)
- Archery (FITA, IPC) (also prohibited *Out-of-Competition*)

- Automobile (FIA)
- Billiards (WCBS)
- Bobsleigh (FIBT)
- Boules (CMSB, IPC bowls)
- Bridge (FMB)
- Curling (WCF)
- Gymnastics (FIG)
- Motorcycling (FIM)
- Modern Pentathlon (UIPM) for disciplines involving shooting
- Nine-pin bowling (FIQ)
- Powerboating (UIM)
- Sailing (ISAF) for match race helms only
- Shooting (ISSF, IPC) (also prohibited *Out-of-Competition*)
- Skiing/Snowboarding (FIS) in ski jumping, freestyle aerials/halfpipe and snowboard halfpipe/big air
- Wrestling (FILA)

WADA Class: Specified Substances

Also listed as a specified substance.

"*The prohibited List may identify specified substances which are particularly susceptible to unintentional anti-doping rule violations because of their general availability in medicinal products or which are less likely to be successfully abused as doping agents.*"

A doping violation involving such substances may result in a reduced sanction provided that the "*...Athlete can establish that the Use of such a specfied substance was not intended to enhance sport performance...*"

E

Esmolol Hydrochloride

Other names: ASL-8052; Esmolol, Chlorhydrate d'; Esmolol Hidroklorür; Esmololi Hydrochloridum; Hidrocloruro de esmolol.

Эсмолола Гидрохлорид

Clinical profile: Esmolol is a cardioselective short-acting beta blocker used in the management of supraventricular arrhythmias and for the control of hypertension and tachycardia during the perioperative period.

WADA Status: Banned in and out of competition as specified below

WADA Class: Beta-Blockers

Unless otherwise specified, beta-blockers are prohibited *In-Competition* only in the following sports.

- Aeronautics (FAI)
- Archery (FITA, IPC) (also prohibited *Out-of-Competition*)
- Automobile (FIA)
- Billiards (WCBS)
- Bobsleigh (FIBT)
- Boules (CMSB, IPC bowls)
- Bridge (FMB)
- Curling (WCF)
- Gymnastics (FIG)
- Motorcycling (FIM)
- Modern Pentathlon (UIPM) for disciplines involving shooting
- Nine-pin bowling (FIQ)
- Powerboating (UIM)
- Sailing (ISAF) for match race helms only
- Shooting (ISSF, IPC) (also prohibited *Out-of-Competition*)
- Skiing/Snowboarding (FIS) in ski jumping, freestyle aerials/halfpipe and snowboard halfpipe/big air
- Wrestling (FILA)

WADA Class: Specified Substances

Also listed as a specified substance.

"The prohibited List may identify specified substances which are particularly susceptible to unintentional anti-doping rule violations because of their general availability in medicinal products or which are less likely to be successfully abused as doping agents."

A doping violation involving such substances may result in a reduced sanction provided that the "*...Athlete can establish that the Use of such a specfied substance was not intended to enhance sport performance...*"

Preparations

Single ingredient: ***Arg.:*** Dublon; ***Austral.:*** Brevibloc; ***Austria:*** Brevibloc; ***Belg.:*** Brevibloc; ***Braz.:*** Brevibloc; ***Canad.:*** Brevibloc; ***Cz.:*** Brevibloc; ***Denm.:*** Brevibloc; ***Fin.:*** Brevibloc; ***Ger.:*** Brevibloc; ***Gr.:*** Brevibloc; ***Hung.:*** Brevibloc; ***India:*** Miniblock; ***Irl.:*** Brevibloc; ***Ital.:*** Brevibloc; ***Neth.:*** Brevibloc; ***NZ:*** Brevibloc; ***S.Afr.:*** Brevibloc; ***Spain:*** Brevibloc; ***Swed.:*** Brevibloc; ***Switz.:*** Brevibloc; ***Turk.:*** Brevibloc; ***UK:*** Brevibloc; ***USA:*** Brevibloc.

Etacrynic Acid

Other names: Acide étacrynique; Ácido etacrínico; Acidum etacrynicum; Etacrynsäure; Etakrino rūgštis; Etakrinsav; Etakrynsyra; Etakryynihappo; Ethacrynic Acid; Kwas etakrynowy; Kyselina etakrynová; MK-595; NSC-85791.

Этакриновая Кислота

Sodium Etacrynate

Other names: Etacrinato sódico; Étacrynate de Sodium; Etacrynate Sodium; Ethacrynate Sodium; Natrii Etacrynas; Sodium Ethacrynate.

Натрий Этакринат

Clinical profile: Etacrynic acid is a loop diuretic. The acid and its sodium salt are used in the treatment of oedema associated with heart failure and with renal and hepatic disorders.

WADA Status: Banned in and out of competition

WADA Class: Diuretics and Other Masking Agents

Includes diuretics or substances with a similar chemical structure or similar biological effect(s).

Preparations

Single ingredient: ***Austral.:*** Edecrin; ***Austria:*** Edecrin; ***Canad.:*** Edecrin; ***Cz.:*** Uregyt; ***Hung.:*** Uregyt; ***Ital.:*** Reomax; ***Rus.:*** Uregyt (Урегит); ***USA:*** Edecrin.

Etafedrine Hydrochloride

Other names: Étafédrine, Chlorhydrate d'; Etafedrini Hydrochloridum; Ethylephedrine Hydrochloride; Hidrocloruro de etafedrina.

Этафедрина Гидрохлорид

Clinical profile: Etafedrine hydrochloride is a sympathomimetic used in combination preparations for the relief of cough and associated respiratory-tract disorders.

WADA Status: Banned in competition

WADA Class: Stimulants

Includes stimulants or substances with a similar chemical structure or similar biological effect(s).

WADA Class: Specified Substances

Also listed as a specified substance.

"The prohibited List may identify specified substances which are particularly susceptible to

unintentional anti-doping rule violations because of their general availability in medicinal products or which are less likely to be successfully abused as doping agents."

A doping violation involving such substances may result in a reduced sanction provided that the "*...Athlete can establish that the Use of such a specfied substance was not intended to enhance sport performance...*"

Preparations
Multi-ingredient: ***Braz.:*** Broncolex; EMS Expectorante; Revenil Dospan; Revenil Expectorante; Revenil; ***Canad.:*** Dalmacol; ratio-Calmydone; ***Indon.:*** Decolsin; ***S.Afr.:*** Nethaprin Dospan; Nethaprin Expectorant; ***Thai.:*** Brondil.

Etamivan

Other names: Etamivaani; Étamivan; Etamiván; Etamivanum; Ethamivan; NSC-406087; Vanillic Acid Diethylamide; Vanillic Diethylamide.

Этамиван

Clinical profile: Etamivan was formerly used as a respiratory stimulant. It is available in compound preparations for cerebrovascular and circulatory disorders and hypotension, but such use is not recommended.

WADA Status: Banned in competition

WADA Class: Stimulants

Includes etamivan and any optical isomers.

WADA Class: Specified Substances

Also listed as a specified substance.

"The prohibited List may identify specified substances which are particularly susceptible to unintentional anti-doping rule violations because of their general availability in medicinal products or which are less likely to be successfully abused as doping agents."

A doping violation involving such substances may result in a reduced sanction provided that the "*...Athlete can establish that the Use of such a specfied substance was not intended to enhance sport performance...*"

Preparations
Multi-ingredient: ***Arg.:*** Dosulfin Bronquial; ***Austria:*** Cinnarplus; Instenon; ***Hong Kong:*** Instenon; ***Rus.:*** Instenon (Инстенон).

Etherified Starches

Other names: Almidón, éteres de; HES; Hydroxyethyl Starch; Hydroxyéthylamidon; Hydroxyethylamylum.

Clinical profile: Etherified starches are used for short-term plasma expansion. They increase the erythrocyte sedimentation rate when added to whole blood and are used in leucapheresis procedures to increase the yield of granulocytes.

WADA Status: Banned in and out of competition

WADA Class: Diuretics and Other Masking Agents

Masking agents including alpha-reductase inhibitors or plasma expanders or substances with similar biological effect(s).

Preparations
Single ingredient: ***Arg.:*** Hessico; Infukoll HES; Venofundin; Voluven; ***Austria:*** Elohast; Expafusin; Expahes; HAES-steril; Hyperhes; Isohes; Osmohes; Plasmasteril; Varihes; Voluven; ***Canad.:*** Hextend; Pentaspan; ***Chile:*** HAES-steril; Hemohes; Voluven; ***Cz.:*** Elohast; HAES-steril; Hemohes; ***Denm.:*** HAES-steril; HyperHAES; Venofundin; Voluven; ***Fin.:*** HAES-steril; Hemohes; HyperHAES; Venofundin; Voluven; ***Fr.:*** Hesteril; Hyperhes; Voluven; ***Ger.:*** Expafusin; Haemofusin; HAES-Rheopond; HAES-steril; Hemohes; HyperHAES; Infukoll HES; Rheohes; Serag-HAES;

Venofundin; Vitafusal; VitaHES; Voluven; ***Gr.:*** HAES-steril; Hemohes; Venofundin; Voluven; ***Hong Kong:*** Voluven; ***Hung.:*** HAES-steril; Hemohes; HyperHAES; Tetraspan; Voluven; ***Indon.:*** Expafusin; Fima HES; HAES-Steril; Hemohes; Voluven; WIDAHES; ***Israel:*** HAES-sterile; ***Ital.:*** Amidolite; HAES-steril; HyperHAES; Voluven; ***Jpn:*** Hespander; ***Malaysia:*** HAES-steril; ***Mex.:*** HAES-steril; Hestar; Voluven; ***Neth.:*** Elohaes; HAES-steril; Hemohes; HyperHAES; Venofundin; Voluven; ***Norw.:*** HyperHAES; Voluven; ***NZ:*** Hemohes; ***Philipp.:*** HAES-steril; Voluven; ***Pol.:*** HAES-steril; Hemohes; Voluven; ***Port.:*** Hemohes; ***Rus.:*** HAES-steril (ХАЕС-стерил); HyperHAES (ГиперХАЕС); Infukoll HES (Инфукол ГЭК); Refortan (Рефортан); Stabisol (Стабизол); Voluven (Волювен); ***S.Afr.:*** HAES-steril; Voluven; ***Singapore:*** HAES-steril; ***Spain:*** Elohes; HAES Esteril; Hes Grifols; Hesteril; Voluven; ***Swed.:*** HAES-steril; HyperHAES; Venofundin; Voluven; ***Switz.:*** HAES-steril; Hemohes; HyperHAES; Venofundin; Voluven; ***Thai.:*** HAES-steril; Hemohes; Voluven; ***Turk.:*** Biohes; Bioplazma; Expahes; HAES-steril; Hemohes; Isohes; Plasmasteril; Varihes; Voluven; ***UK:*** HAES-steril; Hemohes; HyperHAES; Infukoll; Venofundin; Voluven; ***USA:*** Hespan; Pentaspan.

Multi-ingredient: ***Norw.:*** Hemohes; ***Spain:*** Hemohes.

Ethylestrenol

Other names: Éthylestrénol; Ethylestrenolum; Ethyloestrenol; Etilestrenol; Etylestrenol; Etyyliestrenoli.

Этилэстренол

Clinical profile: Ethylestrenol has anabolic properties with little androgenic or progestational activity. It has been given for the promotion of growth in boys with short stature or delayed bone growth. It is used in veterinary medicine.

WADA Status: Banned in and out of competition

WADA Class: Anabolic; Androgenic Steroids (exogenous)

Includes exogenous anabolic androgenic steroids or other substances with a similar chemical structure or similar biological effect(s).

Ethylnoradrenaline Hydrochloride

Other names: Ethylnorepinephrine Hydrochloride.

Clinical profile: Ethylnoradrenaline is a sympathomimetic with predominantly beta-adrenergic activity that has been used as a bronchodilator.

WADA Status: Banned in competition

WADA Class: Stimulants

Includes stimulants or substances with a similar chemical structure or similar biological effect(s).

WADA Class: Specified Substances

Also listed as a specified substance.

"The prohibited List may identify specified substances which are particularly susceptible to unintentional anti-doping rule violations because of their general availability in medicinal products or which are less likely to be successfully abused as doping agents."

A doping violation involving such substances may result in a reduced sanction pro

vided that the "*...Athlete can establish that the Use of such a specfied substance was not intended to enhance sport performance...*"

Etifelmine

Other names: Etifelmina; Étifelmine; Etifelminum.

Этифелмин

Etifelmine Hydrochloride

Other names: Étifelmine, Chlorhydrate d'; Etifelmini Hydrochloridum; Hidrocloruro de etifelmina.

Этифелмина Гидрохлорид

Clinical profile: Etifelmine is a sympathomimetic agent that has been used in the treatment of hypotensive states.

WADA Status: Banned in competition

WADA Class: Stimulants

Includes stimulants or substances with a similar chemical structure or similar biological effect(s).

WADA Class: Specified Substances

Also listed as a specified substance.

"*The prohibited List may identify specified substances which are particularly susceptible to unintentional anti-doping rule violations because of their general availability in medicinal products or which are less likely to be successfully abused as doping agents.*"

A doping violation involving such substances may result in a reduced sanction provided that the "*...Athlete can establish that the Use of such a specfied substance was not intended to enhance sport performance...*"

Etilamfetamine Hydrochloride

Other names: Ethylamphetamine Hydrochloride; Étilamfétamine, Chlorhydrate d'; Etilamfetamini Hydrochloridum; Hidrocloruro de etilanfetamina.

Этиламфетамина Гидрохлорид

Clinical profile: Etilamfetamine hydrochloride has been used as an anorectic in the treatment of obesity.

WADA Status: Banned in competition

WADA Class: Stimulants

Includes etilamfetamine and any optical isomers.

Etilefrine Hydrochloride

Other names: Ethyladrianol Hydrochloride; Ethylnorphenylephrine Hydrochloride; Etilefriinihydrokloridi; Étiléfrine, chlorhydrate d'; Etilefrin-hidroklorid; Etilefrinhydrochlorid; Etilefrinhydroklorid; Etilefrini hydrochloridum; Etilefrino hidrochloridas;

Hidrocloruro de etilefrina; M-I-36.

Этилэфрина Гидрохлорид

Clinical profile: Etilefrine is a direct-acting sympathomimetic used as the hydrochloride for the treatment of hypotensive states. Etilefrine has been used as the polistirex in the management of rhinitis.

WADA Status: Banned in competition

WADA Class: Stimulants

Includes etilefrine and any optical isomers.

Preparations
Single ingredient: ***Arg.:*** Effortil; ***Austria:*** Circupon; Effortil; ***Belg.:*** Effortil; ***Braz.:*** Efortil; ***Chile:*** Effortil; ***Fin.:*** Effortil; ***Fr.:*** Effortil; ***Ger.:*** Bioflutin; Cardanat; Etil; Pholdyston; Thomasin; ***Gr.:*** Effortil; ***Ital.:*** Effortil; ***Jpn:*** Effortil; ***Mex.:*** Effortil; ***Pol.:*** Effortil; ***Port.:*** Effortil; ***S.Afr.:*** Effortil; ***Spain:*** Efortil; ***Swed.:*** Effortil; ***Switz.:*** Effortil; ***Thai.:*** Effortil; Hyprosia; ***Venez.:*** Effontil.
Multi-ingredient: ***Austria:*** Agilan; Amphodyn; Effortil comp; Hypodyn; Influbene; ***Ger.:*** Dihydergot plus; Effortil plus; Ergolefrin; ***Switz.:*** Dihydergot plus; Effortil plus.

Etozolin

Other names: Etozolina; Étozoline; Etozolinum; Gö-687; W-2900A.

Этозолин

Clinical profile: Etozolin is a loop diuretic used in the treatment of oedema and hypertension.

WADA Status: Banned in and out of competition

WADA Class: Diuretics and Other Masking Agents

Includes diuretics or substances with a similar chemical structure or similar biological effect(s).

Exemestane

Other names: Eksemestaani; Eksemestan; Exemestan; Exémestane; Exemestano; Exemestanum; FCE-24304.

Эксеместан

Clinical profile: Exemestane is an aromatase inhibitor that is used for the treatment of breast cancer.

WADA Status: Banned in and out of competition

WADA Class: Hormone Antagonists and Modulators

Includes aromatase inhibitors.

Preparations
Single ingredient: ***Arg.:*** Aromasin; ***Austral.:*** Aromasin; ***Austria:*** Aromasin; ***Belg.:*** Aromasin; ***Braz.:*** Aromasin; ***Canad.:*** Aromasin; ***Chile:*** Aromasin; ***Cz.:*** Aromasin; ***Denm.:*** Aromasin; ***Fin.:*** Aromasin; ***Fr.:*** Aromasine; ***Ger.:*** Aromasin; ***Gr.:*** Aromasin; ***Hong Kong:*** Aromasin; ***Hung.:*** Aromasin; ***Indon.:*** Aromasin; ***Irl.:*** Aromasin; ***Israel:*** Aromasin; ***Ital.:*** Aromasin; ***Malaysia:*** Aromasin; ***Neth.:*** Aromasin; ***Norw.:*** Aromasin; ***NZ:*** Aromasin; ***Philipp.:*** Aromasin; ***Pol.:*** Aromasin; ***Port.:*** Aromasin; ***Rus.:*** Aromasin (Аромазин); ***S.Afr.:*** Aromasin; ***Singapore:*** Aromasin; ***Spain:*** Aromasil; ***Swed.:*** Aromasin; ***Switz.:*** Aromasin; ***Thai.:*** Aromasin; ***Turk.:*** Aromasin; ***UK:*** Aromasin; ***USA:*** Aromasin; ***Venez.:*** Aromasin.

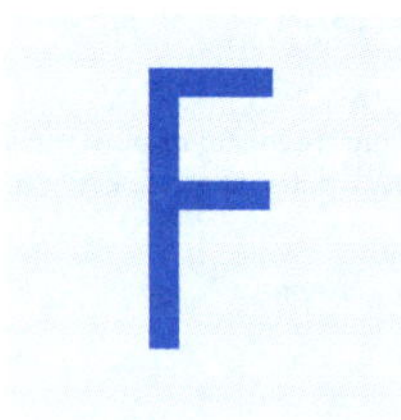

Fadrozole Hydrochloride

Other names: CGS-16949 (fadrozole); CGS-16949A; Fadrozole, Chlorhydrate de; Fadrozoli Hydrochloridum; Hidrocloruro de fadrozol.

Фадрозола Гидрохлорид

Clinical profile: Fadrozole hydrochloride is a selective nonsteroidal aromatase inhibitor used for the treatment of breast cancer.

WADA Status: Banned in and out of competition

WADA Class: Hormone Antagonists and Modulators
Includes aromatase inhibitors.

Famprofazone

Other names: Famprofazona; Famprofazonum.

Фампрофазон

Clinical profile: Famprofazone has analgesic and antipyretic properties and has been given by mouth, usually with other analgesics.

WADA Status: Banned in competition

WADA Class: Stimulants
Includes famprofazone and any optical isomers.

WADA Class: Specified Substances
Also listed as a specified substance.
"The prohibited List may identify specified substances which are particularly susceptible to unintentional anti-doping rule violations because of their general availability in medicinal products or which are less likely to be successfully abused as doping agents."
A doping violation involving such substances may result in a reduced sanction pro-

vided that the "*...Athlete can establish that the Use of such a specfied substance was not intended to enhance sport performance...*"

Fenbutrazate Hydrochloride

Other names: Fenbutrazate, Chlorhydrate de; Fenbutrazati Hydrochloridum; Hidrocloruro de fenbutrazato; Phenbutrazate Hydrochloride; R-381.

Фенбутразата Гидрохлорид

Clinical profile: Fenbutrazate hydrochloride has been used as an anorectic.

WADA Status: Banned in competition

WADA Class: Stimulants

Includes fenbutrazate and any optical isomers.

Fencamfamin Hydrochloride

Other names: Fencamfamine, Chlorhydrate de; Fencamfamini Hydrochloridum; H-610; Hidrocloruro de fencanfamina.

Фенкамфамина Гидрохлорид

Clinical profile: Fencamfamin hydrochloride has been used as a central stimulant.

WADA Status: Banned in competition

WADA Class: Stimulants

Includes fencamfamin and any optical isomers.

Preparations
Multi-ingredient: ***S.Afr.:*** Reactivan.

F

Fenetylline Hydrochloride

Other names: Amfetyline Hydrochloride; 7-Ethyltheophylline Amphetamine Hydrochloride; Fenethylline Hydrochloride; Fénétylline, Chlorhydrate de; Fenetyllini Hydrochloridum; H-814; Hidrocloruro de fenetilina; R-720-11.

Фенетиллина Гидрохлорид

Clinical profile: Fenetylline is a theophylline derivative of amfetamine that has been used in the treatment of hyperactivity disorders.

WADA Status: Banned in competition

WADA Class: Stimulants

Includes fenetylline and any optical isomers.

Preparations
Single ingredient: ***Belg.:*** Captagon

Fenfluramine Hydrochloride

Other names: AHR-3002; Fenfluramine, Chlorhydrate de; Fenfluramini Hydrochloridum; Hidrocloruro de fenfluramina; S-768.

Фенфлюрамина Гидрохлорид

Clinical profile: Fenfluramine hydrochloride is an indirect-acting sympathomimetic that also has serotonergic activity. It was formerly used as an anorectic in the treatment of obesity but was withdrawn worldwide following reports of valvular heart defects.

WADA Status: Banned in competition

WADA Class: Stimulants
Includes fenfluramine and any optical isomers.

Fenoterol

Other names: Fénotérol; Fenoteroli; Fenoterolum.

Фенотерол

Fenoterol Hydrobromide

F

Other names: Fénotérol, bromhydrate de; Fenoterol-hidrobromid; Fenoterolhydrobromid; Fenoterol-hydrobromid; Fenoteroli hydrobromidum; Fenoterolihydrobromidi; Fenoterolio hidrobromidas; Fenoterolu bromowodorek; Hidrobromuro de fenoterol; TH-1165a.

Фенотерола Гидробромид

Clinical profile: Fenoterol is a direct-acting sympathomimetic with beta-adrenoceptor stimulant activity and high selectivity for beta$_2$ receptors. The hydrobromide is used as a bronchodilator in the management of disorders of reversible airways obstruction. It has also been given to arrest premature labour.

WADA Status: Banned in and out of competition

WADA Class: Beta-2 Agonists
Includes beta-2 agonists or their isomers.

WADA Class: Specified Substances
Also listed as a specified substance.
"The prohibited List may identify specified substances which are particularly susceptible to unintentional anti-doping rule violations because of their general availability in medicinal products or which are less likely to be successfully abused as doping agents."
A doping violation involving such substances may result in a reduced sanction provided that the "*...Athlete can establish that the Use of such a specfied substance was not intended to enhance sport performance...*"

Preparations
Single ingredient: ***Arg.:*** Alveofen; Asmopul; Berotec; ***Austria:*** Berotec; ***Belg.:*** Berotec; ***Braz.:*** Berotec; Bromifen; Bromotec; Febiotec; Fenozan; ***Canad.:*** Berotec; ***Cz.:*** Berotec; Partusisten; ***Denm.:*** Berotec; ***Ger.:*** Berotec; Partusisten; ***Hung.:*** Berotec; ***Indon.:*** Berotec; ***Ital.:*** Dosberotec; ***Jpn:*** Berotec; ***Malaysia:*** Berotec; Feno; ***Mex.:*** Partusisten; ***Neth.:*** Berotec; Partusisten; ***Norw.:*** Berotec; ***Philipp.:*** Berotec; ***Pol.:*** Berotec; ***Port.:*** Berotec; ***Rus.:*** Berotec (Беротек); Partusisten (Партусистен); ***S.Afr.:*** Berotec; ***Singapore:*** Berotec; ***Switz.:*** Berotec; ***Thai.:*** Berotec; ***Venez.:*** Segamol.

Multi-ingredient: ***Arg.:*** Berodual; Ipradual; ***Austria:*** Berodual; Berodualin; Ditec; ***Belg.:*** Duovent; ***Braz.:*** Duovent; Fymnal; ***Canad.:*** Duovent; ***Chile:*** Berodual; ***Cz.:*** Berodual; Ditec; ***Denm.:*** Berodual; ***Fin.:*** Atrovent Comp; ***Fr.:*** Bronchodual; ***Ger.:*** Berodual; ***Gr.:*** Berodual; ***Hung.:*** Berodual; ***India:*** Fenovent; ***Indon.:*** Berodual; ***Irl.:*** Duovent; ***Ital.:*** Duovent; Iprafen; ***Malaysia:*** Berodual; Duovent; ***Mex.:*** Berodual; Berosolvon; ***Neth.:*** Berodual; ***Philipp.:*** Berodual; ***Pol.:*** Berodual; ***Port.:*** Berodual; ***Rus.:*** Berodual (Беродуал); Ditec (Дитек); ***S.Afr.:*** Atrovent Beta; Berodual; Duovent; Sabax Nebrafen; ***Singapore:*** Berodual; Duovent; ***Switz.:*** Berodual; ***Thai.:*** Berodual; Inhalex; Punol; ***UK:*** Duovent; ***Venez.:*** Berodual; Duovent; Respidual.

Fenoxazoline Hydrochloride

Other names: Fénoxazoline, Chlorhydrate de; Fenoxazolini Hydrochloridum; Hidrocloruro de fenoxazolina.

Феноксазолина Гидрохлорид

Clinical profile: Fenoxazoline hydrochloride is a sympathomimetic that has been used topically as a nasal decongestant.

WADA Status: Banned in competition

WADA Class: Stimulants

Includes stimulants or substances with a similar chemical structure or similar biological effect(s). Fenoxazoline is an imidazole derivative. Imidazole derivatives for topical use are exempt.

Preparations
Single ingredient: ***Arg.:*** Nebulicina; ***Braz.:*** Nasofelin.

Fenozolone

Other names: Fenozolona; Fénozolone; Fenozolonum; LD-3394; Phenozolone.

Фенозолон

Clinical profile: Fenozolone is a central stimulant and indirect-acting sympathomimetic that has been used in the treatment of symptoms of mental function impairment.

WADA Status: Banned in competition

WADA Class: Stimulants

Includes stimulants or substances with a similar chemical structure or similar biological effect(s).

WADA Class: Specified Substances

Also listed as a specified substance.
"The prohibited List may identify specified substances which are particularly susceptible to unintentional anti-doping rule violations because of their general availability in medicinal products or which are less likely to be successfully abused as doping agents."
A doping violation involving such substances may result in a reduced sanction provided that the *"...Athlete can establish that the Use of such a specfied substance was not intended to enhance sport performance..."*

Fenproporex Hydrochloride

Other names: *N*-2-Cyanoethylamphetamine Hydrochloride; Fenproporex, Chlorhydrate de; Fenproporexi Hydrochloridum; Hidrocloruro de fenproporex.

Фенпропорекса Гидрохлорид

Clinical profile: Fenproporex is a central stimulant and indirect-acting sympathomimetic. It has been used as an anorectic in the treatment of obesity.

WADA Status: Banned in competition

WADA Class: Stimulants

Includes fenproporex and any optical isomers.

Preparations
Single ingredient: ***Braz.:*** Desobesi-M; Lipomax; ***Chile:*** Salcal; ***Mex.:*** Feprorex; Ifa-Diety.
Multi-ingredient: ***Arg.:*** Tratobes; ***Mex.:*** Esbelcaps.

Fenquizone

Other names: Fenquizona; Fenquizonum; MG-13054.
Фенхизон

Fenquizone Potassium

Other names: Fenquizona potásica; Fenquizone Potassique; Kalii Fenquizonum.
Калия Фенхизон

Clinical profile: Fenquizone is a diuretic used as the potassium salt in the treatment of oedema and hypertension.

WADA Status: Banned in and out of competition

WADA Class: Diuretics and Other Masking Agents

Includes diuretics or substances with a similar chemical structure or similar biological effect(s).

Preparations
Single ingredient: ***Ital.:*** Idrolone.

Fentanyl

Other names: Fentanil; Fentanilis; Fentanilo; Fentanylum; Fentanyyli.
Фентанил

Fentanyl Citrate

Other names: Citrato de fentanilo; Fentanil-citrát; Fentanilio citratas; Fentanyl, citrate de; Fentanylcitrat; Fentanyl-citrát; Fentanyli citras; Fentanylu cytrynian; Fentanyylisitraatti; McN-JR-4263-49; Phentanyl Citrate; R-4263.
Фентанила Цитрат

Fentanyl Hydrochloride

Other names: Fentanyl, Chlorhydrate de; Fentanyli Hydrochloridum; Hidrocloruro de fentanilo.
Фентанила Гидрохлорид

Clinical profile: Fentanyl, a phenylpiperidine derivative, is a potent opioid analgesic, chemically related to pethidine. It is primarily a μ-opioid agonist. Fentanyl is used as an analgesic, as an adjunct to general anaesthetics, or for induction and maintenance of anaesthesia. It is also used as a respiratory depressant in the management of mechanically ventilated patients under intensive care. It is used with an antipsychotic such as droperidol to induce neuroleptanalgesia when the patient is required to cooperate during surgery.

WADA Status: Banned in competition

WADA Class: Narcotics

Includes specified narcotics.

Preparations

Single ingredient: ***Arg.:*** Durogesic; Fentax; Gray-F; Nafluvent; Sublimaze; Talnur; ***Austral.:*** Actiq; Durogesic; Sublimaze; ***Austria:*** Durogesic; ***Belg.:*** Durogesic; ***Braz.:*** Durogesic; Fentabbott; Fentanest; Fentatil; ***Canad.:*** Duragesic; ***Chile:*** Durogesic; ***Cz.:*** Durogesic; ***Denm.:*** Actiq; Durogesic; Haldid; ***Fin.:*** Actiq; Durogesic; ***Fr.:*** Actiq; Durogesic; Ionsys; ***Ger.:*** Actiq; Durogesic; ***Gr.:*** Actiq; Durogesic; Fentadur; Matrifen; ***Hong Kong:*** Durogesic; ***Hung.:*** Durogesic; Matrifen; Sedaton; ***India:*** Durogesic; Trofentyl; ***Indon.:*** Durogesic; ***Irl.:*** Actiq; Durogesic; Fental; Sublimaze; ***Israel:*** Durogesic; Tanyl; ***Ital.:*** Actiq; Durogesic; Fentanest; ***Jpn:*** Durotep; ***Malaysia:*** Durogesic; Talgesil; ***Mex.:*** Durogesic; Fenodid; Fentanest; ***Neth.:*** Actiq; Durogesic; ***Norw.:*** Actiq; Durogesic; Leptanal; ***NZ:*** Durogesic; Sublimaze; ***Philipp.:*** Durogesic; Sublimaze; ***Pol.:*** Durogesic; Fentahexal; ***Port.:*** Durogesic; ***Rus.:*** Durogesic (Дюрогезик); ***S.Afr.:*** Durogesic; Sublimaze; Tanyl; ***Singapore:*** Durogesic; ***Spain:*** Actiq; Durogesic; Fentanest; ***Swed.:*** Actiq; Durogesic; Leptanal; Matrifen; ***Switz.:*** Actiq; Durogesic; Sintenyl; ***Thai.:*** Durogesic; ***Turk.:*** Durogesic; ***UK:*** Actiq; Durogesic; Ionsys; Matrifen; Sublimaze; Tilofyl; ***USA:*** Actiq; Duragesic; Fentora; Ionsys; Sublimaze; ***Venez.:*** Durogesic.

Multi-ingredient: ***Arg.:*** Disifelit; ***Austral.:*** Marcain with Fentanyl; Naropin with Fentanyl; ***Braz.:*** Nilperidol; ***Ital.:*** Leptofen; ***NZ:*** Bupafen; Marcain with Fentanyl; Naropin with Fentanyl.

Finasteride

Other names: Finasterid; Finasterida; Finasteridas; Finastéride; Finasteridi; Finasteridum; Finaszterid; MK-906; MK-0906; YM-152.

Финастерид

Clinical profile: Finasteride is an inhibitor of 5α-reductase, the enzyme responsible for conversion of testosterone to dihydrotestosterone in the prostate. It is used in the management of benign prostatic hyperplasia, and in male-pattern baldness (alopecia androgenetica) in men.

WADA Status: Banned in and out of competition

WADA Class: Diuretics and Other Masking Agents

Masking agents including alpha-reductase inhibitors or plasma expanders or substances with similar biological effect(s).

WADA Class: Specified Substances

Also listed as a specified substance.

"The prohibited List may identify specified substances which are particularly susceptible to unintentional anti-doping rule violations because of their general availability in medicinal products or which are less likely to be successfully abused as doping agents."

A doping violation involving such substances may result in a reduced sanction provided that the *"...Athlete can establish that the Use of such a specfied substance was not intended to enhance sport performance..."*

Preparations

Single ingredient: ***Arg.:*** Andropel; Avertex; Daric; Finasterin; Finprostat; Flutiamik; Folcres; HPB; Nasteril; Propecia; Proscar; Prosmin; Prostanil; Prostanovag; Prostene; Renacidin; Sutrico; Tealep; Tricofarma; Urofin; Urototal; Vetiprost; ***Austral.:*** Propecia; Proscar; ***Austria:*** Propecia; Proscar; ***Belg.:*** Proscar; ***Braz.:*** Alfasin; Finalop; Finastec; Finastil; Flaxin; Nasterid A; Nasterid; Pracap; Prohair; Pronasteron; Propecia; Proscar; Prostide; Reduscar; ***Canad.:*** Propecia; Proscar; ***Chile:*** Prohair; Proscar; Saniprostol; Vastus; ***Cz.:*** Finex; Penester; Propecia; Proscar; ***Denm.:*** Propecia; Proscar; ***Fin.:*** Gefina; Propecia; Proscar; ***Fr.:*** Chibro-Proscar; Propecia; ***Ger.:*** Propecia; Proscar; ***Gr.:*** Pervil; Poruxin; Propecia; Proscar; ***Hong Kong:*** Propecia; Proscar; ***Hung.:*** Finpros; Proscar; Prosterid; ***India:*** Fincar; Finpecia; ***Indon.:*** Finaxal; Finpro; Proscar; Prostacom; Reprostom; ***Irl.:*** Proscar; ***Israel:*** Pro-Cure; Propecia; ***Ital.:*** Finastid; Genaprost; Propecia; Proscar; Prostide; ***Malaysia:*** Propecia; Proscar; ***Mex.:*** Propeshia; Proscar; ***Neth.:*** Finaburg; Propecia; Proscar; ***Norw.:*** Proscar; ***NZ:*** Propecia; Proscar; ***Philipp.:*** Propecia; Proscar; ***Pol.:*** Ambulase; Ambulase; Finaride; Finaster; Lifin; Penester; Propecia; Proscar; Zasterid; ***Port.:*** Propecia; Proscar; ***Rus.:*** Finast (Финаст); Penester (Пенестер); Proscar (Проскар); Prosterid (Простерид); ***S.Afr.:*** Propecia; Proscar; ***Singapore:*** Propecia; Proscar; ***Spain:*** Fucoprost; Propecia; Proscar; ***Swed.:*** Propecia; Proscar; ***Switz.:*** Propecia; Proscar; ***Thai.:*** Firide; Harifin; Propecia; Proscar; ***Turk.:***

Dilaprost; Finarid; Propecia; Proscar; Prosterit; ***UK:*** Propecia; Proscar; ***USA:*** Propecia; Proscar; ***Venez.:*** Nasterol; Propecia; Proscar.
Multi-ingredient: ***India:*** Urimax F.

Fipexide Hydrochloride

Other names: BP-662; Fipexide, Chlorhydrate de; Fipexidi Hydrochloridum; Hidrocloruro de fipexida.

Фипексида Гидрохлорид

Clinical profile: Fipexide hydrochloride has been used as a central stimulant.

WADA Status: Banned in competition

WADA Class: Stimulants

Includes stimulants or substances with a similar chemical structure or similar biological effect(s).

WADA Class: Specified Substances

Also listed as a specified substance.

"The prohibited List may identify specified substances which are particularly susceptible to unintentional anti-doping rule violations because of their general availability in medicinal products or which are less likely to be successfully abused as doping agents."

A doping violation involving such substances may result in a reduced sanction provided that the "*...Athlete can establish that the Use of such a specfied substance was not intended to enhance sport performance...*"

F

Flestolol Sulfate

Other names: ACC-9089; Flestolol, Sulfate de; Flestolol Sulphate; Flestololi Sulfas; Sulfato de flestolol.

Флестолола Сульфат

Clinical profile: Flestolol is a short-acting beta blocker.

WADA Status: Banned in and out of competition as specified below

WADA Class: Beta-Blockers

Unless otherwise specified, beta-blockers are prohibited *In-Competition* only in the following sports.

- Aeronautics (FAI)
- Archery (FITA, IPC) (also prohibited *Out-of-Competition*)
- Automobile (FIA)
- Billiards (WCBS)
- Bobsleigh (FIBT)
- Boules (CMSB, IPC bowls)
- Bridge (FMB)
- Curling (WCF)
- Gymnastics (FIG)
- Motorcycling (FIM)
- Modern Pentathlon (UIPM) for disciplines involving shooting
- Nine-pin bowling (FIQ)
- Powerboating (UIM)
- Sailing (ISAF) for match race helms only
- Shooting (ISSF, IPC) (also prohibited *Out-of-Competition*)
- Skiing/Snowboarding (FIS) in ski jumping, freestyle aerials/halfpipe and snowboard halfpipe/big air
- Wrestling (FILA)

WADA Class: Specified Substances

Also listed as a specified substance.

"The prohibited List may identify specified substances which are particularly susceptible to unintentional anti-doping rule violations because of their general availability in medicinal products or which are less likely to be successfully abused as doping agents."

A doping violation involving such substances may result in a reduced sanction provided that the "*...Athlete can establish that the Use of such a specfied substance was not intended to enhance sport performance...*"

Fluazacort

Other names: Fluazacortum; L-6400.

Флуазакорт

Clinical profile: Fluazacort is a corticosteroid that has been used topically in the treatment of various skin disorders.

WADA Status: Banned in competition

WADA Class: Glucocorticosteroids

All glucocorticosteroids are prohibited when administered orally, rectally, intravenously or intramuscularly. Their use requires a Therapeutic Use Exemption approval. Other routes of administration (intraarticular / periarticular / peritendinous / epidural / intradermal injections and inhalation) require an Abbreviated Therapeutic Use Exemption except as noted below.

Topical preparations when used for dermatological (including iontophoresis / phonophoresis), auricular, nasal, ophthalmic, buccal, gingival and perianal disorders are not prohibited and do not require any form of Therapeutic Use Exemption.

WADA Class: Specified Substances

Also listed as a specified substance.

"The prohibited List may identify specified substances which are particularly susceptible to unintentional anti-doping rule violations because of their general availability in medicinal products or which are less likely to be successfully abused as doping agents."

A doping violation involving such substances may result in a reduced sanction provided that the "*...Athlete can establish that the Use of such a specfied substance was not intended to enhance sport performance...*"

Fluclorolone Acetonide

Other names: Acetónido de fluclorolona; Fluclorolone, Acétonide de; Flucloroloni Acetonidum; Flucloronide; Fluklorolonacetonid; Flukloroloniasetonidi; RS-2252.

Флуклоролона Ацетонид

Clinical profile: Fluclorolone acetonide is a corticosteroid used topically in the treatment of various skin disorders.

WADA Status: Banned in competition

WADA Class: Glucocorticosteroids

All glucocorticosteroids are prohibited when administered orally, rectally, intravenously or intramuscularly. Their use requires a Therapeutic Use Exemption approval. Other routes of administration (intraarticular / periarticular / peritendinous / epidural / intradermal injections and inhalation) require an Abbreviated Therapeutic Use Exemption except as noted below.

Topical preparations when used for dermatological (including iontophoresis / phonophoresis), auricular, nasal, ophthalmic, buccal, gingival and perianal disorders are not prohibited and do not require any form of Therapeutic Use Exemption.

WADA Class: Specified Substances

Also listed as a specified substance.

"The prohibited List may identify specified substances which are particularly susceptible to unintentional anti-doping rule violations because of their general availability in medicinal products or which are less likely to be successfully abused as doping agents."

A doping violation involving such substances may result in a reduced sanction provided that the "*...Athlete can establish that the Use of such a specfied substance was not intended to enhance sport performance...*"

Preparations
Single ingredient: ***Spain:*** Cutanit.

Fludroxycortide

Other names: 33379; Fludroksikortidi; Fludroxicortida; Fludroxikortid; Fludroxycortidum; Fluorandrenolone; 6α-Fluoro-16α-hydroxyhydrocortisone 16,17-Acetonide; Flurandrenolide; Flurandrenolone.

Флудроксикортид

F

Clinical profile: Fludroxycortide is a corticosteroid used topically in the treatment of various skin disorders.

WADA Status: Banned in competition

WADA Class: Glucocorticosteroids

All glucocorticosteroids are prohibited when administered orally, rectally, intravenously or intramuscularly. Their use requires a Therapeutic Use Exemption approval. Other routes of administration (intraarticular / periarticular / peritendinous / epidural / intradermal injections and inhalation) require an Abbreviated Therapeutic Use Exemption except as noted below.

Topical preparations when used for dermatological (including iontophoresis / phonophoresis), auricular, nasal, ophthalmic, buccal, gingival and perianal disorders are not prohibited and do not require any form of Therapeutic Use Exemption.

WADA Class: Specified Substances

Also listed as a specified substance.

"The prohibited List may identify specified substances which are particularly susceptible to unintentional anti-doping rule violations because of their general availability in medicinal products or which are less likely to be successfully abused as doping agents."

A doping violation involving such substances may result in a reduced sanction provided that the "*...Athlete can establish that the Use of such a specfied substance was not intended to enhance sport performance...*"

Preparations
Single ingredient: ***Braz.:*** Drenison; ***UK:*** Haelan; ***USA:*** Cordran.
Multi-ingredient: ***Braz.:*** Dreniformio; Drenison N.

Flumetasone Pivalate

Other names: Flumetason pivalát; Flumétasone, pivalate de; Flumetasoni pivalas; Flumetasonipivalaatti; Flumetasonpivalat; Flumetasonum Pivalas; Flumetazon Pivalat; Flumetazono pivalatas; Flumetazon-pivalát; Flumetazonu piwalan; Flumethasone

Pivalate; Flumethasone Trimethylacetate; NSC-107680; Pivalato de flumetasona.

Флуметазона Пивалат

Clinical profile: Flumetasone is a glucocorticoid used by topical application in the treatment of various skin disorders.

WADA Status: Banned in competition

WADA Class: Glucocorticosteroids

All glucocorticosteroids are prohibited when administered orally, rectally, intravenously or intramuscularly. Their use requires a Therapeutic Use Exemption approval. Other routes of administration (intraarticular / periarticular / peritendinous / epidural / intradermal injections and inhalation) require an Abbreviated Therapeutic Use Exemption except as noted below.

Topical preparations when used for dermatological (including iontophoresis / phonophoresis), auricular, nasal, ophthalmic, buccal, gingival and perianal disorders are not prohibited and do not require any form of Therapeutic Use Exemption.

WADA Class: Specified Substances

Also listed as a specified substance.

"The prohibited List may identify specified substances which are particularly susceptible to unintentional anti-doping rule violations because of their general availability in medicinal products or which are less likely to be successfully abused as doping agents."

A doping violation involving such substances may result in a reduced sanction provided that the "*...Athlete can establish that the Use of such a specfied substance was not intended to enhance sport performance...*"

Preparations

Single ingredient: ***Belg.:*** Locacortene; ***Ger.:*** Cerson; Locacorten; ***Neth.:*** Locacorten; ***Pol.:*** Lorinden; ***Switz.:*** Locacorten.

Multi-ingredient: ***Arg.:*** Tresite F; ***Austral.:*** Locacorten Vioform; ***Austria:*** Locacorten mit Neomycin; Locacorten Tar; Locacorten Vioform; Locasalen; ***Belg.:*** Locasalen; ***Braz.:*** Locorten Vioformio; Locorten; Losalen; ***Canad.:*** Locacorten Vioform; ***Cz.:*** Locacorten Tar; Lorinden A; Lorinden C; ***Denm.:*** Locacorten Vioform; ***Fin.:*** Locacorten Vioform; ***Fr.:*** Locacortene Vioforme; Locasalene; Psocortene; ***Ger.:*** Locacorten Vioform; Locasalen; ***Gr.:*** Locasalene; ***Hong Kong:*** Locasalen; ***Hung.:*** Lorinden A; Lorinden C; ***Indon.:*** Locasalen; ***Israel:*** Topicorten V; Topicorten-Tar; Topisalen; ***Ital.:*** Locorten Vioformio; Locorten; Locorten; Losalen; Vasosterone Oto; ***Neth.:*** Locacorten Vioform; Locasalen; ***NZ:*** Locorten Vioform; ***Philipp.:*** Locasalen; ***Pol.:*** Lorinden A; Lorinden C; Lorinden N; ***Port.:*** Locorten Vioformio; Losalen; ***Rus.:*** Lorinden A (Лоринден А); Lorinden C (Лоринден С); ***S.Afr.:*** Locacorten Vioform; ***Spain:*** Losalen; ***Swed.:*** Locacorten Vioform; ***Switz.:*** Locasalen; ***Thai.:*** Flumasalen; Locasalen; ***Turk.:*** Locacortene Vioform; Locasalene; ***UK:*** Locorten Vioform; ***Venez.:*** Locasalen; Locorten Vioformo.

Flunisolide

Other names: Flunisolid; Flunisolida; Flunisolidi; Flunisolidum; RS-3999; RS-1320 (flunisolide acetate).

Флунизолид

Clinical profile: Flunisolide is a glucocorticoid used as a nasal spray for the prophylaxis and treatment of allergic rhinitis and by inhalation in the management of asthma.

WADA Status: Banned in competition

WADA Class: Glucocorticosteroids

All glucocorticosteroids are prohibited when administered orally, rectally, intravenously or intramuscularly. Their use requires a Therapeutic Use Exemption approval. Other routes of administration (intraarticular / periarticular / peritendinous / epidural / intradermal injections and inhalation) require an Abbreviated Therapeutic Use Exemption except as noted below.

Topical preparations when used for dermatological (including iontophoresis / pho-

nophoresis), auricular, nasal, ophthalmic, buccal, gingival and perianal disorders are not prohibited and do not require any form of Therapeutic Use Exemption.

WADA Class: Specified Substances

Also listed as a specified substance.

"The prohibited List may identify specified substances which are particularly susceptible to unintentional anti-doping rule violations because of their general availability in medicinal products or which are less likely to be successfully abused as doping agents."

A doping violation involving such substances may result in a reduced sanction provided that the "*...Athlete can establish that the Use of such a specfied substance was not intended to enhance sport performance...*"

Preparations
Single ingredient: ***Austria:*** Pulmilide; ***Belg.:*** Syntaris; ***Cz.:*** Bronilide; Syntaris; ***Fr.:*** Nasalide; ***Ger.:*** Syntaris; ***Ital.:*** Aerflu; Aerolid; Asmaflu; Assolid; Careflu; Charlyn; Citiflux; Desaflu; Doricoflu; Eliosid; Euroflu; Fluminex; Flunitop; Gibiflu; Givair; Inalcort; Kaimil; Levonis; Lunibron; Lunis; Nebulcort; Nereflun; Nisolid; Nisoran; Plaudit; Pulmist; Syntaris; Turm; Ventoflu; ***Neth.:*** Syntaris; ***Norw.:*** Lokilan; ***UK:*** Syntaris; ***USA:*** AeroBid; AeroSpan; Nasarel.
Multi-ingredient: ***Ital.:*** Plenaer.

Fluocinolone Acetonide

F

Other names: Acetónido de fluocinolona; 6α,9α-Difluoro-16α-hydroxyprednisolone Acetonide; Fluocinolon acetonid; Fluocinolonacetonid; Fluocinolon-acetonid; Fluocinolone, acétonide de; Fluocinoloni acetonidum; Fluocinolono acetonidas; Fluocynolonu acetonid; Fluosinoloniasetonidi; NSC-92339.

Флуоцинолона Ацетонид

Clinical profile: Fluocinolone acetonide is a corticosteroid used topically in the treatment of various eye, ear, nose, and skin disorders.

WADA Status: Banned in competition

WADA Class: Glucocorticosteroids

All glucocorticosteroids are prohibited when administered orally, rectally, intravenously or intramuscularly. Their use requires a Therapeutic Use Exemption approval. Other routes of administration (intraarticular / periarticular / peritendinous / epidural / intradermal injections and inhalation) require an Abbreviated Therapeutic Use Exemption except as noted below.

Topical preparations when used for dermatological (including iontophoresis / phonophoresis), auricular, nasal, ophthalmic, buccal, gingival and perianal disorders are not prohibited and do not require any form of Therapeutic Use Exemption.

WADA Class: Specified Substances

Also listed as a specified substance.

"The prohibited List may identify specified substances which are particularly susceptible to unintentional anti-doping rule violations because of their general availability in medicinal products or which are less likely to be successfully abused as doping agents."

A doping violation involving such substances may result in a reduced sanction provided that the "*...Athlete can establish that the Use of such a specfied substance was not intended to enhance sport performance...*"

Preparations
Single ingredient: ***Arg.:*** Duoflu; Flulone; ***Austria:*** Synalar; ***Belg.:*** Synalar; ***Canad.:*** Capex; Derma-Smoothe/FS; Synalar; ***Chile:*** Adermina; ***Cz.:*** Flucinar; Gelargin; Synalar; ***Denm.:*** Synalar; ***Ger.:*** Flucinar; Jellin; Jellisoft; ***Gr.:*** Synalar; ***Hong Kong:*** Synalar; ***Hung.:*** Flucinar; ***India:*** Flucort-H; Flucort; Luci; ***Indon.:*** Cinolon; Dermasolon; Esinol; Inoderm; Licosolon; ***Israel:*** Dermalar; ***Ital.:*** Atoactive; Dermobeta; Dermolin; Fluocit; Fluomix Same; Fluovitef; Localyn SV; Localyn; Omniderm; Sterolone; Ultraderm; ***Mex.:*** Cortifung-S; Cortilona; Cremisona; Farmacorti; Flumicin; Fluomex; Fusalar; Lonason; Synalar; ***Norw.:*** Synalar; ***NZ:*** Synalar; ***Philipp.:*** Aplosyn; Cynozet; Synalar; Syntopic; ***Pol.:*** Flucinar; ***Port.:*** Synalar; ***Rus.:*** Flucinar (Флуцинар); Sinaflan (Синафлан); ***S.Afr.:*** Cortoderm; Fluoderm; Synalar; ***Singapore:*** Flunolone-V; ***Spain:*** Co Fluocin Fuerte;

Cortiespec; Fluocid Forte; Fluodermo Fuerte; Flusolgen; Gelidina; Synalar Rectal Simple; Synalar; ***Swed.:*** Synalar; ***Switz.:*** Synalar; ***Thai.:*** Cervicum; Flunolone-V; Fulone; Supralan; Synalar; ***UK:*** Synalar; ***USA:*** Capex; Derma-Smoothe/FS; DermOtic; Fluonid; Retisert; Synalar; Synemol; ***Venez.:*** Bratofil; Neo-Synalar.

Multi-ingredient: ***Arg.:*** Tri-Luma; ***Austria:*** Myco-Synalar; Myco-Synalar; Procto-Synalar; Synalar N; ***Belg.:*** Procto-Synalar; Synalar Bi-Otic; ***Braz.:*** Dermobel; Dermoxin; Elotin; Fluo-Vaso; Neocinolon; Otauril; Otocort; Otomixyn; Otosynalar; ***Chile:*** Otoseptil; Tri-Luma; ***Denm.:*** Synalar med Chinoform; ***Fr.:*** Antibio-Synalar; ***Ger.:*** Jellin-Neomycin; ***Gr.:*** Myco-Synalar; Procto-Synalar N; ***Hong Kong:*** Aplosyn-Otic; Flunolone; Fluonid-N; Synalar N; Synco-CFN; Syneolona; Tri-Luma; ***Hung.:*** Flucinar N; ***India:*** Eczo-Wokadine; Flucort-C; Flucort-MZ; Flucort-N; Flucreme NM; Luci-N; Micogel F; Neocip FC; Zole-F; ***Indon.:*** Cinogenta; Cinolon-N; Fasolon; Genolon; Gentasolon; Kalcinol-N; Neosinol; Ociderm-N; Sinobiotik; Zumaderm-N; ***Ital.:*** Cortanest Plus; Doricum; Lauromicina; Localyn-Neomicina; Localyn; Localyn; Mecloderm F; Nefluan; Proctolyn; ***Malaysia:*** Fluonid-N; ***Mex.:*** Acenil; Bentix; Cetoquina Y; Cortifung-N; Cortifung-Y; Cortilona Compuesta; Farmacorti YC; Fluccinol N; Fluo Grin; Gynoclin-V; Lasalar-Y; Luzolona Y; Neoderm-F; Nysmosons-V; Promibasol-Plus; Synalar C; Synalar N; Synalar Neo; Synalar O; Synalar Oftalmico; Tri-Luma; Vagitrol-V; Yderm; ***Norw.:*** Synalar med Chinoform; ***Philipp.:*** Aplosyn C; Aplosyn N; Aplosyn-Otic; Neo-Synalar; Synalar Otic; Tri-Luma; ***Pol.:*** Flucinar N; ***Port.:*** Synalar N; Synalar Rectal; ***Rus.:*** Flucinar N (Флуцинар Н); Simetrid (Симетрид); ***S.Afr.:*** Cortoderm-C; Synalar C; Synalar N; ***Singapore:*** Flunolone; Tri-Luma; ***Spain:*** Abrasone Rectal; Abrasone; Aceoto Plus; Alergical; Artrodesmol Extra; Bazalin; Cetraxal Plus; Creanolona; Flodermol; Fluo Fenic; Midacina; Neo Analsona; Otomidrin; Synalar Nasal; Synalar Neomicina; Synalar Otico; Synalar Rectal; Synalotic; Vinciseptil Otico; ***Switz.:*** Procto-Synalar N; Synalar N; ***Thai.:*** Flunolone; Fluonid-N; Gental-F; Supralan-N; Synalar N; Tri-Luma; ***UK:*** Synalar C; Synalar N; ***USA:*** Tri-Luma; ***Venez.:*** Bratofil c Neomicina; Neo-Synalar con Neomicina; Tri-Luma.

Fluocinonide

F

Other names: Fluocinolide; Fluocinolone Acetonide 21-Acetate; Fluocinonid; Fluocinónida; Fluocinonidum; Fluosinonidi; NSC-101791.

Флуоцинонид

Clinical profile: Fluocinonide is a corticosteroid used topically in the treatment of various skin disorders.

WADA Status: Banned in competition

WADA Class: Glucocorticosteroids

All glucocorticosteroids are prohibited when administered orally, rectally, intravenously or intramuscularly. Their use requires a Therapeutic Use Exemption approval. Other routes of administration (intraarticular / periarticular / peritendinous / epidural / intradermal injections and inhalation) require an Abbreviated Therapeutic Use Exemption except as noted below.

Topical preparations when used for dermatological (including iontophoresis / phonophoresis), auricular, nasal, ophthalmic, buccal, gingival and perianal disorders are not prohibited and do not require any form of Therapeutic Use Exemption.

WADA Class: Specified Substances

Also listed as a specified substance.

"The prohibited List may identify specified substances which are particularly susceptible to unintentional anti-doping rule violations because of their general availability in medicinal products or which are less likely to be successfully abused as doping agents."

A doping violation involving such substances may result in a reduced sanction provided that the "*...Athlete can establish that the Use of such a specfied substance was not intended to enhance sport performance...*"

Preparations

Single ingredient: ***Austria:*** Topsym; Topsymin F; ***Canad.:*** Lidemol; Lidex; Lyderm; Tiamol; Topsyn; ***Denm.:*** Metosyn; ***Ger.:*** Topsym; ***Gr.:*** Lidex; ***Ital.:*** Topsyn; ***Mex.:*** Topsyn; ***Norw.:***

Metosyn; ***Philipp.:*** Lidemol; Lidex; ***Spain:*** Novoter; ***Switz.:*** Topsym; Topsymin; ***UK:*** Metosyn; ***USA:*** Lidex; Vanos.
Multi-ingredient: ***Austria:*** Topsym polyvalent; ***Ger.:*** Jelliproct; Topsym polyvalent; ***Israel:*** Comagis; ***Mex.:*** Topsyn-Y; ***Philipp.:*** Lidex NGN; ***Spain:*** Novoter Gentamicina; ***Switz.:*** Mycolog N; Topsym polyvalent; ***UK:*** Vipsogal.

Fluocortin Butyl

Other names: Butil éster de la fluocortina; Butylis Fluocortinas; Fluocortine Butyle; SH-K-203.

Флуокортин Бутил

Clinical profile: Fluocortin butyl is a corticosteroid used topically in the treatment of various skin disorders. It has been used for the management of allergic rhinitis.

WADA Status: Banned in competition

WADA Class: Glucocorticosteroids

All glucocorticosteroids are prohibited when administered orally, rectally, intravenously or intramuscularly. Their use requires a Therapeutic Use Exemption approval. Other routes of administration (intraarticular / periarticular / peritendinous / epidural / intradermal injections and inhalation) require an Abbreviated Therapeutic Use Exemption except as noted below.

Topical preparations when used for dermatological (including iontophoresis / phonophoresis), auricular, nasal, ophthalmic, buccal, gingival and perianal disorders are not prohibited and do not require any form of Therapeutic Use Exemption.

WADA Class: Specified Substances

Also listed as a specified substance.

"The prohibited List may identify specified substances which are particularly susceptible to unintentional anti-doping rule violations because of their general availability in medicinal products or which are less likely to be successfully abused as doping agents."

A doping violation involving such substances may result in a reduced sanction provided that the "*...Athlete can establish that the Use of such a specfied substance was not intended to enhance sport performance...*"

Preparations
Single ingredient: ***Ital.:*** Vaspit; ***Spain:*** Vaspit.

Fluocortolone

Other names: Fluocortolona; Fluocortolonum; Fluokortolon; Fluokortoloni; 6α-Fluoro-16α-methyl-1-dehydrocorticosterone; SH-742.

Флуокортолон

Fluocortolone Caproate

Other names: Caproato de fluocortolona; Fluocortolone, Caproate de; Fluocortolone Hexanoate; Fluocortoloni Caproas; Fluokortolon Kaproat; Fluokortolon Kapronat; SH-770.

Флуокортолона Капроат

Fluocortolone Pivalate

Other names: Fluocortolone, pivalate de; Fluocortolone Trimethylacetate; Fluocortoloni pivalas; Fluokortolon Pivalat; Fluokortolonipivalaatti; Fluokortolono pivalatas; Fluokortolonpivalat; Fluokortolon-pivalát; Pivalato de fluocortolona.

Флуокортолона Пивалат

Clinical profile: Fluocortolone and its esters are corticosteroids that are mainly used topically in the treatment of various skin disorders, and the local management of anorectal disorders. Fluocortolone is sometimes given orally.

WADA Status: Banned in competition

WADA Class: Glucocorticosteroids

All glucocorticosteroids are prohibited when administered orally, rectally, intravenously or intramuscularly. Their use requires a Therapeutic Use Exemption approval. Other routes of administration (intraarticular / periarticular / peritendinous / epidural / intradermal injections and inhalation) require an Abbreviated Therapeutic Use Exemption except as noted below.

Topical preparations when used for dermatological (including iontophoresis / phonophoresis), auricular, nasal, ophthalmic, buccal, gingival and perianal disorders are not prohibited and do not require any form of Therapeutic Use Exemption.

WADA Class: Specified Substances

Also listed as a specified substance.

"*The prohibited List may identify specified substances which are particularly susceptible to unintentional anti-doping rule violations because of their general availability in medicinal products or which are less likely to be successfully abused as doping agents.*"

A doping violation involving such substances may result in a reduced sanction provided that the "*...Athlete can establish that the Use of such a specfied substance was not intended to enhance sport performance...*"

Preparations

Single ingredient: ***Arg.:*** Ultracur S; ***Austria:*** Ultralan; Ultralan; Ultralan; ***Ger.:*** Ultralan; ***Hong Kong:*** Ultralan; ***Israel:*** Ultralan; ***Ital.:*** Ultralan; Ultralan; Ultralan; ***Philipp.:*** Ultralan; ***Spain:*** Ultralan M; ***Turk.:*** Ultralan; Ultralan.

Multi-ingredient: ***Arg.:*** Ultraproct; ***Austral.:*** Ultraproct; ***Austria:*** Pilison; Ultraproct; ***Belg.:*** Ultraproct; ***Braz.:*** Ultraproct; ***Chile:*** Ultraproct; ***Denm.:*** Doloproct Comp; Doloproct; ***Fin.:*** Neoproct; ***Fr.:*** Ultralan; Ultraproct; ***Ger.:*** Doloproct; ***Gr.:*** Doloproct; ***Hong Kong:*** Ultraproct N; ***Indon.:*** Ultraproct N; Ultraproct; ***Irl.:*** Ultraproct; ***Ital.:*** Doloproct; Ultraproct; ***Mex.:*** Ultraproct; ***NZ:*** Ultraproct; ***Philipp.:*** Ultraproct; ***Port.:*** Ultraproct; ***Rus.:*** Ultraproct (Ультрапрокт); ***Thai.:*** Scheriproct N; ***Turk.:*** Ultralan Crilane; Ultraproct; ***UK:*** Ultralanum Plain; Ultraproct.

Fluorometholone

Other names: Fluorométholone; Fluorometholonum; Fluorometolon; Fluorometolona; Fluorometoloni.

Флуорометолон

Fluorometholone Acetate

Other names: Acetato de fluorometolona; Fluorométholone, Acétate de; Fluorometholoni Acetas; Fluorometolon Asetat; U-17323.

Флуорометолона Ацетат

Clinical profile: Fluorometholone is a glucocorticoid corticosteroid employed in the topical treatment of various eye and skin disorders.

WADA Status: Banned in competition

WADA Class: Glucocorticosteroids

All glucocorticosteroids are prohibited when administered orally, rectally, intravenously or intramuscularly. Their use requires a Therapeutic Use Exemption approval. Other routes of administration (intraarticular / periarticular / peritendinous / epidural / intradermal injections and inhalation) require an Abbreviated Therapeutic

Use Exemption except as noted below.

Topical preparations when used for dermatological (including iontophoresis / phonophoresis), auricular, nasal, ophthalmic, buccal, gingival and perianal disorders are not prohibited and do not require any form of Therapeutic Use Exemption.

WADA Class: Specified Substances

Also listed as a specified substance.

"The prohibited List may identify specified substances which are particularly susceptible to unintentional anti-doping rule violations because of their general availability in medicinal products or which are less likely to be successfully abused as doping agents."

A doping violation involving such substances may result in a reduced sanction provided that the "*...Athlete can establish that the Use of such a specfied substance was not intended to enhance sport performance...*"

Preparations

Single ingredient: ***Arg.:*** Flarex; FML; ***Austral.:*** Flarex; Flucon; FML; ***Belg.:*** Fluacort; Flucon; FML; ***Braz.:*** Florate; Flumex; ***Canad.:*** Flarex; FML; ***Chile:*** Aflarex; Fluforte; ***Cz.:*** Efflumidex; Flarex; Flucon; Flumetol S; Fluoropos; ***Denm.:*** Flurolon; ***Fin.:*** FML; ***Fr.:*** Flucon; ***Ger.:*** Efflumidex; Fluoro-Ophtal; Fluoropos; ***Gr.:*** Flucon; Fluxinam; FML; ***Hong Kong:*** Flarex; Flucon; Flumetholon; FML; ***Hung.:*** Efflumidex; Flarex; Flucon; ***India:*** Flomex; Flosef; ***Indon.:*** Flumetholon; ***Irl.:*** FML; ***Israel:*** Flarex; FML; ***Ital.:*** Flarex; Fluaton; Flumetol; ***Malaysia:*** Flarex; FML; ***Mex.:*** Flarex; Fluforte; Flumetol NF; ***Neth.:*** Flarex; FML; ***NZ:*** Flucon; FML; ***Philipp.:*** Flarex; Flulon; FML; ***Pol.:*** Flarex; Flucon; ***Port.:*** Flurop; FML; ***Rus.:*** Flarex (Фларекс); ***S.Afr.:*** Flucon; FML; ***Singapore:*** FML; ***Spain:*** FML; Isopto Flucon; ***Switz.:*** FML; ***Thai.:*** Flarex; Flu Oph; Flucon; FML; ***Turk.:*** Flarex; FML; ***UK:*** FML; ***USA:*** Eflone; Flarex; FML; ***Venez.:*** Aflarex; Flumetol.

Multi-ingredient: ***Arg.:*** Delisan; Efemolina; FML Neo; Larsimal; ***Belg.:*** Infectoflam; ***Braz.:*** Flumex N; ***Cz.:*** Infectoflam; ***Ger.:*** Cibaflam; Efemolin; ***Gr.:*** Efemoline; FML Neo; Luzin; ***Hong Kong:*** Efemoline; ***India:*** Flomex N; ***Ital.:*** Efemoline; Flumeciclina; Flumezina; Gentacort; ***Malaysia:*** Efemoline; Infectoflam; ***Mex.:*** Fluforte N; Fluorometil; ***Philipp.:*** Efemoline; Infectoflam; ***Port.:*** Neo-Preocil; ***S.Afr.:*** Efemoline; FML Neo; ***Singapore:*** Efemoline; Infectoflam; ***Spain:*** Bexicortil; Cortisdin Urea; Flugen; Fluorvas; ***Switz.:*** Efemoline; FML Neo; Infectoflam; ***Thai.:*** Efemoline; Infectoflam; ***Turk.:*** Efemoline; Flumetol; ***USA:*** FML-S.

Fluoxymesterone

Other names: Fluoksimesteroni; Fluoximesteron; Fluoximesterona; Fluoxymestérone; Fluoxymesteronum; Fluximesterona; NSC-12165.

Флуоксиместерон

Clinical profile: Fluoxymesterone has androgenic properties and has been used in the treatment of male hypogonadism and delayed puberty, and the palliation of inoperable neoplasms of the breast in postmenopausal women.

WADA Status: Banned in and out of competition

WADA Class: Anabolic; Androgenic Steroids (exogenous)

Includes exogenous anabolic androgenic steroids or other substances with a similar chemical structure or similar biological effect(s).

Preparations

Single ingredient: ***Mex.:*** Stenox; ***USA:*** Androxy.

Multi-ingredient: ***Arg.:*** Ferona.

Fluprednidene Acetate

Other names: Acetato de fluprednideno; Fluprednidène, Acétate de; Fluprednideni Acetas; Fluprednylidene 21-Acetate.

Флупреднидена Ацетат

Clinical profile: Fluprednidene acetate is a corticosteroid used topically in the treatment of various skin disorders.

WADA Status: Banned in competition

WADA Class: Glucocorticosteroids

All glucocorticosteroids are prohibited when administered orally, rectally, intravenously or intramuscularly. Their use requires a Therapeutic Use Exemption approval. Other routes of administration (intraarticular / periarticular / peritendinous / epidural / intradermal injections and inhalation) require an Abbreviated Therapeutic Use Exemption except as noted below.

Topical preparations when used for dermatological (including iontophoresis / phonophoresis), auricular, nasal, ophthalmic, buccal, gingival and perianal disorders are not prohibited and do not require any form of Therapeutic Use Exemption.

WADA Class: Specified Substances

Also listed as a specified substance.

"The prohibited List may identify specified substances which are particularly susceptible to unintentional anti-doping rule violations because of their general availability in medicinal products or which are less likely to be successfully abused as doping agents."

A doping violation involving such substances may result in a reduced sanction provided that the "*...Athlete can establish that the Use of such a specfied substance was not intended to enhance sport performance...*"

Preparations

Single ingredient: ***Austria:*** Decoderm; ***Belg.:*** Decoderm; ***Ger.:*** Decoderm; ***Indon.:*** Decoderm; ***Switz.:*** Decoderm.

Multi-ingredient: ***Austria:*** Decoderm Compositum; Decoderm trivalent; ***Belg.:*** Decoderm Compositum; ***Ger.:*** Candio-Hermal Plus; Crinohermal fem; Decoderm Comp; Decoderm tri; Sali-Decoderm; Vobaderm; ***Gr.:*** Antimycotic; Catrigel; Combi; Conazol; Domycotin; Edmudo; Expectein; Feminella; Finicort; Flenazole; Fluniprol; Flunovon; Fosemyk; Fumicon; Micoflup; Micogen; Mifler; Oxigon; Panderm; Panmyk; Sarmel; Verdal; ***Indon.:*** Decoderm 3; Gentacortin; ***Switz.:*** Decoderm bivalent; ***UK:*** Acorvio Plus.

F

Fluprednisolone

Other names: 6α-Fluoroprednisolone; Fluprednisolon; Fluprednisolona; Fluprednisoloni; Fluprednisolonum; NSC-47439; U-7800.

Флупреднизолон

Clinical profile: Fluprednisolone is a glucocorticoid corticosteroid.

WADA Status: Banned in competition

WADA Class: Glucocorticosteroids

All glucocorticosteroids are prohibited when administered orally, rectally, intravenously or intramuscularly. Their use requires a Therapeutic Use Exemption approval. Other routes of administration (intraarticular / periarticular / peritendinous / epidural / intradermal injections and inhalation) require an Abbreviated Therapeutic Use Exemption except as noted below.

Topical preparations when used for dermatological (including iontophoresis / phonophoresis), auricular, nasal, ophthalmic, buccal, gingival and perianal disorders are not prohibited and do not require any form of Therapeutic Use Exemption.

WADA Class: Specified Substances

Also listed as a specified substance.

"The prohibited List may identify specified substances which are particularly susceptible to unintentional anti-doping rule violations because of their general availability in medicinal products or which are less likely to be successfully abused as doping agents."

A doping violation involving such substances may result in a reduced sanction pro

vided that the "*...Athlete can establish that the Use of such a specfied substance was not intended to enhance sport performance...*"

Flurotyl

Other names: Flurothyl; Flurotilo; Flurotylum; Hexafluorodiethyl Ether; SKF-6539.
Флуротил

Clinical profile: Flurotyl stimulates the CNS and induces convulsions. It was formerly used as an alternative to electroconvulsive therapy in the treatment of severe depression.

WADA Status: Banned in competition

WADA Class: Stimulants

Includes stimulants or substances with a similar chemical structure or similar biological effect(s).

WADA Class: Specified Substances

Also listed as a specified substance.
"*The prohibited List may identify specified substances which are particularly susceptible to unintentional anti-doping rule violations because of their general availability in medicinal products or which are less likely to be successfully abused as doping agents.*"
A doping violation involving such substances may result in a reduced sanction provided that the "*...Athlete can establish that the Use of such a specfied substance was not intended to enhance sport performance...*"

F

Fluticasone

Other names: Fluticasona; Fluticasonum.
Флутиказон

Fluticasone Furoate

Other names: Fluticasonum Furoas; Furoate de Fluticasone; Furoato de Fluticasona; GW-685698X.
Флутиказон Фуроат

Fluticasone Propionate

Other names: CCI-18781; Fluticasone, propionate de; Fluticasoni propionas; Flutikasonipropionaatti; Flutikasonpropionat; Flutikason-propionát; Flutikazon Propiyonat; Flutikazono propionatas; Propionato de fluticasona.
Флутиказона Пропионат

Clinical profile: Fluticasone is a corticosteroid used by inhalation in the management of asthma and chronic obstructive pulmonary disease. It is also given intranasally in allergic rhinitis and for nasal polyps. It is applied topically in the treatment of various skin disorders.

WADA Status: Banned in competition

WADA Class: Glucocorticosteroids

All glucocorticosteroids are prohibited when administered orally, rectally, intravenously or intramuscularly. Their use requires a Therapeutic Use Exemption approval. Other routes of administration (intraarticular / periarticular / peritendinous / epidural / intradermal injections and inhalation) require an Abbreviated Therapeutic

Use Exemption except as noted below.

Topical preparations when used for dermatological (including iontophoresis / phonophoresis), auricular, nasal, ophthalmic, buccal, gingival and perianal disorders are not prohibited and do not require any form of Therapeutic Use Exemption.

WADA Class: Specified Substances

Also listed as a specified substance.

"The prohibited List may identify specified substances which are particularly susceptible to unintentional anti-doping rule violations because of their general availability in medicinal products or which are less likely to be successfully abused as doping agents."

A doping violation involving such substances may result in a reduced sanction provided that the "*...Athlete can establish that the Use of such a specfied substance was not intended to enhance sport performance...*"

Preparations

Single ingredient: ***Arg.:*** Cutivate; Flixonase; Flixotide; Fluti-K; Fluticort; Lidil Cort; Proair; Rinisona; ***Austral.:*** Beconase Allergy; Flixonase; Flixotide; ***Austria:*** Cutivate; Flixonase; Flixotide; ***Belg.:*** Cutivate; Flixonase; Flixotide; ***Braz.:*** Flixonase; Flixotide; Fluticaps; Flutivate; Plurair; ***Canad.:*** Cutivate; Flonase; Flovent; ***Chile:*** Albeoler; Brexonase; Brexovent; Flixonase; Flixotide; Flusona; Flutivate; Nebulex; Raffonin; ***Cz.:*** Cutivate; Flixonase; Flixotide; ***Denm.:*** Cutivat; Flixonase; Flixotide; ***Fin.:*** Flixonase; Flixotide; ***Fr.:*** Flixonase; Flixotide; Flixovate; ***Ger.:*** Atemur; Flutide; Flutivate; ***Gr.:*** Alerxem; Cortixide; Dermocort; Flicazen; Flihaler; Flixocort; Flixoderm; Flixotide; Flixotide; Flucortis; Flutinasal; Flutizal; Ybecor; ***Hong Kong:*** Cutivate; Flixonase; Flixotide; ***Hung.:*** Cutivate; Flixonase; Flixotide; Flutirin; ***India:*** Flohale; Flomist; Zoflut; ***Indon.:*** Cutivate; Flixonase; Flixotide; Medicort; ***Irl.:*** Flixonase; Flixotide; Nasofan; ***Israel:*** Allegro; Flixonase; Flixotide; ***Ital.:*** Flixoderm; Flixonase; Flixotide; Fluspiral; Ticavent; ***Jpn:*** Flonase; ***Malaysia:*** Cutivate; Flixonase; Flixotide; ***Mex.:*** Cutivate; Flixonase; Flixotide; ***Neth.:*** Cutivate; Flixonase; Flixotide; Flutide; ***Norw.:*** Flutide; Flutivate; ***NZ:*** Flixonase; Flixotide; Nasaclear; ***Philipp.:*** Cutivate; Flixotide; ***Pol.:*** Cutivate; Flixonase; Flixotide; ***Port.:*** Asmatil; Asmo-Lavi; Brisovent; Cutivate; Eustidil; Flixotaide; Flutaide; Rontilona; Ubizol; ***Rus.:*** Cutivate (Кутивейт); Flixonase (Фликсоназе); Flixotide (Фликсотид); Seretide (Серетид); ***S.Afr.:*** Cutivate; Flixonase; Flixotide; Flohale DP; Flomist; ***Singapore:*** Cutivate; Flixonase; Flixotide; ***Spain:*** Flixonase; Flixotide; Fluinol; Flusonal; Inalacor; Rinosone; Rontilona; Trialona; ***Swed.:*** Flutide; Flutivate; ***Switz.:*** Axotide; Cutivate; Flutinase; ***Thai.:*** Flixonase; Flixotide; ***Turk.:*** Brethal; Cutivate; Flixonase; Flixotide; ***UAE:*** Potencort; ***UK:*** Cutivate; Flixonase; Flixotide; Nasofan; ***USA:*** Cutivate; Flonase; Flovent; Veramyst; ***Venez.:*** Cutivate; Flixonase; Flixotide; Fluticort.

Multi-ingredient: ***Arg.:*** Flutivent; Neumotide; Seretide; ***Austral.:*** Seretide; ***Austria:*** Seretide; Viani; ***Belg.:*** Seretide; ***Braz.:*** Seretide; ***Canad.:*** Advair; ***Chile:*** Aerometrol Plus; Aurituss; Brexotide; Seretide; ***Cz.:*** Seretide; ***Denm.:*** Seretide; ***Fin.:*** Seretide; ***Fr.:*** Seretide; ***Ger.:*** Atmadisc; Viani; ***Gr.:*** Seretide; ***Hong Kong:*** Seretide; ***Hung.:*** Seretide; Thoreus; ***India:*** Duonase; Forair; Seretide; Seroflo; ***Indon.:*** Seretide; ***Irl.:*** Seretide; ***Israel:*** Seretide; ***Ital.:*** Aliflus; Seretide; ***Malaysia:*** Seretide; ***Mex.:*** Seretide; ***Neth.:*** Seretide; Viani; ***Norw.:*** Seretide; ***NZ:*** Seretide; ***Philipp.:*** Seretide; ***Pol.:*** Seretide; ***Port.:*** Brisomax; Maizar; Seretaide; Veraspir; ***S.Afr.:*** Seretide; ***Singapore:*** Seretide; ***Spain:*** Anasma; Brisair; Inaladuo; Plusvent; Seretide; ***Swed.:*** Seretide; ***Switz.:*** Seretide; ***Thai.:*** Seretide; ***Turk.:*** Seretide; ***UK:*** Seretide; ***USA:*** Advair; ***Venez.:*** Seretide.

F

Follicle-stimulating Hormone

Other names: Folitropina; FSH.

Clinical profile: Follicle-stimulating hormone (FSH) is a gonadotrophic hormone secreted by the anterior lobe of the pituitary gland with luteinising hormone (LH). Gonadotrophic substances with LH and/or FSH activity are used in the treatment of fertility disorders, chiefly in females but also in males.

Follitropin Alfa

Other names: Folitropin Alfa; Folitropina alfa; Follitropine Alfa; Follitropinum Alfa.

Фоллитропин Альфа

Clinical profile: Follitropin alfa is a recombinant form of follicle-stimulating hormone (FSH).

Follitropin Beta

Other names: Folitropin Beta; Folitropina beta; Follitropine Bêta; Follitropinum Beta; Org-32489.

Фоллитропин Бета

Clinical profile: Follitropin beta is a recombinant form of follicle-stimulating hormone (FSH).

WADA Status: Banned in and out of competition

WADA Class: Hormones and Related Substances: Gonadotrophins

Includes gonadotrophin or a substance with a similar chemical structure or similar biological effect(s), or one of their releasing factors. Prohibited in males only.

Preparations

Single ingredient: ***Arg.:*** Gonal-F; Puregon; ***Austral.:*** Gonal-F; Puregon; ***Austria:*** Gonal-F; Puregon; ***Belg.:*** Gonal-F; Puregon; ***Braz.:*** Puregon; ***Canad.:*** Gonal-F; Puregon; ***Chile:*** Puregon; ***Cz.:*** Gonal-F; Puregon; ***Denm.:*** Gonal-F; Puregon; ***Fin.:*** Gonal-F; Puregon; ***Fr.:*** Gonal-F; Puregon; ***Ger.:*** Gonal-F; Puregon; ***Gr.:*** Gonal-F; Puregon; ***Hong Kong:*** Gonal-F; Puregon; ***Hung.:*** Gonal-F; Puregon; ***India:*** Gonal-F; ***Indon.:*** Gonal-F; Puregon; ***Irl.:*** Gonal-F; Puregon; ***Israel:*** Gonal-F; Puregon; ***Ital.:*** Gonal-F; Puregon; ***Malaysia:*** Gonal-F; Puregon; ***Mex.:*** Gonal-F; Puregon; ***Neth.:*** Gonal-F; Puregon; ***Norw.:*** Gonal-F; Puregon; ***NZ:*** Gonal-F; Puregon; ***Philipp.:*** Gonal-f; Puregon; ***Pol.:*** Gonal-F; Puregon; ***Port.:*** Gonal-F; Puregon; ***Rus.:*** Gonal-F (Гонал-Ф); Puregon (Пурегон); ***S.Afr.:*** Gonal-F; ***Singapore:*** Gonal-F; Puregon; ***Spain:*** Gonal-F; Puregon; ***Swed.:*** Gonal-F; Puregon; ***Switz.:*** Gonal-F; Puregon; ***Thai.:*** Gonal-F; Puregon; ***Turk.:*** Gonal-F; Puregon; ***UK:*** Gonal-F; Puregon; ***USA:*** Follistim; Gonal-F; ***Venez.:*** Gonal-F; Puregon.

Multi-ingredient: ***UK:*** Pergoveris.

F

Formebolone

Other names: Formebolona; Formébolone; Formebolonum; Formyldienolone.

Формеболон

Clinical profile: Formebolone has been used for its anabolic properties.

WADA Status: Banned in and out of competition

WADA Class: Anabolic; Androgenic Steroids (exogenous)

Includes exogenous anabolic androgenic steroids or other substances with a similar chemical structure or similar biological effect(s).

Formestane

Other names: CGP-32349; Formestaani; Formestan; Formestano; Formestanum; 4-Hydroxyandrostenedione; 4-OHA; 4-OHAD.

Форместан

Clinical profile: Formestane is an aromatase inhibitor used for its anti-oestrogenic properties in the endocrine treatment of breast cancer.

WADA Status: Banned in and out of competition

WADA Class: Hormone Antagonists and Modulators

Includes aromatase inhibitors.

Preparations
Single ingredient: ***Austria:*** Lentaron; ***Braz.:*** Lentaron; ***Cz.:*** Lentaron; ***Turk.:*** Lentaron.

Formocortal

Other names: FI-6341; Fluoroformylon; Formocortalum.

Формокортал

Clinical profile: Formocortal is a corticosteroid used in the topical treatment of inflammatory eye disorders.

WADA Status: Banned in competition

WADA Class: Glucocorticosteroids

All glucocorticosteroids are prohibited when administered orally, rectally, intravenously or intramuscularly. Their use requires a Therapeutic Use Exemption approval. Other routes of administration (intraarticular / periarticular / peritendinous / epidural / intradermal injections and inhalation) require an Abbreviated Therapeutic Use Exemption except as noted below.

Topical preparations when used for dermatological (including iontophoresis / phonophoresis), auricular, nasal, ophthalmic, buccal, gingival and perianal disorders are not prohibited and do not require any form of Therapeutic Use Exemption.

WADA Class: Specified Substances

Also listed as a specified substance.

"The prohibited List may identify specified substances which are particularly susceptible to unintentional anti-doping rule violations because of their general availability in medicinal products or which are less likely to be successfully abused as doping agents."

A doping violation involving such substances may result in a reduced sanction provided that the "...*Athlete can establish that the Use of such a specfied substance was not intended to enhance sport performance...*"

Preparations
Single ingredient: ***Ital.:*** Formoftil.
Multi-ingredient: ***Ital.:*** Formomicin.

Formoterol Fumarate

Other names: BD-40A; CGP-25827A; Eformoterol Fumarat; Eformoterol Fumarate; Formoterol Fumarat; Formotérol, fumarate de; Formoterolfumarat; Formoterol-fumarát; Formoteroli fumaras; Formoterolifumaraatti; Formoterolio fumaratas; Formoterolu fumaran; Fumarato de formoterol; YM-08316.

Формотерола Фумарат

Clinical profile: Formoterol fumarate is a long-acting selective beta$_2$-adrenoceptor agonist used for its bronchodilator properties in respiratory disorders such as asthma and chronic obstructive pulmonary disease.

WADA Status: Banned in and out of competition

WADA Class: Beta-2 Agonists

Includes beta-2 agonists or their isomers. Formoterol when administered by inhalation requires an abbreviated Therapeutic Use Exemption.

WADA Class: Specified Substances

Also listed as a specified substance.

"The prohibited List may identify specified substances which are particularly susceptible to

unintentional anti-doping rule violations because of their general availability in medicinal products or which are less likely to be successfully abused as doping agents."

A doping violation involving such substances may result in a reduced sanction provided that the "*...Athlete can establish that the Use of such a specfied substance was not intended to enhance sport performance...*"

Preparations
Single ingredient: ***Arg.:*** Fordilen; Oxis; Xanol; ***Austral.:*** Foradile; Oxis; ***Austria:*** Foradil; Oxis; ***Belg.:*** Foradil; Oxis; ***Braz.:*** Fluir; Foradil; Formocaps; Oxis; ***Canad.:*** Foradil; Oxeze; ***Cz.:*** Foradil; Oxis; ***Denm.:*** Delnil; Foradil; Oxis; ***Fin.:*** Foradil; Oxis; ***Fr.:*** Foradil; ***Ger.:*** Foradil; Forair; Formatris; FormoLich; Formotop; Oxis; ***Gr.:*** Broncoteril; Foradil; Forair; Forcap; Formopen; Formotil; Imotec; Oxez; ***Hong Kong:*** Oxis; ***Hung.:*** Atimos; Diffumax; Foradil; Fortofan; Oxis; ***India:*** Foratec; ***Irl.:*** Foradil; Oxis; ***Israel:*** Foradil; Oxis; ***Ital.:*** Atimos; Eolus; Foradil; Liferol; Oxis; ***Jpn:*** Atock; ***Malaysia:*** Foradil; Oxis; ***Mex.:*** Foradil; Oxis; ***Neth.:*** Foradil; Oxis; ***Norw.:*** Foradil; Oxis; ***NZ:*** Foradil; Oxis; ***Philipp.:*** Atock; Foradil; Oxis; ***Pol.:*** Atimos; Diffumax; Foradil; Forastmin; Oxis; Oxodil; Zafiron; ***Port.:*** Asmatec; Foradil; Oxis; ***Rus.:*** Atimos (Атимос); Foradil (Форадил); Oxis (Оксис); ***S.Afr.:*** Foradil; Foratec; Oxis; ***Singapore:*** Foradil; Oxis; ***Spain:*** Broncoral; Foradil; Neblik; Oxis; ***Swed.:*** Foradil; Oxis; ***Switz.:*** Foradil; Oxis; ***Turk.:*** Foradil; Oxis; ***UK:*** Atimos Modulite; Foradil; Oxis; ***USA:*** Foradil; Perforomist; ***Venez.:*** Fluir; Foradil; Formotec.

Multi-ingredient: ***Arg.:*** Neumoterol; Symbicort; ***Austral.:*** Symbicort; ***Austria:*** Symbicort; ***Belg.:*** Symbicort; ***Braz.:*** Alenia; Foraseq; Symbicort; ***Canad.:*** Symbicort; ***Chile:*** Symbicort; ***Cz.:*** Symbicort; ***Denm.:*** Symbicort; ***Fin.:*** Symbicort; ***Fr.:*** Symbicort; ***Ger.:*** Symbicort; ***Gr.:*** Symbicort; ***Hong Kong:*** Symbicort; ***Hung.:*** Symbicort; ***India:*** Duova; Foracort; ***Indon.:*** Symbicort; ***Irl.:*** Symbicort; ***Israel:*** Symbicort; ***Ital.:*** Assieme; Sinestic; Symbicort; ***Malaysia:*** Symbicort; ***Mex.:*** Symbicort; ***Neth.:*** Assieme; Sinestic; Symbicort; ***Norw.:*** Symbicort; ***NZ:*** Symbicort; ***Philipp.:*** Symbicort; ***Pol.:*** Symbicort; ***Port.:*** Assieme; Symbicort; ***Rus.:*** Simbicort (Симбикорт); ***S.Afr.:*** Symbicord; ***Singapore:*** Symbicort; ***Spain:*** Rilast; Symbicort; ***Swed.:*** Symbicort; ***Switz.:*** Symbicort; ***Thai.:*** Symbicort; ***Turk.:*** Symbicort; ***UK:*** Fostair; Symbicort; ***USA:*** Symbicort; ***Venez.:*** Foraseq; Symbicort.

Fulvestrant

Other names: Fulvestrantum; ICI-182780; ZD-9238.

Фульвестрант

Clinical profile: Fulvestrant is an oestrogen antagonist that downregulates the oestrogen receptor and is used for the treatment of locally advanced or metastatic breast cancer in postmenopausal women.

WADA Status: Banned in and out of competition

WADA Class: Hormone Antagonists and Modulators: Other Anti-estrogenic Substances
Includes other anti-estrogenic substances not listed elsewhere.

Preparations
Single ingredient: ***Arg.:*** Faslodex; ***Belg.:*** Faslodex; ***Braz.:*** Faslodex; ***Canad.:*** Faslodex; ***Denm.:*** Faslodex; ***Fin.:*** Faslodex; ***Fr.:*** Faslodex; ***Ger.:*** Faslodex; ***Gr.:*** Faslodex; ***Hung.:*** Faslodex; ***Irl.:*** Faslodex; ***Israel:*** Faslodex; ***Ital.:*** Faslodex; ***Mex.:*** Faslodex; ***Neth.:*** Faslodex; ***Norw.:*** Faslodex; ***NZ:*** Faslodex; ***Pol.:*** Faslodex; ***Port.:*** Faslodex; ***Rus.:*** Faslodex (Фазлодекс); ***Spain:*** Faslodex; ***Swed.:*** Faslodex; ***Switz.:*** Faslodex; ***UK:*** Faslodex; ***USA:*** Faslodex; ***Venez.:*** Faslodex.

Furazabol

Other names: Androfurazanol; Furazabolum.

Фуразабол

Clinical profile: Furazabol has been used for its anabolic properties.

WADA Status: Banned in and out of competition

WADA Class: Anabolic; Androgenic Steroids (exogenous)

Includes exogenous anabolic androgenic steroids or other substances with a similar chemical structure or similar biological effect(s).

Furosemide

Other names: Frusemide; Furosemid; Furosemida; Furosémide; Furosemidi; Furosemidum; Furoszemid; Furozemidas; LB-502.

Фуросемид

Clinical profile: Furosemide is a potent loop diuretic. It is used in the treatment of oedema associated with heart failure and with renal and hepatic disorders, in the management of oliguria due to renal failure or insufficiency, and in the treatment of hypertension.

WADA Status: Banned in and out of competition

WADA Class: Diuretics and Other Masking Agents

Includes diuretics or substances with a similar chemical structure or similar biological effect(s).

Preparations

Single ingredient: ***Arg.:*** Errolon; Fabofurox; Furagrand; Furital; Furix; Fursemida; Furtenk; Kolkin; Lasix; Nuriban; Retep; ***Austral.:*** Frusehexal; Frusid; Lasix; Uremide; Urex; ***Austria:*** Fural; Furohexal; Furon; Furostad; Lasix; ***Belg.:*** Docfurose; Furotop; Lasix; ***Braz.:*** Diuremida; Diuret; Diurit; Diurix; Fluxil; Furesin; Furosan; Furosecord; Furosem; Furosen; Furosetron; Furosix; Furozix; Fursemida; Lasix; Neosemid; Normotensor; Urasix; ***Canad.:*** Lasix; Novo-Semide; ***Chile:*** Asax; ***Cz.:*** Dryptal; Furanthril; Furon; Furorese; Lasix; ***Denm.:*** Diural; Furese; Furix; Lasix; ***Fin.:*** Furesis; Furomin; Lasix; Vesix; ***Fr.:*** Lasilix; ***Ger.:*** Diurapid; Furanthril; Furo-Puren; Furo; Furobeta; Furogamma; Furomed; Furorese; Furosal; Fusid; Jufurix; Lasix; ***Gr.:*** Hydroflux; Lasix; Semid; ***Hong Kong:*** CP-Furo; Lasix; Naqua; Urex; ***Hung.:*** Furon; ***India:*** Diucontin-K; Frusemix; Frusenex; Frusix; Lasix; ***Indon.:*** Cetasix; Classic; Diurefo; Edemin; Farsix; Furosix; Impugan; Lasix; Uresix; ***Irl.:*** Fruside; Lasix; ***Israel:*** Fusid; Miphar; ***Ital.:*** Lasix; ***Malaysia:*** Dirine; Furmide; Lasix; Rasitol; ***Mex.:*** Butosali; Diurmessel; Edenol; Furosan; Henexal; Lasix; Osemin; Selectofur; Zafimida; ***Neth.:*** Lasiletten; Lasix; ***Norw.:*** Diural; Furix; Lasix; ***NZ:*** Diurin; Frusid; Lasix; ***Philipp.:*** Diuril; Diuspec; Edemann; Fremid; Fretic; Frusema; Furoscan; Fusimex; Lasix; Pharmix; Rofunil; ***Port.:*** Aquedux; Lasix; Naqua; ***Rus.:*** Lasix (Лазикс); ***S.Afr.:*** Aquarid; Beurises; Lasix; Puresis; Uretic; ***Singapore:*** Dirine; Furmide; Lasix; ***Spain:*** Seguril; ***Swed.:*** Furix; Impugan; Lasix; ***Switz.:*** Furodrix; Fursol; Lasix; Oedemex; ***Thai.:*** Dirine; Furetic; Furide; Furine; Fuseride; H-Mide; Lasiven; Lasix; ***Turk.:*** Desal; Furomid; Lasix; Lizik; Urex; ***UAE:*** Salurin; ***UK:*** Froop; Frusid; Frusol; Lasix; Rusyde; ***USA:*** Lasix; ***Venez.:*** Biosemida; Edemid; Inclens; Lasix; Lifurox; Salca; Terysol.

Multi-ingredient: ***Arg.:*** Aldactone-D; Diflux; Errolon A; Lasilacton; Lasiride; Nuriban A; ***Austria:*** Furo-Aldopur; Furo-Spirobene; Furolacton; Hydrotrix; Lasilacton; Lasitace; Spirono comp; ***Belg.:*** Frusamil; ***Braz.:*** Diurana; Diurisa; Hidrion; Lasilactona; ***Chile:*** Furdiuren; Hidrium; Hidropid; ***Cz.:*** Spiro Compositum; ***Denm.:*** Frusamil; ***Fin.:*** Furesis comp; ***Fr.:*** Aldalix; Logirene; ***Ger.:*** Betasemid; Diaphal; Furo-Aldopur; Furorese Comp; Hydrotrix; Osyrol Lasix; Spiro comp; Spiro-D; ***Gr.:*** Frumil; ***India:*** Frumil; Lasilactone; Spiromide; ***Irl.:*** Diumide-K Continus; Fru-Co; Frumil; ***Ital.:*** Fluss 40; Lasitone; Spirofur; ***Mex.:*** Lasilacton; ***NZ:*** Frumil; ***Philipp.:*** Diumide-K; ***Spain:*** Salidur; ***Switz.:*** Furocombin; Furospir; Lasilactone; ***UK:*** Aridil; Fru-Co; Frumil; Frusene; Komil; Lasikal; Lasilactone; ***Venez.:*** Furdiuren.

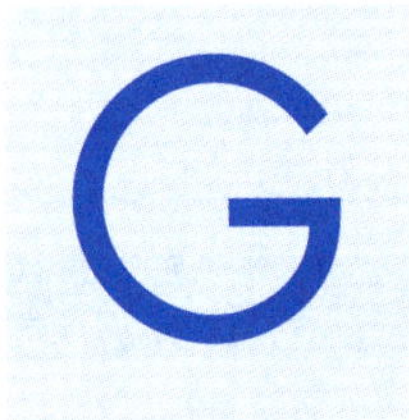

Gelatin

Other names: Gelatina; Gélatine; Liivate; Modifiye Jelatin; Želatina; Żelatyna; Zselatin.

Clinical profile: Gelatin is a protein used as a haemostatic in surgical procedures and as a plasma volume expander. It is an ingredient of preparations used for the protection of stoma and lesions. Gelatin is used in the preparation of pastes, pastilles, suppositories, tablets, and hard and soft capsule shells. It is also used for the microencapsulation of drugs and other industrial materials.

WADA Status: Banned in and out of competition

WADA Class: Diuretics and Other Masking Agents

Masking agents including alpha-reductase inhibitors or plasma expanders or substances with similar biological effect(s).

Preparations

Single ingredient: ***Arg.:*** Gelafundin; Geloplasma; Infukoll; ***Austral.:*** Gelfilm; Gelfoam; Gelofusine; ***Austria:*** Gelofusin; ***Braz.:*** Colagenan; Gelfoam; ***Canad.:*** Gelfilm; Gelfoam; ***Chile:*** Gelfoam; Gelofusine; Geloplasma; ***Cz.:*** Gelofusine; ***Fin.:*** Gelofusine; ***Fr.:*** Bloxang; Gel-Phan; Gelodiet; Hydrocoll; ***Ger.:*** Gelafundin; Gelafusal; Gelaspon; Gelastypt; Spongostan; stypro; ***Gr.:*** Gelofusine; ***Hong Kong:*** Gelofusine; ***Hung.:*** Gelofusine; ***Indon.:*** Gelafundin; ***Israel:*** Gelfoam; ***Ital.:*** Cutanplast; Eufusin; Gelofusine; Spongostan; ***Malaysia:*** Gelfoam; ***Neth.:*** Gelofusine; Geloplasma; ***NZ:*** Gelfilm; Gelfoam; Gelofusine; ***Philipp.:*** Gelfoam; ***Pol.:*** Gelofusine; ***Port.:*** Gelofusine; ***S.Afr.:*** Gelofusine; ***Singapore:*** Gelfoam; ***Switz.:*** Physiogel; ***Thai.:*** Gelafundin; Gelofusine; ***Turk.:*** Gelofusin; ***UK:*** Gelofusine; Volplex; ***USA:*** Gelfilm; Gelfoam; ***Venez.:*** Gelfoam; Gelofusine.
Multi-ingredient: ***Arg.:*** Megaplus; Mucobase; ***Austral.:*** Orabase; Orahesive; Stomahesive; ***Austria:*** Gelacet; ***Canad.:*** Tegasorb; ***Fr.:*** Plasmion; Rectopanbiline; ***Irl.:*** Orabase; ***Ital.:*** Solecin; ***Mex.:*** Gelafundin; ***NZ:*** Orabase; Stomahesive; ***Port.:*** Dagragel; Varihesive; ***S.Afr.:*** Granuflex; Orabase; ***UK:*** Orabase; Orahesive; Stomahesive; ***USA:*** Dome-Paste.

Gepefrine Tartrate

Other names: Gépéfrine, Tartrate de; Gepefrini Tartras; Tartrato de gepefrina. Гепефрина Тартрат

Clinical profile: Gepefrine tartrate is a sympathomimetic that has been used in the treatment of hypotensive states.

WADA Status: Banned in competition

WADA Class: Stimulants

Includes stimulants or substances with a similar chemical structure or similar biological effect(s).

WADA Class: Specified Substances

Also listed as a specified substance.

"The prohibited List may identify specified substances which are particularly susceptible to unintentional anti-doping rule violations because of their general availability in medicinal products or which are less likely to be successfully abused as doping agents."

A doping violation involving such substances may result in a reduced sanction provided that the "*...Athlete can establish that the Use of such a specfied substance was not intended to enhance sport performance...*"

Gestrinone

Other names: A-46745; Ethylnorgestrienone; Gestrinon; Gestrinona; Gestrinoni; Gestrinonum; R-2323; RU-2323.

Гестринон

Clinical profile: Gestrinone is a synthetic steroidal hormone reported to have androgenic, anti-oestrogenic, and anti-progestogenic properties. It is used in the treatment of endometriosis.

WADA Status: Banned in and out of competition

WADA Class: Anabolic; Androgenic Steroids (exogenous)

Includes exogenous anabolic androgenic steroids or other substances with a similar chemical structure or similar biological effect(s).

Preparations

Single ingredient: ***Arg.:*** Nemestran; ***Austral.:*** Dimetriose; ***Braz.:*** Dimetrose; ***Cz.:*** Nemestran; ***Ital.:*** Dimetrose; ***Malaysia:*** Dimetriose; ***Mex.:*** Nemestran; ***Neth.:*** Nemestran; ***NZ:*** Dimetriose; ***Port.:*** Dimetriose; ***S.Afr.:*** Tridomose; ***Singapore:*** Dimetriose; ***Switz.:*** Nemestran; ***Thai.:*** Dimetriose; ***UK:*** Dimetriose.

G

Gonadorelin

Other names: Follicle Stimulating Hormone-releasing Factor; GnRH; Gonadoliberin; Gonadoreliini; Gonadorelina; Gonadoréline; Gonadorelinum; Gonadotrophin-releasing Hormone; Hoe-471; LH/FSH-RF; LH/FSH-RH; LH-RF; LH-RH; Luliberin; Luteinising Hormone-releasing Factor.

Гонадорелин

Gonadorelin Acetate

Other names: Abbott-41070; Acetato de gonadorelina; Gonadolrelin-acetát; Gonadoreliiniasetaatti; Gonadorelinacetat; Gonadorelin-acetát; Gonadoréline, acétate de; Gonadorelini acetas; Gonadorelino acetatas.

Гонадорелина Ацетат

Gonadorelin Hydrochloride

Other names: AY-24031; Gonadoréline, Chlorhydrate de; Gonadorelini Hydrochloridum; Hidrocloruro de gonadorelina.

Гонадорелина Гидрохлорид

Clinical profile: Gonadorelin is a synthetic form of gonadotrophin-releasing hormone, used in the diagnosis of hypothalamic-pituitary-gonadal dysfunction and in the treatment of amenorrhoea and infertility associated with hypogonadotrophic hypogonadism.

WADA Status: Banned in and out of competition

WADA Class: Hormones and Related Substances: Gonadotrophins

Includes gonadotrophin or a substance with a similar chemical structure or similar biological effect(s), or one of their releasing factors. Prohibited in males only.

Preparations
Single ingredient: ***Arg.:*** Luteoliberina; ***Austria:*** Kryptocur; Lutrelef; Relefact LH-RH; ***Belg.:*** HRF; ***Braz.:*** Parlib; ***Canad.:*** Lutrepulse; ***Cz.:*** Relefact LH-RH; ***Fr.:*** Lutrelef; Stimu-LH; ***Ger.:*** Kryptocur; Lutrelef; Relefact LH-RH; ***Gr.:*** Relefact LH-RH; ***Irl.:*** HRF; ***Israel:*** Relefact LH-RH; ***Ital.:*** Kryptocur; Lutrelef; ***Neth.:*** Cryptocur; HRF; Lutrelef; Relefact LH-RH; ***S.Afr.:*** HRF; ***Swed.:*** Lutrelef; ***Switz.:*** Kryptocur; Lutrelef; ***UK:*** HRF; ***USA:*** Factrel.

Goserelin

Other names: Gosereliini; Goserelina; Goserelinas; Goséréline; Goserelinum; Goszerelin; ICI-118630.

Гозерелин

Goserelin Acetate

Other names: Acetato de goserelina; Goséréline, Acétate de; Goserelini Acetas; D-Ser $(Bu^t)^6$ $Azgly^{10}$-LHRH Acetate.

Гозерелина Ацетат

Clinical profile: Goserelin is an analogue of gonadorelin used in the treatment of malignant neoplasms of the prostate, in breast cancer in pre- and peri-menopausal women, in the management of endometriosis and uterine fibroids, and as an adjunct to ovulation induction in the treatment of infertility.

G

WADA Status: Banned in and out of competition

WADA Class: Hormones and Related Substances: Gonadotrophins

Includes gonadotrophin or a substance with a similar chemical structure or similar biological effect(s), or one of their releasing factors. Prohibited in males only.

Preparations
Single ingredient: ***Arg.:*** Larmadex; Zoladex; ***Austral.:*** Zoladex; ***Austria:*** Zoladex; ***Belg.:*** Zoladex; ***Braz.:*** Zoladex; ***Canad.:*** Zoladex; ***Chile:*** Vacromil; Zoladex; ***Cz.:*** Zoladex; ***Denm.:*** Zoladex; ***Fin.:*** Zoladex; ***Fr.:*** Zoladex; ***Ger.:*** Zoladex; ***Gr.:*** Zoladex; ***Hong Kong:*** Zoladex; ***Hung.:*** Zoladex; ***Indon.:*** Zoladex; ***Irl.:*** Zoladex; ***Israel:*** Zoladex; ***Ital.:*** Zoladex; ***Malaysia:*** Zoladex; ***Mex.:*** Zoladex; ***Neth.:*** Zoladex; ***Norw.:*** Zoladex; ***NZ:*** Zoladex; ***Philipp.:*** Zoladex; ***Pol.:*** Zoladex; ***Port.:*** Zoladex; ***Rus.:*** Zoladex (Золадекс); ***S.Afr.:*** Zoladex; ***Singapore:*** Zoladex; ***Spain:*** Zoladex; ***Swed.:*** Zoladex; ***Switz.:*** Zoladex; ***Thai.:*** Zoladex; ***Turk.:*** Zoladex; ***UK:*** Zoladex; ***USA:*** Zoladex; ***Venez.:*** Zoladex.

Growth Hormone

Other names: GH; Phyone; Somatotrophin; Somatotropin; Somatotropina; STH.

Гормон Роста; Соматотропин

Clinical profile: Growth hormone is an anabolic hormone secreted by the anterior lobe of the pituitary. It promotes growth of skeletal, muscular, and other tissues, stimulates protein anabolism, and affects fat and mineral metabolism. The hormone has a diabetogenic action on carbohydrate metabolism. The synthetic forms somatrem and somatropin are used in the treatment of growth retardation of various causes, and in adult growth hormone deficiency and HIV-associated cachexia.

Somatrem

Other names: Met-HGH; Methionyl Human Growth Hormone; Somatremum.

Соматрем

Clinical profile: Somatrem is a biosynthetic form of human growth hormone used in children with open epiphyses for the treatment of short stature due to pituitary dwarfism.

Somatropin

Other names: CB-311; HGH; Human Growth Hormone; LY-137998; Somatropiini; Somatropina; Somatropinas; Somatropine; Somatropinum; Szomatropin.

Соматропин

Clinical profile: Somatropin is a biosynthetic form of human growth hormone used in children with open epiphyses for the treatment of short stature due to pituitary dwarfism. It is also used in children with some other forms of growth retardation, for example in Turner's syndrome, SHOX (short stature homeobox-containing gene) deficiency, or due to chronic renal insufficiency, in short children born small for gestational age and in idiopathic short stature, as well as for Prader-Willi syndrome, adult growth hormone deficiency, and HIV-associated cachexia.

WADA Status: Banned in and out of competition

WADA Class: Hormones and Related Substances: Growth Hormone, Insulin-like Growth Factors, Mechano Growth Factors
Includes growth hormone or insulin-like growth factors or mechano growth factor or substances with a similar chemical structure or similar biological effect(s), or one of their releasing factors.

G

Preparations
Single ingredient: ***Arg.:*** Biotropin; Genotropin; HHT; Hutrope; Norditropin; Saizen; ***Austral.:*** Genotropin; Humatro-Pen; Humatrope; Norditropin; Omnitrope; Saizen; Scitropin; ***Austria:*** Genotropin; Humatrope; Norditropin; NutropinAq; Saizen; Zomacton; ***Belg.:*** Genotonorm; Humatrope; Norditropin; NutropinAq; Zomacton; ***Braz.:*** Genotropin; Hormotrop; Humatrope; Norditropin; Saizen; Somatrop; ***Canad.:*** Humatrope; Nutropin; Saizen; Serostim; ***Chile:*** Genotonorm; HHT; Humatrope; Hutrope; Norditropin; ***Cz.:*** Genotropin; Humatrope; Norditropin; Saizen; Zomacton; ***Denm.:*** Genotropin; Humatrope; Norditropin; NutropinAq; Zomacton; ***Fin.:*** Genotropin; Humatrope; Norditropin; NutropinAq; Saizen; Zomacton; ***Fr.:*** Genotonorm; Maxomat; Norditropine; NutropinAq; Saizen; Umatrope; Zomacton; ***Ger.:*** Genotropin; Humatrope; Norditropin; NutropinAq; Saizen; Zomacton; ***Gr.:*** Genotropin; Humatrope; Norditropin; Nutropin; Saizen; Zomacton; ***Hong Kong:*** Genotropin; Humatrope; Norditropin; Saizen; Scitropin; Serostim; ***Hung.:*** Genotropin; Humatrope; Norditropin; Nutropin; ***India:*** Saizen; ***Indon.:*** Eutropin; Genotropin; Norditropin; Saizen; ***Irl.:*** Genotropin; Norditropin; Saizen; Zomacton; ***Israel:*** Bio-Tropin; Genotropin; Norditropin; ***Ital.:*** Genotropin; Humatrope; Norditropin; Nutropin; Saizen; Zomacton; ***Jpn:*** Growject; Norditropin; ***Malaysia:*** Genotropin; Norditropin; Saizen; ***Mex.:*** Cryo-Tropin; Genotropin; HHT; Humatrope; Norditropin; Saizen; Serostim; ***Neth.:*** Genotropin; Humatrope; Norditropin; Nutropin; Zomacton; ***Norw.:*** Genotropin; Humatrope; Norditropin; NutropinAq; Saizen; Zomacton; ***NZ:*** Genotropin; Norditropin; Saizen; ***Philipp.:*** Gen-Heal; Humatrope; Norditropin; Saizen; SciTropin; ***Pol.:*** Genotropin; ***Port.:*** Genotropin; Humatrope; Norditropin; Saizen; ***Rus.:*** Genotropin (Генотропин); Humatrope (Хуматроп); Norditropin (Нордитропин); Saizen (Сайзен); ***S.Afr.:*** Genotropin; Humatrope; Norditropin; ***Singapore:*** Genotropin; Norditropin; Saizen; ***Spain:*** Genotonorm; Humatrope; Norditropin; Nutropin; Saizen; Zomacton; ***Swed.:*** Genotropin; Humatrope; Norditropin; NutropinAq; Saizen; Zomacton; ***Switz.:*** Genotropin; Humatrope; Norditropine; Saizen; ***Thai.:*** Saizen; ***Turk.:*** Genotropin; Humatrope; Norditropin; Saizen; Zomacton; ***UK:*** Genotropin; Humatrope; Norditropin; Nutropin; Saizen; Zomacton; ***USA:*** Genotropin; Humatrope; Norditropin; Nutropin; Omnitrope; Saizen; Serostim; Tev-Tropin; Zorbtive; ***Venez.:*** Genotropin; Humatrope; Saizen.

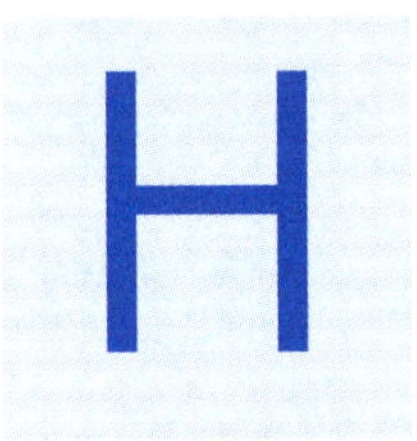

Haemoglobin

Other names: Hemoglobina.

Hemoglobin Glutamer

Other names: Haemoglobin Glutamer; Hemoglobina glutámero; Hémoglobine Glutamère; Hemoglobinum Glutamerum.

Гемоглобин Глутамер

Clinical profile: Haemoglobin has the property of reversible oxygenation and is the respiratory pigment of blood. Solutions of haemoglobin or modified haemoglobin are being investigated as blood substitutes.

WADA Status: Banned in and out of competition

WADA Class: Enhancement of Oxygen Transfer: Artificial Enhancers

Includes products that may be used to artificially enhance the uptake, transport, or delivery of oxygen.

Preparations
Single ingredient: ***S.Afr.:*** Hemopure.
Multi-ingredient: ***India:*** Blosyn; Haem Up.

Halcinonide

Other names: Alcinonide; Halcinonid; Halcinónida; Halcinonidum; Halsinonid; Halsinonidi; SQ-18566.

Гальцинонид

Clinical profile: Halcinonide is a corticosteroid used topically in the treatment of various skin disorders.

WADA Status: Banned in competition

WADA Class: Glucocorticosteroids

All glucocorticosteroids are prohibited when administered orally, rectally, intravenously or intramuscularly. Their use requires a Therapeutic Use Exemption approval. Other routes of administration (intraarticular / periarticular / peritendinous / epidural / intradermal injections and inhalation) require an Abbreviated Therapeutic Use Exemption except as noted below.

Topical preparations when used for dermatological (including iontophoresis / pho-

nophoresis), auricular, nasal, ophthalmic, buccal, gingival and perianal disorders are not prohibited and do not require any form of Therapeutic Use Exemption.

WADA Class: Specified Substances

Also listed as a specified substance.

"The prohibited List may identify specified substances which are particularly susceptible to unintentional anti-doping rule violations because of their general availability in medicinal products or which are less likely to be successfully abused as doping agents."

A doping violation involving such substances may result in a reduced sanction provided that the "*...Athlete can establish that the Use of such a specfied substance was not intended to enhance sport performance...*"

Preparations

Single ingredient: ***Austria:*** Halog; ***Braz.:*** Halog; ***Canad.:*** Halog; ***Cz.:*** Betacorton; ***Hong Kong:*** Halog; ***India:*** Cortilate; ***Indon.:*** Halog; ***Ital.:*** Halciderm; ***Mex.:*** Dermalog; ***Spain:*** Halog; ***Switz.:*** Betacortone; ***Turk.:*** Volog; ***USA:*** Halog; ***Venez.:*** Halog.

Multi-ingredient: ***Cz.:*** Betacorton S; Betacorton U; ***India:*** Cobederm-H; Cortilate-S; ***Ital.:*** Anfocort; Halciderm Combi; Halciderm; ***Mex.:*** Dermalog-C; ***Switz.:*** Betacortone S; Betacortone; ***Turk.:*** Betacorton; ***Venez.:*** Halcicomb; Halog.

Halometasone

Other names: C-48401-Ba; Halometason; Halometasona; Halométasone; Halometasoni; Halometasonum; Halometazon; Halomethasone.

Галометазон

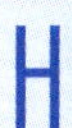

Clinical profile: Halometasone is a corticosteroid used topically in the treatment of various skin disorders.

WADA Status: Banned in competition

WADA Class: Glucocorticosteroids

All glucocorticosteroids are prohibited when administered orally, rectally, intravenously or intramuscularly. Their use requires a Therapeutic Use Exemption approval. Other routes of administration (intraarticular / periarticular / peritendinous / epidural / intradermal injections and inhalation) require an Abbreviated Therapeutic Use Exemption except as noted below.

Topical preparations when used for dermatological (including iontophoresis / phonophoresis), auricular, nasal, ophthalmic, buccal, gingival and perianal disorders are not prohibited and do not require any form of Therapeutic Use Exemption.

WADA Class: Specified Substances

Also listed as a specified substance.

"The prohibited List may identify specified substances which are particularly susceptible to unintentional anti-doping rule violations because of their general availability in medicinal products or which are less likely to be successfully abused as doping agents."

A doping violation involving such substances may result in a reduced sanction provided that the "*...Athlete can establish that the Use of such a specfied substance was not intended to enhance sport performance...*"

Preparations
Single ingredient: ***Austria:*** Sicorten; ***Hong Kong:*** Sicorten; ***Port.:*** Sicorten; ***Spain:*** Sicorten; ***Switz.:*** Sicorten; ***Turk.:*** Sicorten.
Multi-ingredient: ***Ger.:*** Sicorten Plus; ***Port.:*** Sicorten Plus; ***Spain:*** Sicorten Plus; ***Switz.:*** Sicorten Plus.

Heptaminol Hydrochloride

Other names: Heptaminol, Chlorhydrate d'; Heptaminol, chlorhydrate de; Heptaminol hydrochlorid; Heptaminol-hidroklorid; Heptaminolhydroklorid; Heptaminoli hydrochloridum; Heptaminolihydrokloridi; Heptaminolio hidrochloridas; Hidrocloruro de heptaminol; RP-2831.

Гептаминола Гидрохлорид

Clinical profile: Heptaminol hydrochloride is a cardiac stimulant and vasodilator and has been used in the treatment of cardiovascular disorders.

WADA Status: Banned in competition

WADA Class: Stimulants

Includes heptaminol and any optical isomers.

WADA Class: Specified Substances

Also listed as a specified substance.

"The prohibited List may identify specified substances which are particularly susceptible to unintentional anti-doping rule violations because of their general availability in medicinal products or which are less likely to be successfully abused as doping agents."

A doping violation involving such substances may result in a reduced sanction provided that the "*...Athlete can establish that the Use of such a specfied substance was not intended to enhance sport performance...*"

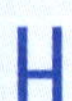

Preparations
Single ingredient: ***Fr.:*** Ampecyclal; Hept-A-Myl; ***Indon.:*** Hept-a-myl.
Multi-ingredient: ***Arg.:*** Flebitol; ***Cz.:*** Ginkor Fort; ***Fr.:*** Debrumyl; Ginkor Fort; ***Hong Kong:*** Ginkor Fort; ***Hung.:*** Ginkor Fort; ***Malaysia:*** Ginkor Fort; ***Port.:*** Debrumyl; Forticol; ***Rus.:*** Ginkor Fort (Гинкор Форт); ***Spain:*** Denubil; ***Thai.:*** Ginkor Fort.

Hexoprenaline Hydrochloride

Other names: Hexoprénaline, Chlorhydrate d'; Hexoprenalini Hydrochloridum; Hidrocloruro de hexoprenalina; ST-1512.

Гексопреналина Гидрохлорид

Hexoprenaline Sulfate

Other names: Hexoprénaline, Sulfate d'; Hexoprenaline Sulphate; Hexoprenalini Sulfas; Sulfato de hexoprenalina.

Гексопреналина Сульфат

Clinical profile: Hexoprenaline is a direct-acting sympathomimetic with a selective action on beta$_2$ adrenoceptors. It has been used as a bronchodilator in the management of respiratory disorders such as asthma and chronic obstructive pulmonary disease. It has also been given to arrest premature labour.

WADA Status: Banned in and out of competition

WADA Class: Beta-2 Agonists

Includes beta-2 agonists or their isomers.

WADA Class: Specified Substances

Also listed as a specified substance.

"The prohibited List may identify specified substances which are particularly susceptible to unintentional anti-doping rule violations because of their general availability in medicinal products or which are less likely to be successfully abused as doping agents."

A doping violation involving such substances may result in a reduced sanction provided that the *"...Athlete can establish that the Use of such a specfied substance was not intended to enhance sport performance..."*

Preparations
Single ingredient: ***Arg.:*** Argocian; ***Austria:*** Gynipral; Ipradol; ***Cz.:*** Gynipral; ***Hong Kong:*** Ipradol; ***Rus.:*** Gynipral (Гинипрал); ***S.Afr.:*** Ipradol; ***Switz.:*** Gynipral.

Histrelin

Other names: Histrelina; Histréline; Histrelinum; ORF-17070; RWJ-17070.
Гистрелин

Histrelin Acetate

Other names: Acetato de histrelina; Histréline, Acétate d'; Histrelini Acetas.
Гистрелина Ацетат

Clinical profile: Histrelin is a synthetic analogue of gonadorelin used in the treatment of precocious puberty and malignant neoplasms of the prostate. It has been investigated in various other disorders, including menstrual disorders and acute porphyrias.

WADA Status: Banned in and out of competition

WADA Class: Hormones and Related Substances: Gonadotrophins

Includes gonadotrophin or a substance with a similar chemical structure or similar biological effect(s), or one of their releasing factors. Prohibited in males only.

Preparations
Single ingredient: ***USA:*** Supprelin; Vantas.

Human Menopausal Gonadotrophins

Other names: Gonadotropina menopáusica humana; HMG; Org-31338; Urogonadotrophin.

Clinical profile: Human menopausal gonadotrophins such as menotrophin are extracted from the urine of postmenopausal women and have both luteinising hormone and follicle-stimulating hormone activity. They are given in the treatment of male and female infertility.

Menotrophin

Other names: Menotropiini; Menotropin; Menotropina; Menotropins; Menotropinum.

Clinical profile: Menotrophin is a gonadotrophin extracted from the urine of postmenopausal women and having both luteinising hormone and follicle-stimulating hormone activity. It is used in the treatment of male and female infertility.

WADA Status: Banned in and out of competition

WADA Class: Hormones and Related Substances: Gonadotrophins

Includes gonadotrophin or a substance with a similar chemical structure or similar biological effect(s), or one of their releasing factors. Prohibited in males only.

Preparations

Single ingredient: ***Arg.:*** HMG Ferring; Lifecell; Menopur; ***Austral.:*** Humegon; ***Austria:*** Menopur; ***Belg.:*** Menopur; ***Braz.:*** Menogon; Menopur; Pergonal; ***Canad.:*** Repronex; ***Chile:*** Menopur; ***Cz.:*** Humegon; Menogon; Merional; ***Denm.:*** Menopur; ***Fin.:*** Menopur; ***Fr.:*** Menopur; ***Ger.:*** Menogon; ***Gr.:*** Altermon; Menogon; Menopur; Merional; ***Hong Kong:*** Menogon; Menopur; Merional; Pergonal; ***Hung.:*** Menopur; Merional; ***India:*** Eventin; Pergonal; Pregnorm; ***Irl.:*** Humegon; Menopur; ***Israel:*** Menogon; Menopur; ***Ital.:*** Menogon; Meropur; ***Jpn:*** Gonadoryl; ***Mex.:*** Merapur HP; Merional; ***Neth.:*** Humegon; Menogon; Menopur; ***Norw.:*** Menopur; ***Pol.:*** Menopur; ***Port.:*** Humegon; ***Rus.:*** Menogon (Меногон); Menopur (Менопур); Pergonal (Пергонал); ***Singapore:*** Menogon; ***Spain:*** HMG; Menopur; ***Swed.:*** Menopur; ***Switz.:*** Menopur; Merional; ***Thai.:*** IVF-M; Menogon; ***Turk.:*** Menogon; Pergonal; ***UK:*** Menopur; ***USA:*** Humegon; Menopur; Repronex.

Hydrochlorothiazide

Other names: Hidrochlorotiazidas; Hidroclorotiazida; Hidroklorotiazid; Hydrochlorothiazid; Hydrochlorothiazidum; Hydrochlorotiazyd; Hydroklooritiatsidi; Hydroklortiazid.

Гидрохлоротиазид

Clinical profile: Hydrochlorothiazide is a thiazide diuretic used in the treatment of oedema, including that associated with heart failure and with renal and hepatic disorders, in the treatment of hypertension, in the treatment of nephrogenic diabetes insipidus, and in the prevention of renal calculus formation in patients with hypercalciuria.

WADA Status: Banned in and out of competition

WADA Class: Diuretics and Other Masking Agents

Includes diuretics or substances with a similar chemical structure or similar biological effect(s).

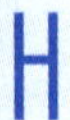

Preparations

Single ingredient: ***Arg.:*** Diural; Diurex; Tandiur; ***Austral.:*** Dithiazide; ***Austria:*** Esidrex; ***Braz.:*** Clorana; Clorizin; Co-Enaprotec; Diurepina; Diuretic; Diuretil; Diurezin; Drenol; Hidroclorana; Hidroclorozil; Hidrofall; Hidrolan; Mictrin; Neo Hidroclor; ***Canad.:*** Apo-Hydro; Novo-Hydrazide; ***Chile:*** Hidroronol; ***Fin.:*** Hydrex; ***Fr.:*** Esidrex; ***Ger.:*** Disalunil; diu-melusin; Esidrix; HCT-Beta; HCT-gamma; HCT-ISIS; HCT; HCTad; ***Hong Kong:*** Hydrozide; ***Hung.:*** Hypothiazid; ***India:*** Aquazide; BPzide; Hydrazide; Selopres; ***Indon.:*** HCT; Lodoz; ***Israel:*** Disothiazide; ***Ital.:*** Esidrex; ***Malaysia:*** Apo-Hydro; Hydrozide; ***Mex.:*** Rofucal; ***Norw.:*** Esidrex; ***Port.:*** Dichlotride; ***Rus.:*** Hypothiazid (Гипотиазид); ***S.Afr.:*** Hexazide; Ridaq; ***Singapore:*** Apo-Hydro; Di-Ertride; Hydrozide; ***Spain:*** Acuretic; Esidrex; Hidrosaluretil; ***Swed.:*** Esidrex; ***Switz.:*** Esidrex; ***Thai.:*** Dichlotride; Hychlozide; Hydrozide; ***USA:*** HydroDiuril; Microzide; Mictrin; ***Venez.:*** Di-Eudrin.

Multi-ingredient: ***Arg.:*** Accuretic; Adana Plus; Aldazida; Atacand-D; Avapro HCT; Carvedil D; Co-Renitec; CoAprovel; Corbis D; Cozaarex D; Dacten D; Defluin Plus; Diovan D; Diovan Triple; Diur Pot; Diurex A; Fabotensil D; Fensartan D; Gadopril D; Gliosartan Plus; Gliotenzide; Hidrenox A; Kinfil D; Klosartan D; Loctenk D; Loplac-D; Losacor D; Lotrial D; Maxen D; Micardis Plus; Moduretic; Niten D; Paxon-D; Plenacor D; Presi Regul D; Presinor D; Ren-Ur; Simultan D; Tacardia D; Tencas D; Tensopril D; Tiadyl Plus; Tritace-HCT; Vapresan Diur; Vericordin Compuesto; Zestoretic; Ziac; ***Austral.:*** Accuretic; Amizide; Atacand Plus; Avapro HCT; Hydrene; Karvezide; Micardis Plus; Moduretic; Monoplus; Olmetec Plus; Renitec Plus; Teveten Plus; ***Austria:*** Accuzide; Acecomb; Acelisino comp; Aceplus; Aldoretic; Amiloral/HCT; Amiloretik; Amilorid comp; Amilostad HCT; Atacand Plus; Beloc comp; Bisocombin; Bisoprolol comp; Bisoprolol-HCT; Bisostad plus; Blopress Plus; Capozide; Captohexal Comp; Captopril Compositum; Captopril-HCT; Co-Acetan; Co-Angiosan; Co-Captopril; Co-Dilatrend; Co-Diovan; Co-Enac; Co-Enalapril; Co-Enaran; Co-Hypomed; Co-Lisinostad; Co-Mepril; Co-Renitec; Concor Plus; Confit; Corenistad; Cosaar Plus; Darbalan Plus; Deverol mit Thiazid; Dilaplus; Dytide H; Enalapril Comp; Enalapril/HCT; Fempress Plus; Fosicomb; Hypren plus; Inhibace Plus; Lannapril plus; Lanuretic; Lisihexal comb; Lisinocomp; Lisinopril comp; Loradur; Metoprolol compositum; MicardisPlus; Moducrin; Moduretic; Nanalan Plus; Ramicomp; Ramipharm comb; Renitec Plus; Rivacor Plus; Salodiur; Seloken retard Plus; Supracid; Synerpril; Teveten Plus; Triamteren comp; Triastad HCT; Triloc; Trioral/HCT; Tritazide; Zestoretic; ***Belg.:*** Accuretic; Atacand Plus; Co-Amiloride; Co-Bisoprolol; Co-Diovane; Co-Enalapril; Co-Inhibace; Co-Lisinopril; Co-Quinapril; Co-Renitec; CoAprovel; Cozaar Plus; Docspirochlor; Dytenzide; Emcoretic; Kinzalkomb; Lodoz; Loortan Plus; Maxsoten; Merck-Co-Bisoprolol; Merck-Co-Lisinopril; Micardis Plus; Moduretic; Olmetec Plus; Sectrazide; Selozide;

Teveten Plus; Tritazide; Zestoretic; Zok-Zid; **Braz.:** Ablok Plus; Adelfan-Esidrex; Aldazida; Amiretic; Aprozide; Aradois H; Atacand HCT; Atens H; Biconcor; Capox H; Captotec + HCT; Co-Pressoless; Co-Pressotec; Co-Renitec; Corus H; Cotareg; Diovan HCT; Duopril; Enatec F; Eupressin H; Gliotenzide; Hidropril; Hydromet; Hyzaar; Iguassina; Lisinoretic; Lisoclor; Lisonotec; Lopril; Lorsar + HCT; Lotensin H; Micardis HCT; Moduretic; Monoplus; Naprix D; Neopress; Polol-H; Prinzide; Pritor HCT; Pryltec-H; Selopress; Tenadren; Torlos H; Triatec D; Vascase Plus; Vasopril Plus; Zestoretic; **Canad.:** Accuretic; Aldactazide; Apo-Amilzide; Apo-Methazide; Apo-Triazide; Atacand Plus; Avalide; Diovan HCT; Gen-Amilazide; Hyzaar; Inhibace Plus; Micardis Plus; Moduret; Novamilor; Novo-Spirozine; Novo-Triamzide; Nu-Amilzide; Nu-Triazide; PMS-Dopazide; Prinzide; Teveten Plus; Vaseretic; Viskazide; Zestoretic; **Chile:** Accuretic; Acerdil-D; Aratan D; Bajaten D; Bilaten-D; Blopress D; Blox-D; CoAprovel; Corodin D; Drinamil; Enalten D; Enalten DN; Esalfon-D; Grifopril-D; Hidroronol T; Hiperson-D; Hyzaar; Inhibace Plus; Losapres-D; Lotrial D; Micardis Plus; Monopril Plus; Normaten Plus; Normaten; Sanipresin-D; Simperten-D; Tareg-D; Tonotensil D; Uren; Valaplex-D; Vartalan D; Ziac; **Cz.:** Accuzide; Amilorid/HCT; Apo-Amilzide; Atacand Plus; Captohexal Comp; Co-Diovan; CoAprovel; Concor Plus; Enap-H; Enap-HL; Hyzaar; Limorid; Loradur; Moduretic; Rhefluin; Tritazide; **Denm.:** Amilco; AtacandZid; Atazid; Capozid; CoAprovel; Corodil Comp; Cozaar Comp; Diovan Comp; Enacozid; Fortzaar; Lisinoplus; MicardisPlus; Sparkal; Synerpril; Teveten Comp; Triatec Comp; Zestoretic; Zok-Zid; **Fin.:** Accupro Comp; Amitrid; Atacand Plus; Bisoprolol Comp; Cardace Comp; Cozaar Comp; Diovan Comp; Diuramin; Diurex; Emconcor Comp; Enalapril Comp; Kinzalkomb; Linatil Comp; Lisipril Comp; MicardisPlus; Miloride; Moduretic; Orloc Comp; Renitec Comp; Renitec Plus; Selocomp ZOC; Sparkal; Teveten Comp; Vivatec Comp; **Fr.:** Acuilix; Alteisduo; Briazide; Captea; Cibadrex; Co-Renitec; CoAprovel; Cokenzen; Coolmetec; Cotareg; Coteveten; Cotriatec; Ecazide; Fortzaar; Foziretic; Hytacand; Hyzaar; Koretic; Lodoz; MicardisPlus; Moducren; Moduretic; Nisisco; Prestole; Prinzide; PritorPlus; Wytens; Zestoretic; Zofenilduo; **Ger.:** Accuzide; ACE-Hemmer comp; Acercomp; Adocomp; Amilocomp beta; Amiloretik; Amilorid comp; Amilorid/HCT; Atacand Plus; Beloc-Zok comp; Benalapril Plus; Benazeplus; Benazepril comp; Benazepril HCT; Beta-Turfa; Biso comp; Biso-Puren comp; Bisobeta comp; Bisohexal plus; BisoLich comp; Bisomerck Plus; Bisoplus; Bisoprolol Comp; Bisoprolol HCT; Bisoprolol Plus; Blopress Plus; Capozide; Capto Comp; Capto Plus; Captobeta Comp; Captodoc Comp; Captogamma HCT; Captohexal Comp; Captopril Comp; Captopril HCT; Captopril Plus; Cardiagen HCT; Cibadrex; Co-Diovan; CoAprovel; Concor Plus; Cordinate plus; Coric Plus; Corvo HCT; Delix Plus; Diu Venostasin; Diuretikum Verla; Diursan; Dociteren; Dynacil comp; Dynorm Plus; Dytide H; Emestar plus; Enabeta comp; Enadura Plus; Enahexal comp; Enala-Q comp; Enalagamma HCT; Enalapril Comp; Enalapril HCT; Enalapril plus; Enalapril-saar Plus; EnaLich comp; Enaplus; Fempress Plus; Fondril HCT; Fortzaar; Fosinorm comp; Isoptin plus; Jutacor comp; Karvezide; Kinzalkomb; Lisi-Puren comp; Lisibeta comp; Lisigamma HCT; LisiLich comp; Lisinopril comp; Lisinopril HCT; Lisiplus; Lisodura plus; Lorzaar plus; Meprolol Comp; Metobeta comp; Metodura comp; Metohexal comp; Metoprolol comp; Metostad Comp; MicardisPlus; Moducrin; Moduretik; Nephral; Olmetec Plus; Pres plus; Propra comp; Provas comp; QuinaLich comp; Quinaplus; Quinapril comp; Rami-Q comp; Ramicard Plus; Ramigamma HCT; RamiLich comp; Ramiplus; Ramipril comp; Ramipril HCT; Ramipril HCTad; Ramipril Plus; Renacor; Spironothiazid; Tensobon comp; Teveten Plus; Thiazid-comp; Treloc; Tri-Thiazid; Triampur Compositum; Triamteren comp; Triamteren HCT; Triamteren tri-comp; Triarese; Triniton; Turfa; Veratide; Vesdil plus; Votum Plus; **Gr.:** Accuretic; Anastol; Atacand Plus; Bumeftyl; Captopress; Captospes+H; Cibadrex; Co-Dalzad; Co-Diovan; Co-Renitec; CoAprovel; Coredopril; Dosturel; Empirol; Fetylan; Fozide; Hyzaar; Iperton; Ividol; Karvezide; Kifarol; Micardis Plus; Moduretic; Nolarmin; Normolose-H; Olartan Plus; Olmetec Plus; Penopril; Pentatec; Piesital; Prinzide; Pritor Plus; Protal complex; Quimea; Return; Sancazid; Savosan; Sedapressin; Siberian; Stibenyl HCT; Superace; Teveten Plus; Tiaden; Triatec Plus; Uresan; Vascase Plus; Z-Bec Plus; Zestoretic; Zidepril; Zofepril Plus; Zopranol Plus; **Hong Kong:** Adelphane-Esidrex; Amithiazide; Apo-Amilzide; Apo-Triazide; Betaloc Comp; Blopress Plus; Co-Diovan; Co-Renitec; CoAprovel; CP-Metolol Co; Dyazide; Hyzaar; Lodoz; Micardis Plus; Moducren; Moduretic; Sefaretic; Teveten Plus; Zestoretic; **Hung.:** Accuzide; Acepril PlusZ; Amilorid Comp; Amilozid-B; Amprilan HD; Amprilan HL; Atacand Plus; Co-Enalapril; Co-Renitec; CoAprovel; Concor Plus; Diovan HCT; Duopril; Ednyt HCT; Ednyt Plus; Enalapril Hexal Plus; Enalapril-HCT; Enap-HL; Hartil HCT; Hyzaar; Inhibace Plus; Lodoz; Lotensin HCT; Meramyl HCT; MicardisPlus; PritorPlus; Ramace Plusz; Ramiwin HCT; Renapril Plus; Renitec Plus; Tritace-HCT; Varexan HCT; **India:** Adelphane-Esidrex; Alsartan-H; Arkamin-H; Beptazine-H; Biduret; Ciplar-H; Cipril-H; Covance-D; EnAce-D; Hipres-D; Invozide; Lisoril-5HT; Lodoz; Losacar-H; Metolar-H; Ramcor H; Ramipres H; Telpres-H; Xarb-H; Zaart-H; **Indon.:** Blopress Plus; Capozide; Co-Diovan; CoAprovel; Dellasidrex; Irtan Plus; Lorinid; Micardis Plus; Sectrazide; Ser-Ap-Es; Tenazide; Zestoretic; **Irl.:** Accuretic; Atacand Plus; Capozide; Captor-HCT; Carace Plus; Co-Betaloc; Co-Diovan; CoAprovel; Cozaar Comp; Dyazide; Half Capozide; Innozide; Lispril-hydrochlorothiazide; MicardisPlus; Moducren; Moduret; Teveten Plus; Zesger Plus; Zestoretic; **Israel:** Atacand Plus; Co-Diovan; Kaluril; Naprizide; Ocsaar Plus; Tritace Comp; Vascace Plus; **Ital.:** Accuretic; Acediur; Acceplus; Accuquide; Acesistem; Aldactazide; Bifrizide; Blopresid; Cibadrex; CoAprovel; Combisartan; Condiuren; Corixil; Cotareg; Elidiur; Enulid; Femipres Plus; Forzaar; Fosicombi; Gentipress; Hizaar; Idroquark; Inibace Plus; Initiss Plus; Karvezide; Lodoz; Losazid; Medozide; Micardis Plus; Moduretic; Nalapres; Neo-Lotan Plus; Neoprex; Prinzide; Pritor-Plus; Quinazide; Ratacand Plus; Sinertec; Spiridazide; Tensadiur; Tensozide; Triatec HCT; Uniprildiur; Vasoretic; Zantipride; Zestoretic; Zinadiur; Zoprazide; **Malaysia:** Ami-Hydrotride; Amizide; Apo-Amilzide; Apo-Triazide; Atacand Plus; Co-Diovan; CoAprovel; Fortzaar; Hyzaar; Micardis Plus; **Mex.:** Atacand Plus; Avalide; Biconcor; Blopress Plus; Capozide; Co-Captral; Co-Diovan; Co-Renitec; CoAprovel; Dyazide; Gliotenzide; Hyzaar; Micardis Plus; Moduretic; Predxal Plus; Prinzide; Selopres; Tritazide; Zestoretic; **Neth.:** Acuzide; Atacand Plus; Blopresid; Cibadrex; Co-

Diovan; Co-Renitec; CoAprovel; Cotareg; Cozaar Plus; Delitab-HCT; Diurace; Dytenzide; Emcoretic; Fortzaar; Hyzaar; Karvezide; Kinzalkomb; Lisidigal HCT; Losazid; Micardis Plus; Moduretic; Novazyd; Prilitab-HCT; Prilitaril-HCT; PritorPlus; Ramitab-HCT; Rataril-HCT; Renitec Plus; Selokomb; Teveten Plus; Tritazide; Zestoretic; ***Norw.:*** Atacand Plus; CoAprovel; Cozaar Comp; Diovan Comp; Enalapril Comp; Lodoz; MicardisPlus; Moduretic; Normorix; Renitec Comp; Teveten Comp; Vivatec Comp; Zestoretic; ***NZ:*** Accuretic; Amizide; Capozide; Co-Renitec; Hyzaar; Inhibace Plus; Karvezide; Triamizide; ***Philipp.:*** Accuzide; Betazide; Blopress Plus; Co-Diovan; Co-Renitec; CoAprovel; Combizar; Hyzaar; Micardis Plus; Norplus; PritorPlus; Teveten Plus; Uniretic; Vascace Plus; Vascoride; Zestoretic; Ziac; ***Pol.:*** Accuzide; Co-Diovan; Enap H; Enap HL; Hyzaar; Inhibace Plus; Lorista H; Lotensin HCT; Micardis Plus; Pritor Plus; Ramicor Comb; Tialorid; ***Port.:*** Acuretic; Aldoretic; Amiloride Composto; Blopress 16 mg + 12,5 mg; Co-Diovan; Co-Tareg; CoAprovel; Concor Plus; Cozaar Plus; Diurene; Dyazide; Ecamais; Enatia; Fortzaar; Hytacand; Inibace Plus; Laprilen; Lopiretic; Lortaan Plus; Micardis Plus; Moducren; Moduretic; Ondolen; Prinzide; Pritor Plus; Renidur; Triam-Tiazida R; Triatec Composto; Vascase Plus; Zestoretic; ***Rus.:*** Adelphane-Esidrex (Адельфан-эзидрекс); Apo-Triazide (Апо-триазид); Capozide (Капозид); Co-Diovan (Ко-Диован); Co-Renitec (Ко-Ренитек); Enap-H (Энап Н); Enap-HL (Энап-НЛ); Fosicard H (Фозикард Н); Fozide (Фозид); Hyzaar (Гизаар); Iruzid (Ирузид); Lisoretic (Лизоретик); Lozap Plus (Лозап Плюс); MicardisPlus (МикардисПлюс); Moex Plus (Моэкс Плюс); Renipril HT (Ренитрил ГТ); Sinorezid (Синорезид); Teveten Plus (Теветен Плюс); Triam-Co (Триам-ко); Triampur Compositum (Триампур Композитум); Triresid K (Трирезид К); ***S.Afr.:*** Accuretic; Adco-Retic; Amiloretic; Atacand Plus; Betaretic; Capozide; Captoretic; Cibadrex; Co-Diovan; Co-Micardis; Co-Renitec; CoAprovel; Cozaar Comp; Dyazide; Enap-Co; Fortzaar; Hexaretic; Inhibace Plus; Lisoretic; Moducren; Moduretic; Monozide; Pharmapress Co; Renezide; Servatrin; Sotazide; Urirex-K; Zapto Co; Zestoretic; Zetomax Co; Ziak; ***Singapore:*** Apo-Amilzide; Apo-Triazide; Atacand Plus; Co-Diovan; Co-Renitec; CoAprovel; Enap-HL; Gliotenzide; Hyzaar; Lodoz; Micardis Plus; Olmetec Plus; ***Spain:*** Acediur; Acetensil Plus; Ameride; Atacand Plus; Baripril Diu; Bicetil; Bitensil Diu; Cesplon Plus; Cibadrex; Co-Diovan; Co-Renitec; Co-Vals; CoAprovel; Cozaar Plus; Crinoretic; Dabonal Plus; Dilabar Diu; Ditenside; Diuzine; Doneka Plus; Ecadiu; Ecazide; Emcoretic; Fortzaar; Fositens Plus; Futuran Plus; Hiperlex Plus; Hipoartel Plus; Inhibace Plus; Inocar Plus; Iricil Plus; Kalpress Plus; Kalten; Karvezide; Labodrex; Lidaltrin Diu; Micardis Plus; Miten Plus; Navixen Plus; Neotensin Diu; Parapres Plus; Pressitan Plus; Prinivil Plus; Pritor Plus; Regulaten Plus; Renitecmax; Rulun; Secubar Diu; Tensikey Complex; Tensiocomplet; Tenso Stop Plus; Tevetens Plus; Zestoretic; ***Swed.:*** Accupro Comp; Amiloferm; Atacand Plus; CoAprovel; Cozaar Comp; Diovan Comp; Enalapril Comp; Inhibace comp; Linatil Comp; Micardis Plus; Moduretic; Normorix; Renitec Comp; Sparkal; Synerpril; Teveten Comp; Triatec Comp; Zestoretic; ***Switz.:*** Accuretic; Adelphan-Esidrex; Amiloride/HCTZ; Atacand Plus; Blopress Plus; Capozide; Captosol comp; Cibadrex; Co-Acepril; Co-Diovan; Co-Enalapril; Co-Enatec; Co-Epril; Co-Lisinopril; Co-Reniten; Co-Vasocor; CoAprovel; Comilorid; Concor Plus; Corpriretic; Cosaar Plus; Dyazide; Ecodurex; Elpradil HCT; Epril Plus; Escoretic; Fosicomp; Grodurex; Inhibace Plus; Kalten; Kinzalplus; Lisitril comp; Lisopril plus; Lodoz; MicardisPlus; Moducren; Moduretic; Olmetec Plus; Prinzide; Provas comp; Provas maxx; Reniten Plus; Rhefluin; t/h-basan; Tensobon comp; Teveten Plus; Tobicor Plus; Triatec Comp; Votum Plus; Zestoretic; ***Thai.:*** Bilduretic; Blopress Plus; Co-Diovan; CoAprovel; Dinazide; Dyazide; Fortzaar; Hydrares; Hydrozide Plus; Hyperretic; Hyzaar; Lodoz; Mano-Ap-Es; Micardis Plus; Miretic; Moduretic; Monoplus; Moure-M; Poli-Uretic; Renase; Reser; Sefaretic; Ser-Ap-Es; ***Turk.:*** Accuzide; Adelphan-Esidrex; Aldactazide; Atacand Plus; Cibadrex; Co-Diovan; Delix Plus; Eklips Plus; Hyzaar; Inhibace Plus; Karvezide; Konveril Plus; Micardis Plus; Moduretic; Monopril Plus; Pritor Plus; Rilace Plus; Sinoretik; Triamteril; Zestoretic; ***UK:*** Accuretic; Acezide; Amil-Co; Capozide; Capto-Co; Carace Plus; Caralpha; Co-Diovan; CoAprovel; Cozaar Comp; Dyazide; Innozide; Kalten; Lisicostad; MicardisPlus; Moducren; Moduret; Moduretic; Olmetec Plus; Triamco; Zestoretic; ***USA:*** Accuretic; Aldactazide; Atacand HCT; Avalide; Benicar HCT; Capozide; Diovan HCT; Dyazide; Esimil; Hydra-zide; Hydropres; Hyzaar; Lopressor HCT; Lotensin HCT; Marpres; Maxzide; Micardis HCT; Moduretic; Monopril-HCT; Prinzide; Quinaretic; Teveten HCT; Timolide; Uniretic; Vaseretic; Zestoretic; Ziac; ***Venez.:*** Accuretic; Aldactazida; Altace Plus; Atacand Plus; Biconcor; Blopress Plus; Capozide; Co-Renitec; CoAprovel; Cormatic; Diovan HCT; Hyzaar Plus; Lisiletic; Micardis Plus; Moduretic; Monopril Plus; Nefrotal H; Pritor Plus; Quinaretic; Reminalet; Vasaten HCT; Ziac.

H

Hydrocortamate Hydrochloride

Other names: Ethamicort; Hidrocloruro de hidrocortamato; Hydrocortamate, Chlorhydrate d'; Hydrocortamati Hydrochloridum; Hydrocortisone Diethylaminoacetate Hydrochloride.

Гидрокортамата Гидрохлорид

Clinical profile: Hydrocortamate hydrochloride is a corticosteroid that has been used topically in the treatment of various skin disorders.

WADA Status: Banned in competition

WADA Class: Glucocorticosteroids

All glucocorticosteroids are prohibited when administered orally, rectally, intravenously or intramuscularly. Their use requires a Therapeutic Use Exemption approval. Other routes of administration (intraarticular / periarticular / peritendinous / epidural / intradermal injections and inhalation) require an Abbreviated Therapeutic Use Exemption except as noted below.

Topical preparations when used for dermatological (including iontophoresis / phonophoresis), auricular, nasal, ophthalmic, buccal, gingival and perianal disorders are not prohibited and do not require any form of Therapeutic Use Exemption.

WADA Class: Specified Substances

Also listed as a specified substance.

"The prohibited List may identify specified substances which are particularly susceptible to unintentional anti-doping rule violations because of their general availability in medicinal products or which are less likely to be successfully abused as doping agents."

A doping violation involving such substances may result in a reduced sanction provided that the "*...Athlete can establish that the Use of such a specfied substance was not intended to enhance sport performance...*"

Hydrocortisone

Other names: Anti-inflammatory Hormone; Compound F; Cortisol; Hidrocortisona; Hidrokortizon; Hidrokortizonas; Hydrocortisonum; Hydrokortison; Hydrokortisoni; Hydrokortyzon; 17-Hydroxycorticosterone; NSC-10483.

Гидрокортизон

Hydrocortisone Acetate

Other names: Acetato de hidrocortisona; Cortisol Acetate; Hidrokortizon Asetat; Hidrokortizon-acetát; Hidrokortizono acetatas; Hydrocortisone, acétate d'; Hydrocortisoni acetas; Hydrokortisonacetat; Hydrokortison-acetát; Hydrokortisoniasetaatti; Hydrokortyzonu octan.

Гидрокортизона Ацетат

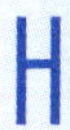

Hydrocortisone Buteprate

Other names: Buteprato de hidrocortisona; Hydrocortisone, Butéprate d'; Hydrocortisone Butyrate Propionate; Hydrocortisone Probutate; Hydrocortisoni Butepras; TS-408.

Гидрокортизона Бутепрат

Hydrocortisone Butyrate

Other names: Butirato de hidrocortisona; Cortisol Butyrate; Hidrokortizon Bütirat; Hydrocortisone, Butyrate d'; Hydrocortisoni Butiras.

Гидрокортизона Бутират

Hydrocortisone Cipionate

Other names: Cipionato de hidrocortisona; Cortisol Cypionate; Hydrocortisone, Cipionate d'; Hydrocortisone Cyclopentylpropionate; Hydrocortisone Cypionate; Hydrocortisoni Cipionas.

Гидрокортизона Ципионат

Hydrocortisone Hydrogen Succinate

Other names: Cortisol Hemisuccinate; Hidrogenosuccinato de hidrocortisona; Hidrokortizon-hidrogén-szukcinát; Hidrokortizono hemisukcinatas; Hydrocortisone Hemisuccinate; Hydrocortisone, Hémisuccinate d'; Hydrocortisone, hydrogénosuccinate d'; Hydrocortisone Succinate; Hydrocortisoni Hemisuccinas; Hydrocortisoni hydrogenosuccinas; Hydrokortison-hydrogen-sukcinát; Hydrokortisonivetysuksinaatti; Hydrokortisonvätesuccinat.

Гидрокортизона Гемисукцинат

Hydrocortisone Sodium Phosphate

Other names: Cortisol Sodium Phosphate; Fosfato sódico de hidrocortisona; Hydrocortisone, Phosphate Sodique d'; Natrii Hydrocortisoni Phosphas.

Натрия Гидрокортизона Фосфат

Hydrocortisone Sodium Succinate

Other names: Cortisol Sodium Succinate; Hydrocortisone, Succinate Sodique d'; Hydrocortisoni Natrii Succinas; Hydrokortyzonu bursztynianu sól sodowa; Succinato sódico de hidrocortisona.

Гидрокортизона Натрия Сукцинат

Hydrocortisone Valerate

Other names: Cortisol Valerate; Hydrocortisone, Valérate d'; Hydrocortisoni Valeras; Valerato de hidrocortisona.

Гидрокортизона Валерат

Clinical profile: Hydrocortisone (cortisol) is a corticosteroid and is the main glucocorticoid secreted by the adrenal cortex. It also has some mineralocorticoid activity. It is used, either in the form of the free alcohol, or in one of the esterified forms, in the treatment of a wide range of conditions that respond to the anti-inflammatory and immunosuppressant effects of corticosteroid therapy, although drugs with fewer mineralocorticoid effects are preferred for long-term management of inflammatory disease. Hydrocortisone is also used for replacement therapy in acute or chronic adrenocortical insufficiency when it may have its mineralocorticoid activity supplemented by fludrocortisone.

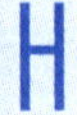

WADA Status: Banned in competition

WADA Class: Glucocorticosteroids

All glucocorticosteroids are prohibited when administered orally, rectally, intravenously or intramuscularly. Their use requires a Therapeutic Use Exemption approval. Other routes of administration (intraarticular / periarticular / peritendinous / epidural / intradermal injections and inhalation) require an Abbreviated Therapeutic Use Exemption except as noted below.

Topical preparations when used for dermatological (including iontophoresis / phonophoresis), auricular, nasal, ophthalmic, buccal, gingival and perianal disorders are not prohibited and do not require any form of Therapeutic Use Exemption.

WADA Class: Specified Substances

Also listed as a specified substance.

"*The prohibited List may identify specified substances which are particularly susceptible to unintentional anti-doping rule violations because of their general availability in medicinal products or which are less likely to be successfully abused as doping agents.*"

A doping violation involving such substances may result in a reduced sanction provided that the "*...Athlete can establish that the Use of such a specfied substance was not intended to enhance sport performance...*"

Preparations

Single ingredient: ***Arg.:*** Alfacort; Anusol-HC; Azuthidrona; Demacort; Fridalit; Hidrotisona; Lactid HC; Locoid; Medrocil; Microsona; Oralsone; Schericur; Sirotamicin HC; Stiefcortil;

Transderma H; **Austral.:** Colifoam; Cortef; Cortic; Derm-Aid; Egocort; Hycor; Hysone; Sigmacort; Siguent Hycor; Solu-Cortef; **Austria:** Colifoam; Ekzemsalbe F; Hydoftal sine neomycino; Hydrocortone; Hydroderm; Locoidon; Retef; **Belg.:** Azacortine; Cremicort-H; Locoid; Nozema; Pannocort; Solu-Cortef; **Braz.:** Berlison; Cortisonal; Cortiston; Cortizol; Cortizon; Hidrocortex; Hidyn H; Locoid; Nutracort; Solu-Cortef; Stiefcortil; Westcort; **Canad.:** Barriere-HC; Claritin Skin Itch Relief; Cortate; Cortef; Cortenema; Cortifoam; Cortoderm; Dermaflex HC; Dermarest Dricort Anti-Itch; Emo-Cort; Hycort; Hyderm; Hydrosone; HydroVal; Novo-Hydrocort; Prevex HC; Sarna HC; Solu-Cortef; Westcort; **Chile:** Aquanil HC; Calmurid; Cortisol; Efficort; Hipoge; Locoid; Nutracort; Pandel; Solu-Cortef; **Cz.:** Laticort; Locoid; Solu-Cortef; **Denm.:** Colifoam; Locoid; Mildison; Solu-Cortef; Uniderm; **Fin.:** Ampikyy; Apocort; Bucort; Colifoam; Kyypakkaus; Locoid; Solu-Cortef; **Fr.:** Aphilan; Colofoam; Cortapaisyl; Cortisedermyl; Dermaspraid Demangeaison; Efficort; Hydracort; Locoid; Mitocortyl; **Ger.:** Alfason; Colifoam; Ebenol; Fenistil Hydrocort; Ficortril; Hydrocutan mild; Hydrocutan; Hydroderm HC; Hydrogalen; Laticort; Linola Cort Hydro; Munitren; Pandel; Posterisan cort; Remederm HC; Sanatison Mono; Soventol HC; Systral Hydrocort; **Gr.:** Colifoam; Filocot; Rolak; Solu-Cortef; **Hong Kong:** Cortef; Derm-Aid; Dhacort; Egocort; Hydrosone; Hytisone; Sigmacort; Solu-Cortef; **Hung.:** Cortef; Laticort; Locoid; Solu-Cortef; **India:** Cipcorlin; Cutisoft; Entofoam; Wycort; **Indon.:** Berlicort; Calacort; Enkacort; Lexacorton; Locoid; Steroderm; **Irl.:** Colifoam; Corlan; Cortopin; Dioderm; Hc45; Hydrocortisyl; Hydrocortone; Locoid; Solu-Cortef; **Israel:** Cortifoam; Cortizone; Efficort; Lanacort; Solu-Cortef; **Ital.:** Colifoam; Cortidro; Cortop; Dermirit; Dermocortal; Flebocortid; Foille Insetti; Idracemi; Lanacort; Lenirit; Locoidon; Sintotrat; Solu-Cortef; **Jpn:** Pandel; **Malaysia:** Derm-Aid; Efficort; Egocort; Hydrocort; Solu-Cortef; **Mex.:** Aquanil HC; Collicort; Efficort; Fadol; Flebocortid; Flemex; Icorsan; Lacticare-HC; Locoid; Microsona; Nositrol; Nutracort; Solhidrol; Westcort; **Neth.:** Buccalsone; Cremicort; Locoid; Mildison; Solu-Cortef; **Norw.:** Colifoam; Locoid; Mildison; Solu-Cortef; **NZ:** BK HC; Colifoam; Derm-Aid; DP Hydrocortisone; Egocort; Lemnis Fatty Cream HC; Lipocort; Locoid; Mildison; Skincalm; Solu-Cortef; **Philipp.:** Cortizan; Droxiderm; Efficort; Hycortil; Hydrotopic; Lacticare-HC; Pharmacort; Solu-Cortef; **Pol.:** Corhydron; Laticort; Locoid; Procortin; **Port.:** Colifoam; Dermimade Hidrocortisona; Hidalone; Hydrocortone; Locoid; Pandel; Pandermil; Solu-Cortef; **Rus.:** Cortef (Кортеф); Laticort (Латикорт); Locoid (Локоид); Sopolcort N (Сополь順корт Н); **S.Afr.:** Biocort; Covocort; Dilucort; Locoid; Mylocort; Procutan; Solu-Cortef; Stopitch; **Singapore:** Derm-Aid; Dhacort; Efficort; Egocort; Hydrocort; Hydroderm; Solu-Cortef; **Spain:** Actocortina; Aftasone; Ceneo; Dermosa Hidrocortisona; Hemodren; Hemorrane; Hidroaltesona; Hidrocisdin; Isdinium; Lactisona; Oralsone; Scalpicin Capilar; Schericur; Suniderma; **Swed.:** Colifoam; Ficortril; Locoid; Mildison; Solu-Cortef; Uniderm; **Switz.:** Alfacortone; Hydrocortone; Locoid; Sanadermil; Solu-Cortef; **Thai.:** Hytisone; Prevex HC; Solu-Cortef; **Turk.:** Cortimycine; Hipokort; Locoid; **UAE:** Alfacort; **UK:** Colifoam; Corlan; Cortopin; Cortropin; Dermacort; Dioderm; Efcortelan; Efcortesol; Exe-Cort; Hc45; Hydrocortistab; Hydrocortone; Lanacort; Locoid; Mildison; Solu-Cortef; Zenoxone; **USA:** A-Hydrocort; Acticort; Ala-Cort; Anucort-HC; Aquanil HC; Bactine; CaldeCort; Carmol HC; Cetacort; Colocort; Cort-Dome; Cortaid; Cortef Feminine Itch; Cortef; Corticaine; Cortifoam; Cortizone; Dermarest Dri-Cort; Dermol HC; Dermolate; EarSol-HC; Gynecort; Hemril-HC; Hi-Cor; Hydrocortone; HydroSkin; Hytone; Lacticare-HC; Lanacort; Locoid; Massengill Medicated; Neutrogena T/Scalp; Nutracort; Orabase HCA; Pandel; Penecort; Procort; Proctocort; Proctocream HC 2.5%; Recort Plus; Solu-Cortef; Synacort; Tegrin-HC; Texacort; U-Cort; Westcort; **Venez.:** Corticina; Efficort; Hidrocort; Hidrozona; Liocort; Nutracort; Solu-Cortef; Stricort.

Multi-ingredient: **Arg.:** Anusol Duo S; Anusol Duo; Atomoderma Plus; Bactisona; Bexon; Cipro HC; Ciprocort; Ciprocort; Ciproflox-Otic; Ciriax Otic L; Ciriax Otic; Colirio Antibiotico CNH; Cristalomicina; Delos Otic; Dercotex; Dermoperative; Disel Hidrocortisona; Epiprocto; Gentacler; Griseoplus; Hipoglos con Hidrocortisona; Irigal; Lidocort Proct; Linfol Dermico; Masivol Urea; Microsona C; Microsona Otica; Monizol Cort; Neo Pelvicillin; Otex HC; Oto Biotaer; Otobiotic; Otocipro; Otoseptil; Otosporin C; Otosporin L; Otosporin; Procto-Ikatral; Proctocrem; Prootocipro; Quemicetina con Hidrocortisona; Terra-Cortril; Tocorectal; Tricur; Tridermal; Vagicural; Xilocler; Xyloprocto; **Austral.:** Ciproxin HC; Hydroform; Hydrozole; Proctosedyl; Rectinol HC; Resolve Plus; Xyloproct; **Austria:** C-Bildz; Calmurid HC; Cortison Kemicetin; Hydoftal; Hydrocortimycin; Ichtho-Cortin; Otosporin; Tropoderm; **Belg.:** Daktacort; Fucidin Hydrocortisone; Onctose a l'Hydrocortisone; Terra-Cortril + Polymyxine B; Terra-Cortril; **Braz.:** Anusol-HC; Cipro HC; Hemodotti; Hidrocorte; Hidroneo; Nitrolerg; Otosporin; Terra-Cortril; Vioformio-Hidrocortisona; Xyloproct; **Canad.:** Anodan-HC; Anugesic-HC; Anusol-HC; Anuzinc HC Plus; Anuzinc HC; Cipro HC; Cortimyxin; Cortimyxin; Cortisporin; Cortisporin; Egozinc-HC; Fucidin H; Pentamycetin-HC; Pramox HC; Proctodan-HC; Proctofoam-HC; Proctol; Proctomyxin HC; Proctosedyl; ratio-Hemcort-HC; ratio-Proctosone; Rectogel HC; Rivasol HC; Sterex Plus; Uremol-HC; Vioform-Hydrocortisone; **Chile:** Fucidin H; Otex HC; **Cz.:** Ciprobay HC Otic; Dobexil Plus; Ophthalmo-Framykoin Compositum; Otosporin; Pimafucort; Proctosedyl; Septomixine; **Denm.:** Brentacort; Ciflox; Fucidin-Hydrocortison; Hydrocortison med Terramycin og Polymyxin-B; Hydrocortison med Terramycin; Locoidol; Proctosedyl; **Fin.:** Ciproxin-Hydrocortison; Daktacort; Duocort; Fucidin-Hydrocortison; Pantyson; Pimafucort; Proctosedyl; Sibicort; Terra-Cortril P; Terra-Cortril; Trosycort; **Fr.:** Bacicoline; **Ger.:** Baycuten HC; Hydrodexan; Ichthocortin; Nystaderm comp; Pigmanorm; Polyspectran HC; **Gr.:** Cortiphenol H; Daktodor; Fucidin H; Hydrofusin; Terra-Cortril; **Hong Kong:** Canesten HC; Cipro HC; Cortiphenol H; Daktacort; Fucidin H; Hydro-Funga; Micosone; Otosporin; Posterisan Forte; Xyloproct; **Hung.:** Fucidin H; Otosporin; Oxycort; Pimafucort; Posterisan Forte; Tetran-Hydrocortison; **India:** Bell Diono Resolvent; Bell Resolvent; Belmycetin-C; Cortola-m; Cortoquinol; Crotorax-HC; Daktacort; Efcorlin; Furacin-S; Keralin; Medithane; Neosporin-H; Neosporin-H; Pino-Cort; Proctosedyl; Shield; Wycort c Neomycin; **Indon.:** Anusol-HC; Brentan; Chloramphecort; Dermacort; Enpicortyn;

H

Haemocaine; Indoson; Kemiderm; Nufacort; Particol; Ramicort; Sancortmycin; Terra-Cortril; Terra-Cortril; Thecort; Viohydrocort; Visancort; Zolacort; ***Irl.:*** Alphaderm; Anugesic-HC; Anugesic-HC; Anusol-HC; Calmurid HC; Canesten HC; Daktacort; Eurax-Hydrocortisone; Fucidin H; Gentisone HC; Locoid C; Otosporin; Perinal; Proctofoam-HC; Proctosedyl; Timodine; Vioform-Hydrocortisone; Xyloproct; ***Israel:*** Benzantine H; Ciproxin HC; Daktacort; Epifoam; Hycocin; Hycomycin; Hydroagisten; Panthisone; Perinal; Procto-Glyvenol; Proctofoam-HC; Proctozorin-N; ***Ital.:*** Argisone; Cort-Inal; Cortison Chemicetina; Emorril; Fucidin H; Idracemi Eparina; Idracemi; Kinogen; Mictasone; Mixotone; Mobilat; Nasomixin; Nevacort; Prepacort H; Proctidol; Proctofoam-HC; Proctosedyl; Proctosedyl; Proctosoll; Reumacort; Scalpicin; Vasosterone Antibiotico; Vasosterone Collirio; Vasosterone; ***Malaysia:*** Candacort; Cipro HC; Crotamiton H; Daktacort; Decocort; Fucidin H; Miconazole H; Pocin H; Proctosedyl; Proctosone; Ucort; Xyloproct; Zaricort; ***Mex.:*** Angenovag; Biotarson N; Ciproxina HC; Clioderm-H; Cortisporin; Daktacort; Dermanol; Hidrofenil; Hidropolicin; Litiset; Ofodex; Orecil NF; Otifar; Oto Eni; Poral; Soldrin; Sulfa Hidro; Ultracortin; Vioformo-Cort; Xyloderm; Xyloproct Plus; ***Neth.:*** Bacicoline-B; Calmurid HC; Daktacort; Otosporin; Pimafucort; Proctosedyl; Terra-Cortril met polymyxine-B; ***Norw.:*** Daktacort; Fucidin-Hydrocortison; Locoidol; Proctosedyl; Terra-Cortril Polymyxin B; Terra-Cortril; Xyloproct; ***NZ:*** Ciproxin HC; Daktacort; DP Lotion - HC; Locoid C; Micreme H; Pimafucort; Proctosedyl; Xyloproct; ***Philipp.:*** Cortisporin; Daktacort; Fucidin H; Hydrospor; Isonep H; Proctosedyl; Trimycin-H; ***Pol.:*** Atecortin; Chlorchinaldin H; Hemcort HC; Laticort-CH; Oxycort; Pimafucort; Posterisan H; Proctosone; ***Port.:*** Anucet; Clorcorticil; Corticil T; Daktacort; Fucidine H; Leuco Hubber; Locoid C; Pimafucort; Proctonostrum; ***Rus.:*** Cortomycetin (Кортомицетин); Fucidin H (Фуцидин Г); Gioxyson (Гиоксизон); Oxycort (Оксикорт); Pimafucort (Пимафукорт); Posterisan Forte (Постеризан Форте); Relief Ultra (Релиф Ультра); ***S.Afr.:*** Ciprobay HC; Daktacort; Fucidin H; Neoderm; Otosporin; Proctosedyl; Terra-Cortril; Terra-Cortril; Viocort; ***Singapore:*** Candacort; Canesten HC; Ciprobay HC; Daktacort; Decocort; Fucidin H; Hydroderm-C; Micon-H; Neo-Hydro; Proctosedyl; Zaricort; ***Spain:*** Aftajuventus; Aftasone B C; Anginovag; Antihemorroidal; Bacisporin; Brentan; Cilinafosal Hidrocortisona; Ciproxina; Cohortan; Cortenema; Cortison Chemicet Topica; Dermo Hubber; Detraine; Edifaringen; Fucidine H; Halibut Hidrocortisona; Hepro; Leuco Hubber; Milrosina Nistatina; Neo Hubber; Otosporin; Roberfarin; Terra-Cortril; Terra-Cortril; Tisuderma; ***Swed.:*** Cortimyk; Daktacort; Fenuril-Hydrokortison; Fucidin-Hydrocortison; Terracortril med polymyxin B; Terracortril; Xyloproct; ***Switz.:*** Ciproxin HC; Cortifluid N; Cortimycine; Cortimycine; Daktacort; Dermacalm-d; Fucidin H; Haemocortin; Haemocortin; Hydrocortisone compositum; Neo-Hydro; Otosporin; Septomixine; ***Thai.:*** Candacort; Daktacort; Decocort; Dermasol; Doproct; Fucidin H; Ladocort; Proctosedyl; ***Turk.:*** Cormisin; Kortos; Kortos; Ma-Ka-Ta; Ureacort; ***UK:*** Actinac; Alphaderm; Alphosyl HC; Anugesic-HC; Anugesic-HC; Anusol-HC; Anusol Plus HC; Calmurid HC; Canesten HC; Daktacort HC; Daktacort; Econacort; Eurax-Hydrocortisone; Fucidin H; Gentisone HC; Germoloids HC; Locoid C; Nystaform-HC; Otosporin; Perinal; Proctofoam-HC; Proctosedyl; Timodine; Uniroid-HC; Vioform-Hydrocortisone; Xyloproct; ***USA:*** I + I-F; Acetasol HC; Alcortin; Analpram-HC; AnaMantle HC; Anumed HC; Cipro HC; Coly-Mycin S Otic; Corque; Cortane-B; Cortatrigen; Cortic ND; Corticaine; Cortimycin; Cortimycin; Cortisporin-TC; Cortisporin; Cortisporin; Cyotic; Dermtex HC with Aloe; Ear-Eze; Emergent-Ez; Enzone; Epifoam; Fungoid HC; HC Derma-Pax; HC Pramoxine; Hysone; LazerSporin-C; LidaMantle HC; Mediotic-HC; Neotricin HC; Novacort; Otic-Care; OtiTricin; Otobiotic; Otocort; Otomar-HC; Otomycin-HPN; Otosporin; Pediotic; Pramosone; Proctofoam-HC; Terra-Cortril; UAD-Otic; Vanoxide-HC; Vytone; Xyralid; Zone-A; Zoto-HC; ***Venez.:*** Otalex; Quinotic HC.

Hydroflumethiazide

Other names: Hidroflumetiazida; Hydrofluméthiazide; Hydroflumethiazidum; Hydroflumetiatsidi; Hydroflumetiazid; Trifluoromethylhydrothiazide.

Гидрофлуметиазид

Clinical profile: Hydroflumethiazide is a thiazide diuretic used for oedema, including that associated with heart failure, and for hypertension.

WADA Status: Banned in and out of competition

WADA Class: Diuretics and Other Masking Agents

Includes diuretics or substances with a similar chemical structure or similar biological effect(s).

Preparations
Single ingredient: ***USA:*** Saluron.

Multi-ingredient: ***Irl.:*** Aldactide; ***S.Afr.:*** Protensin-M; ***UK:*** Aldactide.

Hydromorphone Hydrochloride

Other names: Dihydromorphinone Hydrochloride; Hidrocloruro de hidromorfona; Hidromorfono hidrochloridas; Hydromorfon-hydrochlorid; Hydromorfonhydroklorid; Hydromorfonihydrokloridi; Hydromorphone, chlorhydrate d'; Hydromorphoni hydrochloridum.

Гидроморфона Гидрохлорид

Clinical profile: Hydromorphone hydrochloride, a phenanthrene derivative, is an opioid analgesic related to morphine but with greater analgesic potency. It is used for the relief of moderate to severe pain and for the relief of non-productive cough.

WADA Status: Banned in competition

WADA Class: Narcotics

Includes specified narcotics.

Preparations
Single ingredient: ***Arg.:*** Dolonovag; ***Austral.:*** Dilaudid; ***Austria:*** Dilaudid; Hydal; ***Belg.:*** Palladone; ***Canad.:*** Dilaudid; Hydromorph; ***Denm.:*** Palladon; ***Fin.:*** Palladon; ***Fr.:*** Sophidone; ***Ger.:*** Dilaudid; Palladon; ***Hung.:*** Palladone; ***Irl.:*** Palladone; ***Israel:*** Palladone; ***Mex.:*** Liberaxim; ***Neth.:*** Palladon; ***Norw.:*** Palladon; ***Swed.:*** Palladon; ***Switz.:*** Palladon; ***UK:*** Palladone; ***USA:*** Dilaudid.

Multi-ingredient: ***Swed.:*** Dilaudid-Atropin; ***USA:*** Dilaudid Cough.

Hydroxyamfetamine Hydrobromide

Other names: Bromhidrato de Hidroxianfetamina; Hidrobromuro de hidroxianfetamina; Hydroxyamfétamine, Bromhydrate d'; Hydroxyamfetamini Hydrobromidum; Hydroxyamphetamine Hydrobromide; *p*-Hydroxyamphetamine Hydrobromide; Oxamphetamine Hydrobromide.

Гидроксиамфетамина Гидробромид

Clinical profile: Hydroxyamfetamine hydrobromide is a sympathomimetic that was formerly used as a vasopressor and in the management of some cardiac disorders. In ophthalmology, hydroxyamfetamine hydrobromide has been used as a mydriatic and in the diagnosis of Horner's syndrome.

WADA Status: Banned in competition

WADA Class: Stimulants

Includes hydroxyamfetamine and any optical isomers.

Preparations
Single ingredient: ***Cz.:*** Pedrolon.

Multi-ingredient: ***USA:*** Paremyd.

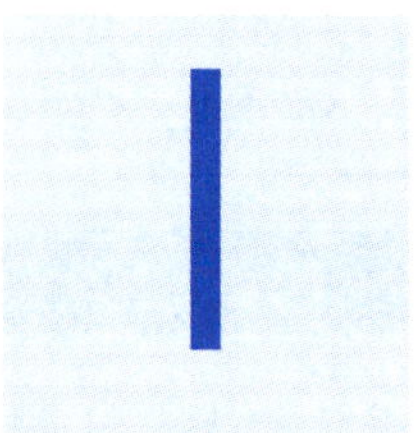

Ibopamine

Other names: Ibopamina; Ibopaminum; SB-7505; SKF-100168.
Ибопамин

Ibopamine Hydrochloride

Other names: Hidrocloruro de ibopamina; Ibopamiinihydrokloridi; Ibopamine, Chlorhydrate d'; Ibopaminhydroklorid; Ibopamini Hydrochloridum.
Ибопамина Гидрохлорид

Clinical profile: Ibopamine is converted in the body to epinine, a peripheral dopamine agonist with vasodilating and weak positive inotropic effects. It is used in the management of mild heart failure. It is also used topically as a mydriatic.

WADA Status: Banned in competition

WADA Class: Stimulants

Includes stimulants or substances with a similar chemical structure or similar biological effect(s).

WADA Class: Specified Substances

Also listed as a specified substance.
"The prohibited List may identify specified substances which are particularly susceptible to unintentional anti-doping rule violations because of their general availability in medicinal products or which are less likely to be successfully abused as doping agents."
A doping violation involving such substances may result in a reduced sanction provided that the "*...Athlete can establish that the Use of such a specfied substance was not intended to enhance sport performance...*"

Preparations
Single ingredient: ***Belg.:*** Scandine; ***Ital.:*** Scandine; Trazyl; ***Neth.:*** Inopamil.

Idoxifene

Other names: CB-7432; Idoxifène; Idoxifeno; Idoxifenum; SB-223030.
Идоксифен

Clinical profile: Idoxifene is an analogue of tamoxifen that has been investigated for the treatment of breast cancer and osteoporosis.

WADA Status: Banned in and out of competition

WADA Class: Hormone Antagonists and Modulators
Includes selective estrogen receptor modulators.

Indacaterol

Other names: Indacatérol; Indacaterolum; QAB-149.

Индакатерол

Clinical profile: Indacaterol is a long-acting beta$_2$ agonist under investigation in asthma and chronic obstructive pulmonary disease.

WADA Status: Banned in and out of competition

WADA Class: Beta-2 Agonists
Includes beta-2 agonists or their isomers.

WADA Class: Specified Substances
Also listed as a specified substance.
"*The prohibited List may identify specified substances which are particularly susceptible to unintentional anti-doping rule violations because of their general availability in medicinal products or which are less likely to be successfully abused as doping agents.*"
A doping violation involving such substances may result in a reduced sanction provided that the "*...Athlete can establish that the Use of such a specfied substance was not intended to enhance sport performance...*"

Indanazoline Hydrochloride

Other names: Hidrocloruro de indanazolina; Indanazolin Hidroklorür; Indanazoline, Chlorhydrate d'; Indanazolini Hydrochloridum.

Инданазолина Гидрохлорид

Clinical profile: Indanazoline is a sympathomimetic related to naphazoline. It has been used as a nasal decongestant.

WADA Status: Banned in competition

WADA Class: Stimulants
Includes stimulants or substances with a similar chemical structure or similar biological effect(s). Indanazoline is an imidazole derivative. Imidazole derivatives for topical use are exempt.

Preparations
Single ingredient: ***Ger.:*** Farial; ***Turk.:*** Farial.

Indapamide

Other names: Indapamid; Indapamida; Indapamidi; Indapamidum; SE-1520.

Индапамид

Clinical profile: Indapamide is a diuretic similar to the thiazide diuretics. It is used for hypertension and for oedema, including that associated with heart failure.

WADA Status: Banned in and out of competition

WADA Class: Diuretics and Other Masking Agents

Includes diuretics or substances with a similar chemical structure or similar biological effect(s).

Preparations

Single ingredient: ***Arg.:*** Bajaten; Duremid; Natrilix; Noranat; ***Austral.:*** Dapa-Tabs; Indahexal; Insig; Napamide; Natrilix; ***Austria:*** Fludex; ***Belg.:*** Docindapa; Fludex; ***Braz.:*** Indapen; Natrilix; ***Canad.:*** Lozide; ***Chile:*** Indapress; Natrilix; ***Cz.:*** Indap; Tertensif; ***Denm.:*** Indacar; Natrilix; ***Fin.:*** Natrilix; ***Fr.:*** Fludex; ***Ger.:*** Inda-Puren; Natrilix; ***Gr.:*** Fludex; Magniton-R; Transipen; ***Hong Kong:*** Dapa-Tabs; Diflerix; Frumeron; Indalix; Millibar; Natrilix; ***Hung.:*** Apadex; Pretanix; Rawel; ***India:*** Indicontin; Inditor; Lorvas; Natrilix; ***Indon.:*** Natrilix; ***Irl.:*** Natrilix; ***Israel:*** Pamid; ***Ital.:*** Damide; Indaflex; Indamol; Ipamix; Millibar; Natrilix; Pressural; Veroxil; ***Malaysia:*** Dapa; Diflerix; Napamide; Natrilix; Rinalix; ***Mex.:*** Natrilix; ***Neth.:*** Fludex; ***NZ:*** Napamide; Natrilix; ***Philipp.:*** Natrilix; ***Pol.:*** Apo-Indap; Diuresin; Indapen; Indapres; Indapsan; Indix; Ipres; Rawel; Tertensif; ***Port.:*** Fludex; Fluidema; Tandix; ***Rus.:*** Akripamide (Акрипамид); Arifon (Арифон); Arindap (Ариндап); Indap (Индап); Indiur (Индиур); Ionik (Ионик); Rawel (Равел); Retapres (Ретапрес); ***S.Afr.:*** Catexan; Dapamax; Daptril; Hydro-Less; Indalix; Lixamide; Natrilix; ***Singapore:*** Dapa-Tabs; Napamide; Natrilix; Rinalix; ***Spain:*** Extur; Tertensif; ***Switz.:*** Fludapamide; Fludex; ***Thai.:*** Frumeron; Inpamide; Napamide; Natrilix; ***Turk.:*** Flubest; Fludex; Fludin; Flupamid; Flutans; Indamid; Indapen; Indurin; ***UAE:*** Indanorm; ***UK:*** Natrilix; ***USA:*** Lozol; ***Venez.:*** Natrilix.

Multi-ingredient: ***Arg.:*** Bipreterax; Preterax; ***Austral.:*** Coversyl Plus; ***Austria:*** Delapride; Predonium; Preterax; ***Belg.:*** Bi Preterax; Coversyl Plus; Preterax; ***Canad.:*** Coversyl Plus; Preterax; ***Cz.:*** Noliprel; ***Denm.:*** Coversyl Comp; ***Fin.:*** Coversyl Comp; ***Fr.:*** Bipreterax; Preterax; ***Ger.:*** Coversum Combi; Preterax; ***Gr.:*** Dinapres; Preterax; ***Hong Kong:*** Predonium; ***Hung.:*** Armix Komb; Armix Prekomb; Co-Prenessa; Coverex Komb; Coverex Prekomb; ***India:*** Coversyl Plus; Perigard D; Perigard DF; ***Irl.:*** Bipreterax; Coversyl Plus; Preterax; ***Ital.:*** Atinorm; Delapride; Dinapres; Nor-Pa; Normopress; Prelectal; Preterax; ***Malaysia:*** Coversyl Plus; ***Mex.:*** Preterax; ***Neth.:*** Coversyl Plus; Predonium; Preterax; ***NZ:*** Coversyl Plus; Predonium; ***Philipp.:*** Bi-Preterax; Preterax; ***Pol.:*** Noliprel; Prestarium Plus; ***Port.:*** Predonium; Preterax; ***Rus.:*** Enzix (Энзикс); Noliprel (Нолипрел); Sonoprel (Сонопрел); ***S.Afr.:*** Bipreterax; Coversyl Plus; Preterax; Prexum Plus; ***Singapore:*** Coversyl Plus; Preterax; ***Spain:*** Bipreterax; Preterax; ***Switz.:*** Coversum Combi; Preterax; ***Turk.:*** Coversyl Plus; Preterax; ***UK:*** Coversyl Plus; ***Venez.:*** Bipreterax; Preterax.

Indenolol Hydrochloride

Other names: Hidrocloruro de indenolol; Indénolol, Chlorhydrate d'; Indenololi Hydrochloridum; Sch-28316Z (indenolol); YB-2.

Инденолола Гидрохлорид

Clinical profile: Indenolol is a non-cardioselective beta blocker that has been used in the management of various cardiovascular disorders.

WADA Status: Banned in and out of competition as specified below

WADA Class: Beta-Blockers

Unless otherwise specified, beta-blockers are prohibited *In-Competition* only in the following sports.

- Aeronautics (FAI)
- Archery (FITA, IPC) (also prohibited *Out-of-Competition*)
- Automobile (FIA)
- Billiards (WCBS)
- Bobsleigh (FIBT)
- Boules (CMSB, IPC bowls)
- Bridge (FMB)
- Curling (WCF)
- Gymnastics (FIG)
- Motorcycling (FIM)
- Modern Pentathlon (UIPM) for disciplines involving shooting
- Nine-pin bowling (FIQ)
- Powerboating (UIM)
- Sailing (ISAF) for match race helms only
- Shooting (ISSF, IPC) (also prohibited *Out-of-Competition*)
- Skiing/Snowboarding (FIS) in ski jumping, freestyle aerials/halfpipe and snowboard halfpipe/big air
- Wrestling (FILA)

WADA Class: Specified Substances

Also listed as a specified substance.

"The prohibited List may identify specified substances which are particularly susceptible to unintentional anti-doping rule violations because of their general availability in medicinal products or which are less likely to be successfully abused as doping agents."

A doping violation involving such substances may result in a reduced sanction provided that the "*...Athlete can establish that the Use of such a specfied substance was not intended to enhance sport performance...*"

Insulin

Other names: Insuliini; Insülin; Insulina; Insuline; Insulinin; Insulinum.

Clinical profile: Insulin is a pancreatic hormone involved in the regulation of blood-glucose concentrations as well as having a role in protein and lipid metabolism. Human, porcine, bovine, mixed porcine-bovine insulin, or insulin analogues, are given to patients with type 1 diabetes mellitus to control their blood-glucose concentrations; insulin may also be necessary in some type 2 diabetics. Insulin is an essential part of the emergency management of diabetic ketoacidosis.

WADA Status: Banned in and out of competition

WADA Class: Hormones and Related Substances: Insulins

Includes insulins or substances with a similar chemical structure or similar biological effect(s), or one of their releasing factors.

Preparations

Single ingredient: ***Arg.:*** Actrapid HM; Apidra; Biohulin C; Biohulin N; Densulin; Humalog Mix 25; Humalog; Humulin 70/30; Humulin NPH; Humulin R; Insulatard HM; Insuman N; Insuman R; Lantus; Levemir; Mixtard 30 HM; NovoMix 30; NovoRapid; ***Austral.:*** Actrapid; Humalog Mix 25; Humalog; Humulin 20/80, 30/70 and 50/50; Humulin L; Humulin NPH; Humulin R; Humulin UL; Hypurin Isophane; Hypurin Neutral; Lantus; Levemir; Mixtard 20/80, 30/70, 50/50; Monotard; NovoMix 30; NovoRapid; Protaphane; Ultratard; ***Austria:*** Actrapid HM; Humalog Mix 25 and 50; Humalog; Huminsulin Basal; Huminsulin Long; Huminsulin Normal; Huminsulin Profil II and III; Huminsulin Ultralong; Insulatard HM; Insuman Basal; Insuman Comb 15, 25, and 50; Insuman Infusat; Insuman Rapid; Mixtard HM 10/90, 20/80, 30/70, 40/60, and 50/50; Monotard HM; Ultratard HM; ***Belg.:*** Actrapid HM; Humalog Mix 25 and 50; Humalog; Humuline 30/70, 50/50; Humuline NPH; Humuline Regular; Insulatard; Lantus; Levemir; Mixtard 10, 20, 30, 40, 50; NovoMix 30; NovoRapid; Velosulin; ***Braz.:*** Actrapid MC; Biohulin 70/30, 80/20, and 90/10; Biohulin Lenta; Biohulin NPH; Biohulin Regular; Biohulin Ultralenta; Humalog Mix 25; Humalog; Humulin 70/30; Humulin Lenta; Humulin NPH; Humulin Regular; Insuman Comb 85N/15R and 75N/25R; Insuman N; Insuman R; Lantus; Monotard MC; Novolin 90/10, 80/20, and 70/30; Novolin L; Novolin N; Novolin R; Novolin U; NovoRapid; Protaphane MC; ***Canad.:*** Humalog Mix 25; Humalog; Humulin 20/80, 30/70; Humulin L; Humulin N; Humulin R; Humulin U; Hypurin NPH; Hypurin Regular; Iletin II Pork Lente; Iletin II Pork NPH; Iletin II Pork Regular; Lantus; Novolin 10/90, 20/80, 30/70, 40/60, 50/50; Novolin NPH; Novolin Toronto; NovoRapid; ***Chile:*** Actrapid HM; Humalog Mix 25; Humalog; Insulatard HM; Insuman N; Insuman R; Lantus; Mixtard 30 HM; NovoMix 30; NovoRapid; Wosulin 30/70; Wosulin-N; Wosulin-R; ***Cz.:*** Actrapid HM; Humalog Mix 25 and 50; Humalog NPL; Humalog; Humulin L; Humulin M3; Humulin N; Humulin R; Humulin U; Hypurin Bovine Isophane; Hypurin Bovine Protamin Zink Sulfat; Hypurin Porcin Neutral; Insulatard HM; Insuman Basal; Insuman Komb Typ 15, Typ 25, and Typ 50; Insuman Rapid; Lantus; Mixtard HM 10, 20, 30, 40, 50; Monotard HM; NovoMix 30; NovoRapid; Ultratard HM; Velosulin HM; ***Denm.:*** Actrapid; Apidra; Humalog Mix 25 and 50; Humalog; Humulin Mix 30/70; Humulin NPH; Humulin Regular; Insulatard; Insuman Basal; Insuman Comb 25; Insuman Rapid; Lantus; Levemir; Mixtard 10, 20, 30, 40, and 50; Monotard; NovoMix 30; NovoRapid; Velosulin; ***Fin.:*** Actrapid; Humalog Mix 25 and 50; Humalog; Humulin NPH; Humulin Regular; Insuman Basal; Insuman Comb 25; Insuman Infusat; Insuman Rapid; Lantus; Levemir; Mixtard 10, 20, 30, and 50; Monotard; NovoMix 30; NovoRapid; Protaphane; ***Fr.:*** Actrapid; Apidra; Exubera; Humalog Mix 25 and 50; Humalog; Insulatard; Insuman Basal; Insuman Comb 15, 25, and 50; Insuman Infusat; Insuman Rapid; Insuplant; Lantus; Levemir; Mixtard 10, 20, 30, 40, and 50; NovoMix 30; NovoRapid; Umuline NPH; Umuline Profil 30; Umuline Rapide; ***Ger.:*** Actraphane 10, 20, 30, 40, 50; Actrapid; Apidra; Berlinsulin H 30/70; Berlinsulin H Basal; Berlinsulin H Normal; Humalog Mix 25 and 50; Humalog; Huminsulin Basal; Huminsulin Normal; Huminsulin Profil III; Insulin Basal; Insulin Comb 30/70; Insulin Novo Semilente MC; Insulin Rapid; Insuman Basal; Insuman Comb 15, 25, and 50; Insuman Infusat; Insuman Rapid; Lantus; Levemir; Liprolog Mix 25 and 50; Liprolog; Monotard; NovoMix 30; NovoRapid; Protaphane; Ultratard; Velosulin; ***Gr.:*** Actrapid, Apidra, Exubera; Humalog Mix 25 and 50; Humalog NPL; Humalog; Humulin Lente; Humulin M2, M3; Humulin NPH; Humulin Regular; Humulin Utralente; Lantus; Levemir; Mixtard 10, 20, 30, 40, and 50; Monotard; NovoMix 30; NovoRapid; Protaphane; Ultratard; ***Hong Kong:*** Actrapid HM; Humalog; Humulin 70/30; Humulin L; Humulin N; Humulin R; Lantus; Mixtard 30 HM; Monotard HM; NovoMix 30; NovoRapid; Protaphane HM; Ultratard HM; ***Hung.:*** Actrapid; Apidra; Humalog Mix25 and Mix50; Humalog; Humulin M3; Humulin N; Humulin R; Insulatard; Lantus; Levemir; Mixtard 10, 20, 30, 40, 50; NovoMix 30; NovoRapid; ***India:*** Actrapid; Human Actrapid; Human Insultard; Human Mixtard 30 and 50; Human Monotard; Insuman Rapid; Insuman 25/75 and 50/50; Lantus; Lentard; Mixulin; Rapidica; Rapimix; Wosulin Biphasic 30/70 and 50/50; Wosulin-N; Wosulin-R; Zinulin; ***Indon.:*** Actrapid HM; Apidra; Humalog Mix 25; Humalog; Humulin 30/70; Humulin N; Humulin R; Insulatard HM; Lantus; Mixtard 30 HM; Monotard HM; ***Irl.:*** Actrapid; Apidra; Humalog Mix 25 and 50; Humalog; Humulin I; Humulin M3; Humulin S; Insulatard; Insuman Basal; Insuman Comb 15, 25, and 50; Insuman Rapid; Lantus; Levemir; Mixtard 10, 20, 30, 40, and 50; NovoMix 30; NovoRapid; ***Israel:*** Humalog Mix 25; Humalog; Humulin 70/30; Humulin N; Humulin R; Lantus; Levemir; NovoMix 30; NovoRapid; ***Ital.:*** Actraphane 10, 20, 30, 40, 50; Actrapid; Apidra; Humalog Mix 25 and 50; Humalog; Humulin 30/70 and 50/50; Humulin I; Humulin R; Lantus; Levemir; Monotard; NovoMix 30; NovoRapid; Protaphane; Ultratard; ***Jpn:*** Humacart 3/7; InnoLet 10R, 20R, 30R, 40R, and 50R; InnoLet N; InnoLet R; Novolin 10R, 20R, 30R, 40R, and 50R; Novolin N; Novolin R; NovoRapid 30 Mix chu; NovoRapid; Penfill N; Penfill R; Penfill 10R, 20R, 30R, 40R, 50R; Velosulin; ***Malaysia:*** Actrapid; Humalog; Humulin 30/70; Humulin L; Humulin N; Humulin R; Insulatard; Lantus; Mixtard 30 HM; NovoRapid; ***Mex.:*** Glinux 70/30; Glinux-N; Humalog Mix 25; Humalog; Humanilusin; Humulin 70/30, 80/20; Humulin L; Humulin N; Humulin R; Insulex; Insuman 100N; Insuman 15R/85N, 25R/75N, and 50R/50N; Insuman R; Lantus; Levemir; Novolin 30/70; Novolin N; Novolin R; NovoMix 30; NovoRapid; Prodiabin-N; ***Neth.:*** Actraphane 10, 20, 30, 40, 50; Actrapid; Apidra; Humalog Mix 25, 50; Humalog NPL; Humalog; Humuline 30/70; Humuline NPH; Humuline; Insulatard; Insuman Basal; Insuman Comb 15, 25, and 50; Insuman Infusat; Insuman Rapid; Lantus; Levemir; Liprolog Mix 25, 50; Liprolog; Mixtard 10, 20, 30, 40, and 50; Monotard; NovoMix 30, 50, 70; NovoRapid; Optisulin; Protaphane; Ultratard; Velosulin; ***Norw.:*** Actrapid; Humalog Mix 25; Humalog; Humulin NPH; Insulatard; Insuman Basal; Insuman Comb 25; Insuman Infusat; Insuman Rapid; Lantus; Levemir; Mixtard 10, 20, 30, 40, and 50; NovoMix 30; NovoRapid; ***NZ:*** Actrapid; Humalog Mix 25 or 50; Humalog; Humulin 70/30; Humulin NPH; Humulin R; Insulatard MC; Lantus; Levemir; Mixtard 30 or 50; Monotard; NovoRapid; PenMix 10, 20, 30, 40, or 50; Protaphane; Ultratard; Velosulin HM; Velosulin MC; ***Philipp.:*** Actrapid HM; Biosulidd L; Humalog; Humulin 70/30; Humulin N (NPH); Humulin R (Regular); Insulatard HM; Lantus; Mixtard 30 HM; NovoMix 30; SciLin M30; SciLin N; SciLin R; ***Pol.:*** Actrapid; Apidra; Gensulin N; Gensulin R; Gensulin M10, M20, M30, M40, or M50; Humalog Mix 25 and 50; Humalog; Humulin M3 (30/70); Humulin N; Humulin R; Insulatard; Insulinum Lente; Insulinum Maxirapid; Insulinum Semilente; Insulinum Ultralente; Insuman Basal; Insuman Comb 25; Insuman Rapid; Lantus; Levemir; Mixtard 10, 20, 30, 40, and 50; NovoMix 30; NovoRapid; Polhumin Mix-3; Polhumin N; Polhumin R; Ultratard HM; ***Port.:*** Actrapid; Humalog; Humulin Lenta; Humulin M1, M2, M3, M4, M5; Humulin NPH; Humulin Regular; Humulin Ultralenta; Insulatard; Isuhuman Basal; Isuhuman Comb 25; Isuhuman Rapid; Mixtard 10, 20, 30, 40, and 50 HM; Monotard; Ultratard; ***Rus.:*** Actrapid HM (Актрапид НМ); Actrapid MC (Актрапид МС); Biosulin N (Биосулин Н); Biosulin R (Биосулин Р); Humalog (Хумалог); Humalog Mix 25 (Хумалог Микс 25); Humulin M3 (Хумулин М3); Humulin NPH (Хумулин НПХ); Humulin Regular (Хумулин Регуляр); Insulidd L (Инсулидд Л); Insulin Lt (Инсулин Лт); Insulin Maxirapid (Инсулин Максирапид); Insuman Basal (Инсуман Базал); Insuman Comb 25 (Инсуман Комб 25); Insuman Rapid (Инсуман Рапид); Lantus (Лантус); Levemir (Левемир); Levulin L (Левулин Л); Mixtard 30 HM (Микстард 30 НМ); Monotard MC (Монотард Нм); NovoMix 30 (НовоМикс 30); NovoRapid (Новорапид); Protaphane HM (Протафан НМ); ***S.Afr.:*** Actraphane HM; Actrapid HM; Apidra; Humalog Mix 25; Humalog; Humulin 30/70; Humulin N; Humulin R; Lantus; Levemir; NovoMix 30; NovoRapid; Protaphane HM; ***Singapore:*** Actrapid HM; Humalog Mix 25; Humalog; Humulin 30/70; Humulin N; Humulin R; Insulatard HM; Lantus; Levemir; Mixtard 30, 50; NovoMix 30; NovoRapid; ***Spain:*** Actrapid; Humalog Mix 25 and 50; Humalog NPL; Humalog; Humulina 30:70; Humulina NPH; Humulina Regular; Insulatard; Lantus; Levemir; Mixtard 30; NovoMix 30; NovoRapid; ***Swed.:*** Actrapid; Apidra; Humalog Mix 25 and 50; Humalog; Humulin Mix 30/70; Humulin NPH; Humulin Regular; Insulatard; Insuman Basal; Insuman Comb 25; Insuman Infusat; Insuman Rapid; Lantus; Levemir; Mixtard 10, 20, 30, 40, and 50; Monotard; NovoMix 30; NovoRapid; Ultratard; ***Switz.:*** Actrapid HM; Actrapid MC; Apidra; Humalog; Huminsulin Basal (NPH); Huminsulin Long; Huminsulin Normal; Huminsulin Profil III; Huminsulin Ultralong; Hypurin 30/70 Mix; Hypurin Isophane; Hypurin Neutral; Insulatard HM; Insulatard MC; Insuman Basal; Insuman Comb 25; Insuman Infusat; Insuman Rapid; Lantus; Levemir; Mixtard 30 MC; Mixtard HM 10, 20, 30, 40, 50; Monotard HM; NovoMix 30; NovoRapid; Semilente MC; Ultratard HM; ***Thai.:*** Actrapid HM; Humalog Mix 25; Humalog; Humulin 70/30; Humulin N; Humulin R; Insulatard; Lantus; Mixtard HM; NovoMix 30; NovoRapid; ***Turk.:*** Humalog Mix 25 and 50; Humalog; Humulin M 70/30 and 80/20; Humulin N; Humulin R; Insulatard; Lantus; Mixtard 10, 20, 30, 40, and 50; NovoMix 30; NovoRapid; Orgasulin Mix 30/70; ***UAE:*** Jusline 70/30; Jusline N; Jusline R; ***UK:*** Actrapid; Apidra; Exubera; Humalog Mix 25 and 50; Humalog; Humulin I; Humulin M3; Humulin S; Hypurin 30/70; Hypurin Isophane; Hypurin Lente; Hypurin Neutral; Hypurin Protamine Zinc; Insulatard; Insuman Basal; Insuman Comb 15, 25, and 50; Insuman Rapid; Lantus; Levemir; Mixtard 30; NovoMix 30; NovoRapid; ***USA:*** Apidra; Exubera; Humalog Mix 75/25 and 50/50; Humalog; Humulin 70/30, 50/50; Humulin N; Humulin R; Lantus; Lente Iletin II; Lente; Levemir; Novolin 70/30; Novolin N;

Novolin R; NovoLog Mix 70/30; NovoLog; Regular Iletin II; Ultralente; ***Venez.:*** Humalog Mix 25; Humalog; Humulin 70/30; Humulin N; Humulin R; Insuman N; Insuman R; Lantus.

Isoetarine

Other names: Isoetariini; Isoetarin; Isoetarina; Isoétarine; Isoetarinum; Isoetharine; Win-3406.

Изоэтарин

Isoetarine Hydrochloride

Other names: Etyprenaline Hydrochloride; Hidrocloruro de isoetarina; Isoétarine, Chlorhydrate d'; Isoetarini Hydrochloridum; Isoetharine Hydrochloride; *N*-Isopropylethylnoradrenaline Hydrochloride.

Изоэтарина Гидрохлорид

Isoetarine Mesilate

Other names: Isoétarine, Mésilate d'; Isoetarini Mesilas; Isoetharine Mesylate; Isoetharine Methanesulphonate; *N*-Isopropylethylnoradrenaline Mesylate; Mesilato de isoetarina.

Изоэтарина Мезилат

Clinical profile: Isoetarine is a sympathomimetic with predominantly beta-adrenergic activity. It has been used as a bronchodilator in reversible airways obstruction.

WADA Status: Banned in and out of competition

WADA Class: Beta-2 Agonists

Includes beta-2 agonists or their isomers.

WADA Class: Specified Substances

Also listed as a specified substance.

"The prohibited List may identify specified substances which are particularly susceptible to unintentional anti-doping rule violations because of their general availability in medicinal products or which are less likely to be successfully abused as doping agents."

A doping violation involving such substances may result in a reduced sanction provided that the "*...Athlete can establish that the Use of such a specfied substance was not intended to enhance sport performance...*"

I

Isoflupredone Acetate

Other names: Acetato de isoflupredona; 9α-Fluoroprednisolone Acetate; Isoflupredone, Acétate d'; Isoflupredoni Acetas; U-6013.

Изофлупредона Ацетат

Clinical profile: Isoflupredone is a glucocorticoid that has been used topically in rhinitis. It is also used in veterinary medicine.

WADA Status: Banned in competition

WADA Class: Glucocorticosteroids

All glucocorticosteroids are prohibited when administered orally, rectally, intravenously or intramuscularly. Their use requires a Therapeutic Use Exemption approval. Other routes of administration (intraarticular / periarticular / peritendinous / epidural / intradermal injections and inhalation) require an Abbreviated Therapeutic

Use Exemption except as noted below.

Topical preparations when used for dermatological (including iontophoresis / phonophoresis), auricular, nasal, ophthalmic, buccal, gingival and perianal disorders are not prohibited and do not require any form of Therapeutic Use Exemption.

WADA Class: Specified Substances

Also listed as a specified substance.

"The prohibited List may identify specified substances which are particularly susceptible to unintentional anti-doping rule violations because of their general availability in medicinal products or which are less likely to be successfully abused as doping agents."

A doping violation involving such substances may result in a reduced sanction provided that the "*...Athlete can establish that the Use of such a specfied substance was not intended to enhance sport performance...*"

Preparations
Multi-ingredient: ***Israel:*** Proaf.

Isometheptene Hydrochloride

Other names: Hidrocloruro de isometepteno; Isométheptène, Chlorhydrate d'; Isomethepteni Hydrochloridum.

Изометептена Гидрохлорид

Isometheptene Mucate

Other names: Isométheptène, Mucate d'; Isomethepteni Mucas; Mucato de isometepteno.

Изометептена Мукат

Clinical profile: Isometheptene is an indirect-acting sympathomimetic given for its vasoconstrictor effect in acute attacks of migraine. It is also used in the management of smooth muscle spasm.

WADA Status: Banned in competition

WADA Class: Stimulants

Includes isometheptene and any optical isomers.

WADA Class: Specified Substances

Also listed as a specified substance.

"The prohibited List may identify specified substances which are particularly susceptible to unintentional anti-doping rule violations because of their general availability in medicinal products or which are less likely to be successfully abused as doping agents."

A doping violation involving such substances may result in a reduced sanction provided that the "*...Athlete can establish that the Use of such a specfied substance was not intended to enhance sport performance...*"

Preparations
Single ingredient: ***Turk.:*** Octinum.
Multi-ingredient: ***Braz.:*** Cefaldina; Doralgina; Doridina; Dorsedin; Migranette; Neomigran; Neosaldina; Neuralgina; Sedalgina; Sedol; Tensaldin; ***UK:*** Midrid; ***USA:*** Midrin.

Isoprenaline

Other names: Isoprenaliini; Isoprenalin; Isoprenalina; Isoprénaline; Isoprenalinum; Isopropylarterenol; Isopropylnoradrenaline; Isoproterenol.

Изопреналин

Isoprenaline Hydrochloride

Other names: Hidrocloruro de isoprenalina; Isoprenaliinihydrokloridi; Isoprénaline, chlorhydrate d'; Isoprenalin-hydrochlorid; Isoprenalinhydroklorid; Isoprenalini hydrochloridum; Isopropylarterenol Hydrochloride; Isopropylnoradrenaline Hydrochloride; Isoproterenol Hydrochloride; Izoprenalin Hidroklorür; Izoprenalin-hidroklorid; Izoprenalino hidrochloridas.

Изопреналина Гидрохлорид

Isoprenaline Sulfate

Other names: Isoprenaliinisulfaatti; Isoprenalin sulfát dihydrát; Isoprénaline, sulfate d'; Isoprenaline Sulphate; Isoprenalini sulfas; Isoprenalini Sulfas Dihydricus; Isoprenalinsulfat; Isopropylarterenol Sulphate; Isopropylnoradrenaline Sulphate; Isoproterenol Sulfate; Izoprenalino sulfatas; Izoprenalin-szulfát; Izoprenaliny siarczan; Sulfato de isoprenalina.

Изопреналина Сульфат

Clinical profile: Isoprenaline is a sympathomimetic acting almost exclusively on beta adrenoceptors. It is used to control bradycardia in selected cardiac disorders. Isoprenaline has been used for its powerful bronchodilator effects in the symptomatic relief of reversible airways obstruction although $beta_2$-selective sympathomimetics, such as salbutamol, are now generally preferred.

WADA Status: Banned in competition

WADA Class: Stimulants

Includes stimulants or substances with a similar chemical structure or similar biological effect(s).

WADA Class: Specified Substances

Also listed as a specified substance.

"The prohibited List may identify specified substances which are particularly susceptible to unintentional anti-doping rule violations because of their general availability in medicinal products or which are less likely to be successfully abused as doping agents."

A doping violation involving such substances may result in a reduced sanction provided that the "*...Athlete can establish that the Use of such a specfied substance was not intended to enhance sport performance...*"

Preparations

Single ingredient: ***Austral.:*** Isuprel; ***Austria:*** Ingelan; ***Belg.:*** Isuprel; ***Fr.:*** Isuprel; ***India:*** Isolin; ***Indon.:*** Isuprel; ***Israel:*** Isuprel; ***NZ:*** Isuprel; ***S.Afr.:*** Imuprel; ***Spain:*** Aleudrina; ***Thai.:*** Isuprel; ***USA:*** Isuprel; Medihaler-Iso.

Multi-ingredient: ***Austria:*** Ingelan; ***Port.:*** Prelus; ***Spain:*** Aldo Asma; Frenal Compositum; ***USA:*** Norisodrine with Calcium Iodide.

Isosorbide

Other names: AT-101; Isosorbida; Isosorbidum; NSC-40725.

Изосорбид

Clinical profile: Isosorbide is an osmotic diuretic used for short-term reduction of intraocular pressure in acute glaucoma or prior to surgery.

WADA Status: Banned in and out of competition

WADA Class: Diuretics and Other Masking Agents

Includes diuretics or substances with a similar chemical structure or similar biological effect(s).

Preparations

Single ingredient: ***Mex.:*** Biordyn; ***USA:*** Ismotic.

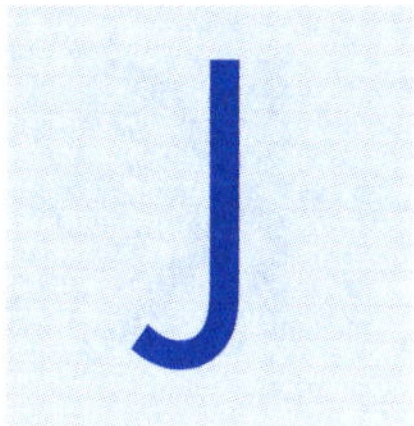

No monographs have been included for drugs beginning with the letter J.

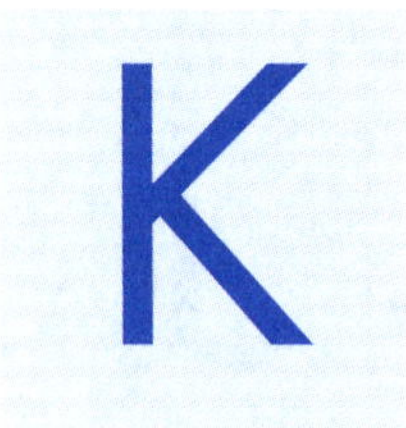

No monographs have been included for drugs beginning with the letter K.

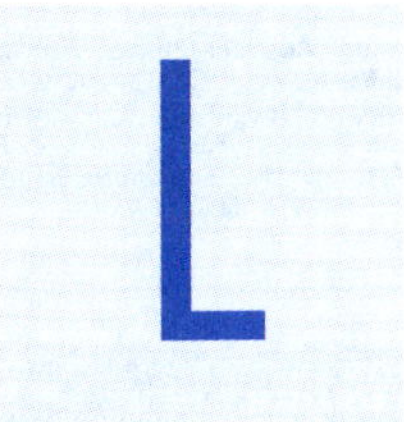

Labetalol Hydrochloride

Other names: AH-5158A; Hidrocloruro de labetalol; Ibidomide Hydrochloride; Labétalol, chlorhydrate de; Labetalol hydrochlorid; Labetalol-hidroklorid; Labetalol-hydroklorid; Labetaloli hydrochloridum; Labetalolihydrokloridi; Labetalolio hidrochloridas; Sch-15719W.

Лабеталола Гидрохлорид

Clinical profile: Labetalol is a non-cardioselective beta blocker with selective alpha$_1$-blocking properties that decrease peripheral vascular resistance. It is used in the management of hypertension and to induce hypotension during surgery.

WADA Status: Banned in and out of competition as specified below

WADA Class: Beta-Blockers

Unless otherwise specified, beta-blockers are prohibited *In-Competition* only in the following sports.

- Aeronautics (FAI)
- Archery (FITA, IPC) (also prohibited *Out-of-Competition*)
- Automobile (FIA)
- Billiards (WCBS)
- Bobsleigh (FIBT)
- Boules (CMSB, IPC bowls)
- Bridge (FMB)
- Curling (WCF)
- Gymnastics (FIG)
- Motorcycling (FIM)
- Modern Pentathlon (UIPM) for disciplines involving shooting
- Nine-pin bowling (FIQ)
- Powerboating (UIM)
- Sailing (ISAF) for match race helms only
- Shooting (ISSF, IPC) (also prohibited *Out-of-Competition*)
- Skiing/Snowboarding (FIS) in ski jumping, freestyle aerials/halfpipe and snowboard halfpipe/big air
- Wrestling (FILA)

WADA Class: Specified Substances

Also listed as a specified substance.

"The prohibited List may identify specified substances which are particularly susceptible to unintentional anti-doping rule violations because of their general availability in medicinal products or which are less likely to be successfully abused as doping agents."

A doping violation involving such substances may result in a reduced sanction provided that the "*...Athlete can establish that the Use of such a specfied substance was not intended to enhance sport performance...*"

Preparations
Single ingredient: ***Arg.:*** Biascor; ***Austral.:*** Presolol; Trandate; ***Austria:*** Trandate; ***Belg.:*** Trandate; ***Canad.:*** Trandate; ***Chile:*** Trandate; ***Cz.:*** Coreton; Trandate; ***Denm.:*** Trandate; ***Fin.:*** Albetol; ***Fr.:*** Trandate; ***Gr.:*** Trandate; ***Hong Kong:*** Trandate; ***Irl.:*** Trandate; ***Israel:*** Trandate; ***Ital.:*** Ipolab; Trandate; ***Malaysia:*** Trandate; ***Neth.:*** Trandate; ***Norw.:*** Trandate; ***NZ:*** Hybloc; Trandate; ***Port.:*** Trandate; ***S.Afr.:*** Trandate; ***Singapore:*** Trandate; ***Spain:*** Trandate; ***Swed.:*** Trandate; ***Switz.:*** Trandate; ***UK:*** Trandate; ***USA:*** Trandate.
Multi-ingredient: ***Ital.:*** Trandiur.

Landiolol Hydrochloride

Other names: Hidrocloruro de landiolol; Landiolol, Chlorhydrate de; Landiololi Hydrochloridum; ONO-1101.

Ландиолола Гидрохлорид

Clinical profile: Landiolol is a short-acting, cardioselective beta blocker given intravenously as the hydrochloride in the management of intra- and postoperative cardiac arrhythmias.

WADA Status: Banned in and out of competition as specified below

WADA Class: Beta-Blockers

Unless otherwise specified, beta-blockers are prohibited *In-Competition* only in the following sports.

- Aeronautics (FAI)
- Archery (FITA, IPC) (also prohibited *Out-of-Competition*)
- Automobile (FIA)
- Billiards (WCBS)
- Bobsleigh (FIBT)
- Boules (CMSB, IPC bowls)
- Bridge (FMB)
- Curling (WCF)
- Gymnastics (FIG)
- Motorcycling (FIM)
- Modern Pentathlon (UIPM) for disciplines involving shooting
- Nine-pin bowling (FIQ)
- Powerboating (UIM)
- Sailing (ISAF) for match race helms only
- Shooting (ISSF, IPC) (also prohibited *Out-of-Competition*)
- Skiing/Snowboarding (FIS) in ski jumping, freestyle aerials/halfpipe and snowboard halfpipe/big air
- Wrestling (FILA)

WADA Class: Specified Substances

Also listed as a specified substance.

"*The prohibited List may identify specified substances which are particularly susceptible to unintentional anti-doping rule violations because of their general availability in medicinal products or which are less likely to be successfully abused as doping agents.*"

A doping violation involving such substances may result in a reduced sanction provided that the "*...Athlete can establish that the Use of such a specfied substance was not intended to enhance sport performance...*"

Preparations
Single ingredient: ***Jpn:*** Onoact.

Letrozole

Other names: CGS-20267; Letrotsoli; Letrozol; Létrozole; Letrozolum.

Летрозол

Clinical profile: Letrozole is a selective nonsteroidal aromatase inhibitor used for the treatment of breast cancer.

WADA Status: Banned in and out of competition

WADA Class: Hormone Antagonists and Modulators

Includes aromatase inhibitors.

Preparations

Single ingredient: ***Arg.:*** Cendalon; Fecinole; Femara; Kebirzol; ***Austral.:*** Femara; ***Austria:*** Femara; ***Belg.:*** Femara; ***Braz.:*** Femara; ***Canad.:*** Femara; ***Chile:*** Femara; ***Cz.:*** Femara; ***Denm.:*** Femar; ***Fin.:*** Femar; ***Fr.:*** Femara; ***Ger.:*** Femara; ***Gr.:*** Femara; ***Hong Kong:*** Femara; ***Hung.:*** Femara; ***India:*** Femara; Fempro; Oncolet; Trozet; ***Indon.:*** Femara; ***Irl.:*** Femara; ***Israel:*** Femara; ***Ital.:*** Femara; ***Jpn:*** Femara; ***Malaysia:*** Femara; ***Mex.:*** Femara; ***Neth.:*** Femara; ***Norw.:*** Femar; ***NZ:*** Femara; ***Philipp.:*** Femara; ***Pol.:*** Aromek; Femara; Lametta; ***Port.:*** Femara; ***Rus.:*** Femara (Фемара); ***S.Afr.:*** Femara; ***Singapore:*** Femara; ***Spain:*** Femara; Insegar; ***Swed.:*** Femar; ***Switz.:*** Femara; ***Thai.:*** Femara; ***Turk.:*** Femara; ***UK:*** Femara; ***USA:*** Femara; ***Venez.:*** Femara.

Leuprorelin

Other names: Leuprolide; Leuproreliini; Leuprorelina; Leuprorelinas; Leuproréline; Leuprorelinum.

Лейпрорелин

Leuprorelin Acetate

Other names: Abbott-43818; Acetato de leuprorelina; Leuprolide Acetate; Leuproreliiniasetaatti; Leuprorelinacetat; Leuproréline, Acétate de; Leuprorelini Acetas; Löprorelin Asetat; TAP-144.

Лейпрорелина Ацетат

Clinical profile: Leuprorelin is an analogue of gonadorelin used for the suppression of testosterone in the treatment of malignant neoplasms of the prostate. It is also used in precocious puberty, endometriosis, and uterine fibroids.

WADA Status: Banned in and out of competition

WADA Class: Hormones and Related Substances: Gonadotrophins

Includes gonadotrophin or a substance with a similar chemical structure or similar biological effect(s), or one of their releasing factors. Prohibited in males only.

Preparations

Single ingredient: ***Arg.:*** Eligard; Lectrum; Lupron; ***Austral.:*** Eligard; Lucrin; ***Austria:*** Enantone; Trenantone; ***Belg.:*** Depo-Eligard; Lucrin; ***Braz.:*** Lectrum; Lupron; Reliser; ***Canad.:*** Eligard; Lupron; ***Chile:*** Lupron; ***Cz.:*** Lucrin; ***Denm.:*** Procren; ***Fin.:*** Eligard; Enanton; Procren; ***Fr.:*** Eligard; Enantone; ***Ger.:*** Eligard; Enantone-Gyn; Enantone; Trenantone; ***Gr.:*** Daronda; Elityran; Leuprol; ***Hong Kong:*** Enantone; Lorelin; ***Hung.:*** Eligard; Lucrin; ***India:*** Lupride; ***Indon.:*** Endrolin; Lectrum; Tapros; ***Irl.:*** Prostap; ***Israel:*** Lucrin; ***Ital.:*** Enantone; ***Jpn:*** Leuplin; Lupron; ***Malaysia:*** Lucrin; ***Mex.:*** Lectrum; Lorelin; Lucrin; ***Neth.:*** Daronda; Eligard; Lucrin; ***Norw.:*** Enanton; Procren; ***NZ:*** Eligard; Lucrin; ***Philipp.:*** Luprolex; ***Pol.:*** Eligard; Lucrin Depot; ***Port.:*** Lucrin; ***Rus.:*** Lucrin (Люкрин); ***S.Afr.:*** Lucrin; ***Singapore:*** Lucrin; ***Spain:*** Eligard; Ginecrin; Procrin; ***Swed.:*** Eligard; Enanton; Procren; ***Switz.:*** Eligard; Lucrin; ***Thai.:*** Enantone; ***Turk.:*** Lucrin; ***UK:*** Prostap; ***USA:*** Eligard; Lupron; ***Venez.:*** Lupron.

Levmetamfetamine

Other names: *l*-Deoxyephedrine; L-Desoxiefedrina; L-Desoxyephedrine; Lesoxyephedrine; Levmétamfétamine; Levmetamfetaminum; Levmetanfetamina; Levometanfetamina; *l*-Methamphetamine; *l*-Methylamphetamine.

Левметамфетамин

Clinical profile: Levmetamfetamine is an isomer of metamfetamine and is used topically in the treatment of nasal congestion.

WADA Status: Banned in competition

WADA Class: Stimulants

Includes levmetamfetamine and any optical isomers.

WADA Class: Specified Substances

Also listed as a specified substance.

"The prohibited List may identify specified substances which are particularly susceptible to unintentional anti-doping rule violations because of their general availability in medicinal products or which are less likely to be successfully abused as doping agents."

A doping violation involving such substances may result in a reduced sanction provided that the "*...Athlete can establish that the Use of such a specified substance was not intended to enhance sport performance...*"

Preparations
Single ingredient: ***USA:*** Vicks Vapor Inhaler.

Levobetaxolol Hydrochloride

Other names: AL-1577A (levobetaxolol or levobetaxolol hydrochloride); Hidrocloruro de levobetaxolol; Lévobétaxolol, Chlorhydrate de; Levobetaxololi Hydrochloridum.

Левобетаксолола Гидрохлорид

Clinical profile: Levobetaxolol is a cardioselective beta blocker that has been used in the management of glaucoma and ocular hypertension.

WADA Status: Banned in and out of competition as specified below

WADA Class: Beta-Blockers

Unless otherwise specified, beta-blockers are prohibited *In-Competition* only in the following sports.

- Aeronautics (FAI)
- Archery (FITA, IPC) (also prohibited *Out-of-Competition*)
- Automobile (FIA)
- Billiards (WCBS)
- Bobsleigh (FIBT)
- Boules (CMSB, IPC bowls)
- Bridge (FMB)
- Curling (WCF)
- Gymnastics (FIG)
- Motorcycling (FIM)
- Modern Pentathlon (UIPM) for disciplines involving shooting
- Nine-pin bowling (FIQ)
- Powerboating (UIM)
- Sailing (ISAF) for match race helms only
- Shooting (ISSF, IPC) (also prohibited *Out-of-Competition*)
- Skiing/Snowboarding (FIS) in ski jumping, freestyle aerials/halfpipe and snowboard halfpipe/big air
- Wrestling (FILA)

WADA Class: Specified Substances

Also listed as a specified substance.

"The prohibited List may identify specified substances which are particularly susceptible to unintentional anti-doping rule violations because of their general availability in medicinal products or which are less likely to be successfully abused as doping agents."

A doping violation involving such substances may result in a reduced sanction pro-

vided that the "*...Athlete can establish that the Use of such a specfied substance was not intended to enhance sport performance...*"

Levobunolol Hydrochloride

Other names: (−)-Bunolol Hydrochloride; *l*-Bunolol Hydrochloride; Hidrocloruro de levobunolol; Lévobunolol, Chlorhydrate de; Levobunolol Hidroklorür; Levobunololhydroklorid; Levobunololi Hydrochloridum; Levobunololihydrokloridi; W-7000A.

Левобунолола Гидрохлорид

Clinical profile: Levobunolol is a non-cardioselective beta blocker used to reduce raised intra-ocular pressure in open-angle glaucoma and ocular hypertension.

WADA Status: Banned in and out of competition as specified below

WADA Class: Beta-Blockers

Unless otherwise specified, beta-blockers are prohibited *In-Competition* only in the following sports.

- Aeronautics (FAI)
- Archery (FITA, IPC) (also prohibited *Out-of-Competition*)
- Automobile (FIA)
- Billiards (WCBS)
- Bobsleigh (FIBT)
- Boules (CMSB, IPC bowls)
- Bridge (FMB)
- Curling (WCF)
- Gymnastics (FIG)
- Motorcycling (FIM)
- Modern Pentathlon (UIPM) for disciplines involving shooting
- Nine-pin bowling (FIQ)
- Powerboating (UIM)
- Sailing (ISAF) for match race helms only
- Shooting (ISSF, IPC) (also prohibited *Out-of-Competition*)
- Skiing/Snowboarding (FIS) in ski jumping, freestyle aerials/halfpipe and snowboard halfpipe/big air
- Wrestling (FILA)

WADA Class: Specified Substances

Also listed as a specified substance.

"*The prohibited List may identify specified substances which are particularly susceptible to unintentional anti-doping rule violations because of their general availability in medicinal products or which are less likely to be successfully abused as doping agents.*"

A doping violation involving such substances may result in a reduced sanction provided that the "*...Athlete can establish that the Use of such a specfied substance was not intended to enhance sport performance...*"

Preparations

Single ingredient: ***Arg.:*** Betagan; Levunolol; ***Austral.:*** Betagan; ***Austria:*** Vistagan; ***Belg.:*** Betagan; ***Braz.:*** Betagan; ***Canad.:*** Betagan; ***Chile:*** Betagen; ***Cz.:*** Vistagan; ***Denm.:*** Betagan; ***Fr.:*** Betagan; ***Ger.:*** Vistagan; ***Gr.:*** Vistagan; ***Hong Kong:*** Betagan; ***Hung.:*** Vistagan; ***Irl.:*** Betagan; ***Israel:*** Betagan; ***Ital.:*** Vistagan; ***Malaysia:*** Betagan; ***Mex.:*** Betagan; ***Neth.:*** Betagan; ***NZ:*** Betagan; ***Port.:*** Betagan; ***S.Afr.:*** Betagan; ***Singapore:*** Betagan; ***Spain:*** Betagan; ***Switz.:*** Vistagan; ***Thai.:*** Betagan; ***Turk.:*** Betagan; ***UK:*** Betagan; ***USA:*** Ak-Beta; Betagan; ***Venez.:*** Vistagan.

L

Levomethadone Hydrochloride

Other names: Hidrocloruro de levometadona; Levometadonhidroklorid; Levometadonhydroklorid; Levometadonihydrokloridi; Levometadono hidrochloridas;

Lévométhadone, chlorhydrate de; Levomethadon-hydrochlorid; Levomethadoni hydrochloridum; (–)-Methadone Hydrochloride.

Левометадона Гидрохлорид

Clinical profile: Levomethadone hydrochloride, an opioid analgesic, is the active isomer of racemic methadone hydrochloride and is used in the treatment of severe pain.

WADA Status: Banned in competition

WADA Class: Narcotics

Includes specified narcotics.

Preparations
Single ingredient: ***Ger.:*** L-Polamidon.

Levomoprolol Hydrochloride

Other names: Hidrocloruro de levomoprolol; Lévomoprolol, Chlorhydrate de; Levomoprololi Hydrochloridum; (–)-(S)-Moprolol Hydrochloride.

Левомопролола Гидрохлорид

Clinical profile: Levomoprolol is a beta blocker. It is the (–)-enantiomer of moprolol and is responsible for moprolol's beta-blocking activity. Both have been given in the management of hypertension.

WADA Status: Banned in and out of competition as specified below

WADA Class: Beta-Blockers

Unless otherwise specified, beta-blockers are prohibited *In-Competition* only in the following sports.

- Aeronautics (FAI)
- Archery (FITA, IPC) (also prohibited *Out-of-Competition*)
- Automobile (FIA)
- Billiards (WCBS)
- Bobsleigh (FIBT)
- Boules (CMSB, IPC bowls)
- Bridge (FMB)
- Curling (WCF)
- Gymnastics (FIG)
- Motorcycling (FIM)
- Modern Pentathlon (UIPM) for disciplines involving shooting
- Nine-pin bowling (FIQ)
- Powerboating (UIM)
- Sailing (ISAF) for match race helms only
- Shooting (ISSF, IPC) (also prohibited *Out-of-Competition*)
- Skiing/Snowboarding (FIS) in ski jumping, freestyle aerials/halfpipe and snowboard halfpipe/big air
- Wrestling (FILA)

WADA Class: Specified Substances

Also listed as a specified substance.

"The prohibited List may identify specified substances which are particularly susceptible to unintentional anti-doping rule violations because of their general availability in medicinal products or which are less likely to be successfully abused as doping agents."

A doping violation involving such substances may result in a reduced sanction pro-

vided that the "*...Athlete can establish that the Use of such a specfied substance was not intended to enhance sport performance...*"

Levosalbutamol

Other names: Levalbuterol; Lévosalbutamol; Levosalbutamolum.

Левосальбутамол

Levosalbutamol Hydrochloride

Other names: Hidrocloruro de levosalbutamol; Levalbuterol Hydrochloride; Lévosalbutamol, Chlorhydrate de; Levosalbutamoli Hydrochloridum.

Левосальбутамола Гидрохлорид

Levosalbutamol Sulfate

Other names: Levalbuterol Sulfate; Lévosalbutamol, Sulfate de; Levosalbutamol Sulphate; Levosalbutamoli Sulfas; Sulfato de levosalbutamol.

Левосальбутамола Сульфат

Levosalbutamol Tartrate

Other names: Levalbuterol Tartrate; Lévosalbutamol, Tartrate de; Levosalbutamoli Tartras; Tartrato de levosalbutamol.

Левосальбутамола Тартрат

Clinical profile: Levosalbutamol, the active isomer of salbutamol, is used for the treatment of asthma.

WADA Status: Banned in and out of competition

WADA Class: Beta-2 Agonists

Includes beta-2 agonists or their isomers.

WADA Class: Specified Substances

Also listed as a specified substance.

"*The prohibited List may identify specified substances which are particularly susceptible to unintentional anti-doping rule violations because of their general availability in medicinal products or which are less likely to be successfully abused as doping agents.*"

A doping violation involving such substances may result in a reduced sanction provided that the "*...Athlete can establish that the Use of such a specfied substance was not intended to enhance sport performance...*"

Preparations

Single ingredient: ***Arg.:*** Albulair; Ventoplus; ***India:*** Levolin; ***USA:*** Xopenex.

Lisdexamfetamine Mesilate

Other names: Lisdexamfetamine Dimesylate; Lisdexamfétamine, Mésilate de; Lisdexamfetamini Mesilas; Mesilato de lisdexanfetamina; NRP-104.

Лисдексамфетамина Мезилат

Clinical profile: Lisdexamfetamine is a prodrug of dexamfetamine used as the mesilate in the treatment of hyperactivity disorders in children.

WADA Status: Banned in competition

WADA Class: Stimulants

Includes stimulants or substances with a similar chemical structure or similar biological effect(s).

WADA Class: Specified Substances

Also listed as a specified substance.

"The prohibited List may identify specified substances which are particularly susceptible to unintentional anti-doping rule violations because of their general availability in medicinal products or which are less likely to be successfully abused as doping agents."

A doping violation involving such substances may result in a reduced sanction provided that the "*...Athlete can establish that the Use of such a specfied substance was not intended to enhance sport performance...*"

Preparations
Single ingredient: ***USA:*** Vyvanse.

Lithium Benzoate

Other names: Litio, benzoato de.

Clinical profile: Lithium benzoate has been used as a diuretic and urinary disinfectant. Its use cannot be recommended because of the pharmacological effect of the lithium ion.

WADA Status: Banned in and out of competition

WADA Class: Diuretics and Other Masking Agents

Includes diuretics or substances with a similar chemical structure or similar biological effect(s).

Lobelia

Other names: Indian Tobacco.

Lobeline Hydrochloride

Other names: Alpha-lobeline Hydrochloride; Hidrocloruro de lobelina; Lobeliinihydrokloridi; Lobéline, chlorhydrate de; Lobelin-hidroklorid; Lobelin-hydrochlorid; Lobelinhydroklorid; Lobelini hydrochloridum; Lobelino hidrochloridas.

Лобелина Гидрохлорид

Lobeline Sulfate

Other names: Lobéline, Sulfate de; Lobeline Sulphate; Lobelini Sulfas; Sulfato de lobelina.

Лобелина Сульфат

Clinical profile: Lobelia is the dried aerial parts of *Lobelia inflata* (Lobeliaceae). Lobeline is the main alkaloidal constituent and has peripheral and central effects similar to those of nicotine. Lobelia has been used in preparations aimed at relieving respiratory-tract disorders. Lobeline has been given by mouth as a smoking deterrent. Lobelia has been used similarly given either by mouth or incorporated into herbal cigarettes.

WADA Status: Banned in competition

WADA Class: Stimulants

Includes stimulants or substances with a similar chemical structure or similar biological effect(s).

WADA Class: Specified Substances

Also listed as a specified substance.

"The prohibited List may identify specified substances which are particularly susceptible to unintentional anti-doping rule violations because of their general availability in medicinal products or which are less likely to be successfully abused as doping agents."

A doping violation involving such substances may result in a reduced sanction provided that the "*...Athlete can establish that the Use of such a specfied substance was not intended to enhance sport performance...*"

Preparations

Single ingredient: ***Austral.:*** Cig-Ridettes; ***Canad.:*** Butt-Out; ***Spain:*** Smokeless.
Multi-ingredient: ***Austral.:*** Potassium Iodide and Stramonium Compound; ***Braz.:*** Asmatiron; Broncofenil; Bronquidex; Brontoss; Expectobron; Expectol; Iodeto de Potassio; Iodeto de Potassio; Iol; Iolin; MM Expectorante; Pulmoforte; ***Chile:*** Paltomiel Plus; Pulmagol; Ramistos; ***Spain:*** Pazbronquial; ***UK:*** Antibron; Asthma & Catarrh Relief; Balm of Gilead; Chest Mixture; Herbelix; Horehound and Aniseed Cough Mixture; Modern Herbals Cold & Congestion; Vegetable Cough Remover; ***Venez.:*** Novacodin.

Loteprednol Etabonate

Other names: CDDD-5604; Etabonato de loteprednol; HGP-1; Lotéprednol, Etabonate de; Loteprednol Ethyl Carbonate; Loteprednoli Etabonas; P-5604.
Лотепреднола Этабонат

Clinical profile: Loteprednol etabonate is a glucocorticoid used in the topical treatment of inflammatory and allergic disorders of the eye.

WADA Status: Banned in competition

WADA Class: Glucocorticosteroids

All glucocorticosteroids are prohibited when administered orally, rectally, intravenously or intramuscularly. Their use requires a Therapeutic Use Exemption approval. Other routes of administration (intraarticular / periarticular / peritendinous / epidural / intradermal injections and inhalation) require an Abbreviated Therapeutic Use Exemption except as noted below.

Topical preparations when used for dermatological (including iontophoresis / phonophoresis), auricular, nasal, ophthalmic, buccal, gingival and perianal disorders are not prohibited and do not require any form of Therapeutic Use Exemption.

WADA Class: Specified Substances

Also listed as a specified substance.

"The prohibited List may identify specified substances which are particularly susceptible to unintentional anti-doping rule violations because of their general availability in medicinal products or which are less likely to be successfully abused as doping agents."

A doping violation involving such substances may result in a reduced sanction provided that the "*...Athlete can establish that the Use of such a specfied substance was not intended to enhance sport performance...*"

Preparations

Single ingredient: ***Arg.:*** Alrex; Lopred; Lotemax; Lotesoft; ***Braz.:*** Alrex; ***Ger.:*** Lotemax; ***Gr.:*** Lotemax; ***Hong Kong:*** Lotemax; ***India:*** Loteflam; ***Ital.:*** Lotemax; ***Mex.:*** Loterex; ***Singapore:*** Lotemax; ***USA:*** Alrex; Lotemax; ***Venez.:*** Lotesoft.
Multi-ingredient: ***Arg.:*** Lotemicin.

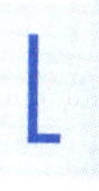

Luteinising Hormone

Other names: Human Interstitial-cell-stimulating Hormone; ICSH; LH; Lutropin; Lutropina.

Clinical profile: Luteinising hormone (LH) is a gonadotrophic hormone secreted by the anterior lobe of the pituitary gland, with another gonadotrophin, follicle-stimulating hormone (FSH). Gonadotrophic substances with LH and/or FSH activity are used in the treatment of fertility disorders, chiefly in females but also in males.

Lutropin Alfa

Other names: Lutropina alfa; Lutropine Alfa; Lutropinum Alfa.

Лутропин Альфа

Clinical profile: Lutropin alfa is a recombinant human luteinising hormone used with follicle-stimulating hormone in the treatment of fertility disorders in women.

WADA Status: Banned in and out of competition

WADA Class: Hormones and Related Substances: Gonadotrophins

Includes gonadotrophin or a substance with a similar chemical structure or similar biological effect(s), or one of their releasing factors. Prohibited in males only.

Preparations

Single ingredient: ***Arg.:*** Luveris; ***Braz.:*** Luveris; ***Cz.:*** Luveris; ***Denm.:*** Luveris; ***Fin.:*** Luveris; ***Fr.:*** Luveris; ***Ger.:*** Luveris; ***Gr.:*** Luveris; ***Hong Kong:*** Luveris; ***Hung.:*** Luveris; ***Indon.:*** Luveris; ***Irl.:*** Luveris; ***Israel:*** Luveris; ***Ital.:*** Luveris; ***Malaysia:*** Luveris; ***Mex.:*** Luveris; ***Neth.:*** Luveris; ***Norw.:*** Luveris; ***NZ:*** Luveris; ***Philipp.:*** Luveris; ***Pol.:*** Luveris; ***Port.:*** Luveris; ***Rus.:*** Luveris (Луверис); ***Singapore:*** Luveris; ***Spain:*** Luveris; ***Swed.:*** Luveris; ***Switz.:*** Luveris; ***Thai.:*** Luveris; ***Turk.:*** Luveris; ***UK:*** Luveris; ***USA:*** Luveris; ***Venez.:*** Luveris.

Multi-ingredient: ***UK:*** Pergoveris.

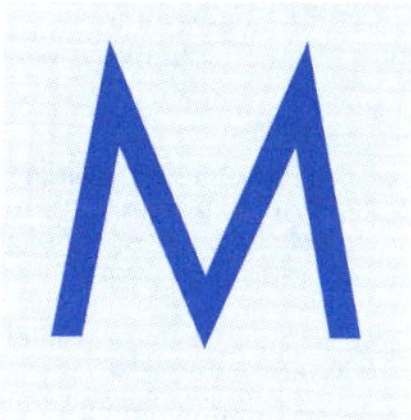

Mabuterol

Other names: KF-868 (mabuterol hydrochloride); Mabutérol; Mabuterolum; PB-868CL (mabuterol hydrochloride).

Мабутерол

Clinical profile: Mabuterol is a sympathomimetic agent that has been used as a bronchodilator.

WADA Status: Banned in competition

WADA Class: Stimulants

Includes stimulants or substances with a similar chemical structure or similar biological effect(s).

WADA Class: Specified Substances

Also listed as a specified substance.

"The prohibited List may identify specified substances which are particularly susceptible to unintentional anti-doping rule violations because of their general availability in medicinal products or which are less likely to be successfully abused as doping agents."

A doping violation involving such substances may result in a reduced sanction provided that the "*...Athlete can establish that the Use of such a specfied substance was not intended to enhance sport performance...*"

Mannitol

Other names: Cordycepic Acid; E421; Manita; Manitol; Manitolis; Manna Sugar; Mannit; Mannite; Mannitoli; Mannitolum.

Clinical profile: Mannitol is an osmotic agent used to increase urine flow in patients with acute renal failure and to reduce raised intracranial pressure and treat cerebral oedema. It is also used to reduce raised intra-ocular pressure, to promote the excretion of toxic substances by forced diuresis, as a bladder irrigation during transurethral resection of the prostate, and as an osmotic laxative for bowel preparation. Mannitol is used as a diluent and excipient in pharmaceutical preparations and as a bulk sweetener. It is under investigation for bronchiectasis and cystic fibrosis.

WADA Status: Banned in and out of competition

WADA Class: Diuretics and Other Masking Agents

Includes diuretics or substances with a similar chemical structure or similar biological effect(s).

Preparations

Single ingredient: ***Austral.:*** Mede-Prep; Osmitrol; ***Canad.:*** Osmitrol; ***Cz.:*** Ardeaosmosol MA; Mannisol; Osmofundin 15% N; ***Ger.:*** Deltamannit; Mannit-Losung; Osmofundin 15% N; Osmosteril 20%; ***Hung.:*** Mannisol; ***Ital.:*** Isotol; ***Mex.:*** Osmorol; ***Neth.:*** Osmosteril; ***Port.:*** Osmofundina; ***Spain:*** Osmofundina Concentrada; ***Switz.:*** Mannite; ***Turk.:*** Resectisol; Rezosel; ***USA:*** Osmitrol; Resectisol.

Multi-ingredient: ***Austria:*** Osmofundin 10%; Resectal; ***Chile:*** Gelsolets; ***Denm.:*** Pharmalgen Albumin; ***Fin.:*** Somanol + Ethanol; ***Ger.:*** Flacar; Freka-Drainjet Purisole; Osmosteril 10%; ***Ital.:*** Levoplus; Naturalass; ***Mex.:*** Jarabe de Manzanas; ***Pol.:*** Purisole SM; ***Port.:*** Xarope de Macas Rainetas; ***Rus.:*** Rheogluman (Реоглюман); ***Spain:*** Salmagne.

Mazindol

Other names: 42-548; AN-448; Matsindoli; Mazindolum; SaH-42548.

Мазиндол

Clinical profile: Mazindol is a central stimulant that has been used as an anorectic in the treatment of obesity. Mazindol has been investigated in the treatment of Duchenne muscular dystrophy.

WADA Status: Banned in competition

WADA Class: Stimulants

Includes stimulants or substances with a similar chemical structure or similar biological effect(s).

WADA Class: Specified Substances

Also listed as a specified substance.

"*The prohibited List may identify specified substances which are particularly susceptible to unintentional anti-doping rule violations because of their general availability in medicinal products or which are less likely to be successfully abused as doping agents.*"

A doping violation involving such substances may result in a reduced sanction provided that the "*...Athlete can establish that the Use of such a specfied substance was not intended to enhance sport performance...*"

Preparations

Single ingredient: ***Arg.:*** Afilan; Dimagrir; Fagolip Plus; Samonter; ***Braz.:*** Absten S; Fagolipo; ***Hong Kong:*** Qualizindol; ***Indon.:*** Teronac; ***Mex.:*** Diestet; Ifa Lose; Ilezol; Obendol; Solucaps; ***Singapore:*** Teronac.

Multi-ingredient: ***Arg.:*** Maxitratobes; ***Braz.:*** Dobesix; Moderine.

Mazipredone

Other names: Mazipredona; Maziprédone; Mazipredonum.

Мазипредон

Clinical profile: Mazipredone is a corticosteroid used with miconazole in the treatment of fungal infections of the skin.

WADA Status: Banned in competition

WADA Class: Glucocorticosteroids

All glucocorticosteroids are prohibited when administered orally, rectally, intravenously or intramuscularly. Their use requires a Therapeutic Use Exemption approval. Other routes of administration (intraarticular / periarticular / peritendinous / epidural / intradermal injections and inhalation) require an Abbreviated Therapeutic

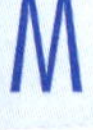

Use Exemption except as noted below.

Topical preparations when used for dermatological (including iontophoresis / phonophoresis), auricular, nasal, ophthalmic, buccal, gingival and perianal disorders are not prohibited and do not require any form of Therapeutic Use Exemption.

WADA Class: Specified Substances

Also listed as a specified substance.

"The prohibited List may identify specified substances which are particularly susceptible to unintentional anti-doping rule violations because of their general availability in medicinal products or which are less likely to be successfully abused as doping agents."

A doping violation involving such substances may result in a reduced sanction provided that the "*...Athlete can establish that the Use of such a specfied substance was not intended to enhance sport performance...*"

Preparations
Single ingredient: ***Cz.:*** Depersolon.
Multi-ingredient: ***Cz.:*** Mycosolon; ***Hung.:*** Mycosolon; ***Pol.:*** Mycosolon; ***Rus.:*** Mycosolon (Микозолон).

Mebutizide

Other names: Mebutizida; Mébutizide; Mebutizidum.

Мебутизид

Clinical profile: Mebutizide is a thiazide diuretic that has been used in the treatment of oedema and hypertension.

WADA Status: Banned in and out of competition

WADA Class: Diuretics and Other Masking Agents

Includes diuretics or substances with a similar chemical structure or similar biological effect(s).

Meclofenoxate Hydrochloride

Other names: Centrophenoxine Hydrochloride; Clofenoxine Hydrochloride; Clophenoxate Hydrochloride; Deanol 4-Chlorophenoxyacetate Hydrochloride; Hidrocloruro de meclofenoxato; Meclofenoxane Hydrochloride; Méclofénoxate, Chlorhydrate de; Meclofenoxati Hydrochloridum.

Меклофеноксата Гидрохлорид

Clinical profile: Meclofenoxate hydrochloride has been claimed to aid cellular metabolism in the presence of diminished oxygen concentrations. It has been given mainly for mental changes in the elderly, or following strokes or head injury.

WADA Status: Banned in competition

WADA Class: Stimulants

Includes meclofenoxate and any optical isomers.

WADA Class: Specified Substances

Also listed as a specified substance.

"The prohibited List may identify specified substances which are particularly susceptible to unintentional anti-doping rule violations because of their general availability in medicinal products or which are less likely to be successfully abused as doping agents."

A doping violation involving such substances may result in a reduced sanction pro-

vided that the "...*Athlete can establish that the Use of such a specfied substance was not intended to enhance sport performance...*"

Preparations
Single ingredient: ***Austria:*** Lucidril.

Medroxalol Hydrochloride

Other names: Hidrocloruro de medroxalol; MDL-81968A; Médroxalol, Chlorhydrate de; Medroxaloli Hydrochloridum; RMI-81968A.

Медроксалола Гидрохлорид

Clinical profile: Medroxalol hydrochloride is reported to have alpha- and beta-blocking activity and has been investigated in the treatment of hypertension.

WADA Status: Banned in and out of competition as specified below

WADA Class: Beta-Blockers

Unless otherwise specified, beta-blockers are prohibited *In-Competition* only in the following sports.

- Aeronautics (FAI)
- Archery (FITA, IPC) (also prohibited *Out-of-Competition*)
- Automobile (FIA)
- Billiards (WCBS)
- Bobsleigh (FIBT)
- Boules (CMSB, IPC bowls)
- Bridge (FMB)
- Curling (WCF)
- Gymnastics (FIG)
- Motorcycling (FIM)
- Modern Pentathlon (UIPM) for disciplines involving shooting
- Nine-pin bowling (FIQ)
- Powerboating (UIM)
- Sailing (ISAF) for match race helms only
- Shooting (ISSF, IPC) (also prohibited *Out-of-Competition*)
- Skiing/Snowboarding (FIS) in ski jumping, freestyle aerials/halfpipe and snowboard halfpipe/big air
- Wrestling (FILA)

WADA Class: Specified Substances

Also listed as a specified substance.

"*The prohibited List may identify specified substances which are particularly susceptible to unintentional anti-doping rule violations because of their general availability in medicinal products or which are less likely to be successfully abused as doping agents.*"

A doping violation involving such substances may result in a reduced sanction provided that the "...*Athlete can establish that the Use of such a specfied substance was not intended to enhance sport performance...*"

Medrysone

Other names: 11β-Hydroxy-6α-methylprogesterone; Medrisona; Médrysone; Medrysonum; NSC-63278; U-8471.

Медризон

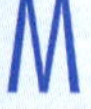

Clinical profile: Medrysone is a glucocorticoid corticosteroid employed in the topical treatment of allergic and inflammatory conditions of the eye.

WADA Status: Banned in competition

WADA Class: Glucocorticosteroids

All glucocorticosteroids are prohibited when administered orally, rectally, intravenously or intramuscularly. Their use requires a Therapeutic Use Exemption approval. Other routes of administration (intraarticular / periarticular / peritendinous / epidural / intradermal injections and inhalation) require an Abbreviated Therapeutic Use Exemption except as noted below.

Topical preparations when used for dermatological (including iontophoresis / phonophoresis), auricular, nasal, ophthalmic, buccal, gingival and perianal disorders are not prohibited and do not require any form of Therapeutic Use Exemption.

WADA Class: Specified Substances

Also listed as a specified substance.

"The prohibited List may identify specified substances which are particularly susceptible to unintentional anti-doping rule violations because of their general availability in medicinal products or which are less likely to be successfully abused as doping agents."

A doping violation involving such substances may result in a reduced sanction provided that the "*...Athlete can establish that the Use of such a specfied substance was not intended to enhance sport performance...*"

Preparations

Single ingredient: ***Austral.:*** HMS; ***Port.:*** Medrisocil.

Mefenorex Hydrochloride

Other names: Hidrocloruro de mefenorex; Méfénorex, Chlorhydrate de; Mefenorexi Hydrochloridum; Ro-4-5282.

Мефенорекса Гидрохлорид

Clinical profile: Mefenorex hydrochloride is a central stimulant and indirect-acting sympathomimetic that has been used as an anorectic in the treatment of obesity.

WADA Status: Banned in competition

WADA Class: Stimulants

Includes mefenorex and any optical isomers.

Mefruside

Other names: Bay-1500; FBA-1500; Mefrusid; Mefrusida; Méfruside; Mefrusidi; Mefrusidum.

Мефрузид

Clinical profile: Mefruside is a diuretic similar to the thiazide diuretics. It is used for oedema, including that associated with heart failure, and for hypertension.

WADA Status: Banned in and out of competition

WADA Class: Diuretics and Other Masking Agents

Includes diuretics or substances with a similar chemical structure or similar biological effect(s).

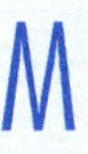

Preparations
Multi-ingredient: ***Ger.:*** Sali-Adalat; Sali-Prent.

Mephentermine Sulfate

Other names: Méphentermine, Sulfate de; Mephentermine Sulphate; Mephentermini Sulfas; Mephetedrine Sulphate; Sulfato de mefentermina.

Мефентермина Сульфат

Clinical profile: Mephentermine sulfate is a sympathomimetic with mainly indirect effects on adrenergic receptors. It has alpha- and beta-adrenergic activity, and a slight stimulating effect on the CNS. It has an inotropic effect on the heart. It is used to maintain blood pressure in hypotensive states, for example following spinal anaesthesia.

WADA Status: Banned in competition

WADA Class: Stimulants

Includes mephentermine and any optical isomers.

Preparations
Single ingredient: ***India:*** Mephentine.
Multi-ingredient: ***USA:*** Emergent-Ez.

Mepindolol Sulfate

Other names: LF-17895 (mepindolol); Mépindolol, Sulfate de; Mepindolol Sulphate; Mepindololi Sulfas; SHE-222; Sulfato de mepindolol.

Мепиндолола Сульфат

Clinical profile: Mepindolol, the methyl analogue of pindolol, is a non-cardioselective beta blocker used in the management of cardiovascular disorders including hypertension.

WADA Status: Banned in and out of competition as specified below

WADA Class: Beta-Blockers

Unless otherwise specified, beta-blockers are prohibited *In-Competition* only in the following sports.

- Aeronautics (FAI)
- Archery (FITA, IPC) (also prohibited *Out-of-Competition*)
- Automobile (FIA)
- Billiards (WCBS)
- Bobsleigh (FIBT)
- Boules (CMSB, IPC bowls)
- Bridge (FMB)
- Curling (WCF)
- Gymnastics (FIG)
- Motorcycling (FIM)
- Modern Pentathlon (UIPM) for disciplines involving shooting
- Nine-pin bowling (FIQ)
- Powerboating (UIM)
- Sailing (ISAF) for match race helms only
- Shooting (ISSF, IPC) (also prohibited *Out-of-Competition*)
- Skiing/Snowboarding (FIS) in ski jumping, freestyle aerials/halfpipe and snowboard halfpipe/big air
- Wrestling (FILA)

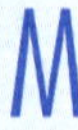

WADA Class: Specified Substances

Also listed as a specified substance.

"The prohibited List may identify specified substances which are particularly susceptible to unintentional anti-doping rule violations because of their general availability in medicinal

products or which are less likely to be successfully abused as doping agents."
A doping violation involving such substances may result in a reduced sanction provided that the "*...Athlete can establish that the Use of such a specfied substance was not intended to enhance sport performance...*"

Preparations
Single ingredient: ***Ger.:*** Corindolan.

Mepitiostane

Other names: Mépitiostane; Mepitiostano; Mepitiostanum; S-10364.

Мепитиостан

Clinical profile: Mepitiostane has androgenic and anabolic properties, and is used in treating neoplasms of the breast and anaemia of renal failure.

WADA Status: Banned in and out of competition

WADA Class: Anabolic; Androgenic Steroids (exogenous)
Includes exogenous anabolic androgenic steroids or other substances with a similar chemical structure or similar biological effect(s).

Preparations
Single ingredient: ***Jpn:*** Thioderon.

Meprednisone

Other names: Meprednisona; Méprednisone; Meprednisonum; 16β-Methylprednisone; NSC-527579; Sch-4358.

Мепреднизон

Clinical profile: Meprednisone is a glucocorticoid corticosteroid.

WADA Status: Banned in competition

WADA Class: Glucocorticosteroids
All glucocorticosteroids are prohibited when administered orally, rectally, intravenously or intramuscularly. Their use requires a Therapeutic Use Exemption approval. Other routes of administration (intraarticular / periarticular / peritendinous / epidural / intradermal injections and inhalation) require an Abbreviated Therapeutic Use Exemption except as noted below.
Topical preparations when used for dermatological (including iontophoresis / phonophoresis), auricular, nasal, ophthalmic, buccal, gingival and perianal disorders are not prohibited and do not require any form of Therapeutic Use Exemption.

WADA Class: Specified Substances
Also listed as a specified substance.
"The prohibited List may identify specified substances which are particularly susceptible to unintentional anti-doping rule violations because of their general availability in medicinal products or which are less likely to be successfully abused as doping agents."
A doping violation involving such substances may result in a reduced sanction provided that the "*...Athlete can establish that the Use of such a specfied substance was not intended to enhance sport performance...*"

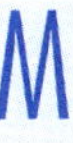

Preparations
Single ingredient: ***Arg.:*** Cortipyren B; Deltisona B; Latisona B; Prednisonal; Prenolone; Rupesona B; ***Mex.:*** Lectan.

Mersalyl Acid

Other names: Acidum Mersalylicum; Mersal. Acid; Mersálico, ácido; Mersalylum Acidum.

Mersalyl Sodium

Other names: Mcrsalyl; Mersalilo; Mersalylum; Mersalyyli.

Мерсалил

Clinical profile: Mersalyl acid is a powerful mercurial diuretic now superseded by thiazide and other diuretics that are both potent and less toxic.

WADA Status: Banned in and out of competition

WADA Class: Diuretics and Other Masking Agents

Includes diuretics or substances with a similar chemical structure or similar biological effect(s).

Mesocarb

Other names: Mésocarb; Mesocarbo; Mesocarbum.

Мезокарб

Clinical profile: Mesocarb is reported to be a central stimulant.

WADA Status: Banned in competition

WADA Class: Stimulants

Includes mesocarb and any optical isomers.

Mesterolone

Other names: Mesterolon; Mesterolona; Mesterolonas; Mestérolone; Mesteroloni; Mesterolonum; Meszterolon; NSC-75054; SH-723.

Местеролон

Clinical profile: Mesterolone has androgenic properties and may be used in the treatment of androgen deficiency or male infertility associated with hypogonadism.

WADA Status: Banned in and out of competition

WADA Class: Anabolic; Androgenic Steroids (exogenous)

Includes exogenous anabolic androgenic steroids or other substances with a similar chemical structure or similar biological effect(s).

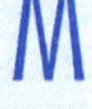

Preparations
Single ingredient: ***Austral.:*** Proviron; ***Austria:*** Proviron; ***Belg.:*** Proviron; ***Braz.:*** Proviron; ***Chile:*** Proviron; ***Cz.:*** Proviron; ***Gr.:*** Proviron; ***Hung.:*** Proviron; ***India:*** Provironum; ***Indon.:*** Androlon; Infelon; Proviron; ***Israel:*** Proviron; ***Ital.:*** Proviron; ***Malaysia:*** Provironum; Vistimon; ***Mex.:*** Proviron; ***Neth.:*** Proviron; ***Philipp.:*** Proviron; ***Pol.:*** Proviron; ***Port.:*** Proviron; ***S.Afr.:***

Proviron; ***Singapore:*** Provironum; ***Spain:*** Proviron; ***Thai.:*** Provironum; ***Turk.:*** Proviron; ***UK:*** Proviron; ***Venez.:*** Proviron.

Metamfepramone Hydrochloride

Other names: Dimepropion Hydrochloride; Hidrocloruro de metanfepramona; Métamfépramone, Chlorhydrate de; Metamfepramoni Hydrochloridum; Metamfepyramone Hydrochloride.

Метамфепрамона Гидрохлорид

Clinical profile: Metamfepramone is a sympathomimetic that has been used in the treatment of hypotension and in preparations for the symptomatic relief of the common cold.

WADA Status: Banned in competition

WADA Class: Stimulants

Includes stimulants or substances with a similar chemical structure or similar biological effect(s).

WADA Class: Specified Substances

Also listed as a specified substance.

"The prohibited List may identify specified substances which are particularly susceptible to unintentional anti-doping rule violations because of their general availability in medicinal products or which are less likely to be successfully abused as doping agents."

A doping violation involving such substances may result in a reduced sanction provided that the "*...Athlete can establish that the Use of such a specfied substance was not intended to enhance sport performance...*"

Preparations
Multi-ingredient: ***Ger.:*** Tempil N.

Metamfetamine Hydrochloride

Other names: *d*-Deoxyephedrine Hydrochloride; *d*-Desoxyephedrine Hydrochloride; Hidrocloruro de metanfetamina; Métamfétamine, Chlorhydrate de; Metamfetamini Hydrochloridum; Methamphetamine Hydrochloride; Methamphetamini Hydrochloridum; Methylamphetamine Hydrochloride; Phenylmethylaminopropane Hydrochloride.

Метамфетамина Гидрохлорид

Clinical profile: Metamfetamine hydrochloride is an amfetamine derivative and an indirect-acting sympathomimetic. It has been used in the treatment of hyperactivity disorders in children. It has also been used as an anorectic in the management of obesity.

WADA Status: Banned in competition

WADA Class: Stimulants

Includes metamfetamine and any optical isomers.

Preparations
Single Ingredient: ***Chile:*** Cidrin; ***USA:*** Desoxyn.

Metaraminol Tartrate

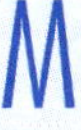

Other names: Hydroxynorephedrine Bitartrate; Metaradrine Bitartrate; Metaraminol Acid Tartrate; Metaraminol Bitartrate; Métaraminol, Tartrate de; Metaraminoli Tartras; Tartrato de metaraminol.

Метараминола Тартрат

Clinical profile: Metaraminol tartrate is a sympathomimetic with direct and indirect effects on adrenergic receptors. It has alpha- and beta-adrenergic activity, the former being predominant. It has an inotropic effect and acts as a peripheral vasoconstrictor. It is used for its pressor action in hypotensive states such as those that may occur following spinal anaesthesia.

WADA Status: Banned in competition

WADA Class: Stimulants

Includes stimulants or substances with a similar chemical structure or similar biological effect(s).

WADA Class: Specified Substances

Also listed as a specified substance.

"The prohibited List may identify specified substances which are particularly susceptible to unintentional anti-doping rule violations because of their general availability in medicinal products or which are less likely to be successfully abused as doping agents."

A doping violation involving such substances may result in a reduced sanction provided that the "*...Athlete can establish that the Use of such a specfied substance was not intended to enhance sport performance...*"

Preparations
Single ingredient: ***Arg.:*** Fadamine; ***Austral.:*** Aramine; ***Braz.:*** Aramin; ***NZ:*** Aramine; ***USA:*** Aramine.

Metenolone

Other names: Metenolon; Metenolona; Méténolone; Metenoloni; Metenolonum; Methenolone.

Метенолон

Metenolone Acetate

Other names: Acetato de metenolona; Acetato de metilandrostenolona; Méténolone, Acétate de; Metenoloni Acetas; Methenolone Acetate; NSC-74226; SH-567; SQ-16496.

Метенолона Ацетат

Metenolone Enantate

Other names: Enantato de metenolona; Enantato de metilandrostenolona; Méténolone, Enantate de; Metenoloni Enantas; Methenolone Enanthate; Methenolone Oenanthate; NSC-64967; SH-601; SQ-16374.

Метенолона Энантат

Clinical profile: Metenolone is an anabolic steroid that has been used in aplastic anaemia, breast cancer in women, and osteoporosis.

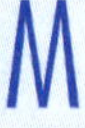

WADA Status: Banned in and out of competition

WADA Class: Anabolic; Androgenic Steroids (exogenous)

Includes exogenous anabolic androgenic steroids or other substances with a similar chemical structure or similar biological effect(s).

Preparations
Single ingredient: ***Austral.:*** Primobolan; ***Mex.:*** Primobolan; ***S.Afr.:*** Primobolan; ***Spain:*** Primobolan Depot.

Methadone Hydrochloride

Other names: Amidine Hydrochloride; Amidone Hydrochloride; Hidrocloruro de metadona; Metadon Hidroklorür; Metadon-hidroklorid; Metadonhydroklorid; Metadonihydrokloridi; Metadono hidrochloridas; Metadonu chlorowodorek; Methadon hydrochlorid; Méthadone, chlorhydrate de; (±)-Methadone Hydrochloride; Methadoni hydrochloridum; Phenadone.

Метадона Гидрохлорид

Clinical profile: Methadone hydrochloride, a diphenylheptane derivative, is an opioid analgesic that is primarily a μ opioid agonist. It is used in the treatment of severe pain and in the management of opioid dependence. Because of methadone's depressant action on the cough centre, it may also be used as a cough suppressant in terminal illness.

WADA Status: Banned in competition

WADA Class: Narcotics

Includes specified narcotics.

Preparations
Single ingredient: ***Arg.:*** Gobbidona; ***Austral.:*** Physeptone; ***Austria:*** Heptadon; ***Belg.:*** Mephenon; ***Braz.:*** Metadon; ***Canad.:*** Metadol; ***Fin.:*** Dolmed; ***Hung.:*** Depridol; Metadon; ***Irl.:*** Phymet DTF; Pinadone DTF; ***Israel:*** Adolan; ***Ital.:*** Eptadone; ***Neth.:*** Symoron; ***NZ:*** Biodone; Methatabs; Pallidone; ***S.Afr.:*** Physeptone; ***Spain:*** Metasedin; ***Switz.:*** Ketalgine; ***UK:*** Eptadone; Martindale Methadone Mixture DTF; Methadose; Physeptone; Synastone; ***USA:*** Diskets; Dolophine; Methadose.

Methandienone

Other names: Metandienone; Metandienon; Metandienona; Métandiénone; Metandienoni; Metandienonum; Methandrostenolone; NSC-42722.

Метандиенон

Clinical profile: Methandienone has been used for its anabolic properties; it has some androgenic properties with little progestogenic activity.

WADA Status: Banned in and out of competition

WADA Class: Anabolic; Androgenic Steroids (exogenous)

Includes exogenous anabolic androgenic steroids or other substances with a similar chemical structure or similar biological effect(s).

Preparations
Single ingredient: ***Pol.:*** Metanabol; ***Thai.:*** Anabol; Melic.

Methandriol

Other names: Mestenediol; Metandriol; Méthandriol; Methandriolum; Methylandrostenediol.

Метандриол

Clinical profile: Methandriol has anabolic and androgenic properties.

WADA Status: Banned in and out of competition

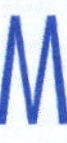

Methazolamide

WADA Class: Anabolic; Androgenic Steroids (exogenous)

Includes exogenous anabolic androgenic steroids or other substances with a similar chemical structure or similar biological effect(s).

Methazolamide

Other names: Metazolamida; Méthazolamide; Methazolamidum.

Метазоламид

Clinical profile: Methazolamide is an inhibitor of carbonic anhydrase used in the treatment of glaucoma.

WADA Status: Banned in and out of competition

WADA Class: Diuretics and Other Masking Agents

Includes diuretics or substances with a similar chemical structure or similar biological effect(s).

Methcathinone

Other names: Ephedrone; Methylcathinone; Monomethylpropion.

Clinical profile: Methcathinone, a methyl derivative of cathinone, produces CNS stimulant effects similar to those of the amfetamines and is subject to abuse.

WADA Status: Banned in competition

WADA Class: Stimulants

Includes stimulants or substances with a similar chemical structure or similar biological effect(s).

WADA Class: Specified Substances

Also listed as a specified substance.

"*The prohibited List may identify specified substances which are particularly susceptible to unintentional anti-doping rule violations because of their general availability in medicinal products or which are less likely to be successfully abused as doping agents.*"

A doping violation involving such substances may result in a reduced sanction provided that the "...*Athlete can establish that the Use of such a specfied substance was not intended to enhance sport performance...*"

Methoxamine Hydrochloride

Other names: Hidrocloruro de metoxamina; Methoxamedrine Hydrochloride; Méthoxamine, Chlorhydrate de; Methoxamini Hydrochloridum.

Метоксамина Гидрохлорид

Clinical profile: Methoxamine hydrochloride is a sympathomimetic with mainly direct effects on adrenergic receptors. It has alpha-adrenergic activity entirely; beta-adrenergic activity is not demonstrable and beta-adrenoceptor blockade has been postulated. It has been used for its pressor action in hypotensive states, notably in general or spinal anaesthesia. It has also been used for paroxysmal supraventricular tachycardia and for nasal congestion.

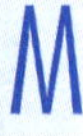

WADA Status: Banned in competition

WADA Class: Stimulants

Includes stimulants or substances with a similar chemical structure or similar biological effect(s).

WADA Class: Specified Substances

Also listed as a specified substance.

"The prohibited List may identify specified substances which are particularly susceptible to unintentional anti-doping rule violations because of their general availability in medicinal products or which are less likely to be successfully abused as doping agents."

A doping violation involving such substances may result in a reduced sanction provided that the "*...Athlete can establish that the Use of such a specfied substance was not intended to enhance sport performance...*"

Methoxyphenamine Hydrochloride

Other names: Hidrocloruro de metoxifenamina; Methoxiphenadrin Hydrochloride; Méthoxyphénamine, Chlorhydrate de; Methoxyphenamini Hydrochloridum; Mexyphamine Hydrochloride.

Метоксифенамина Гидрохлорид

Clinical profile: Methoxyphenamine hydrochloride is a sympathomimetic that has been used as a bronchodilator and in combination preparations for the relief of cough and cold symptoms.

WADA Status: Banned in competition

WADA Class: Stimulants

Includes stimulants or substances with a similar chemical structure or similar biological effect(s).

WADA Class: Specified Substances

Also listed as a specified substance.

"The prohibited List may identify specified substances which are particularly susceptible to unintentional anti-doping rule violations because of their general availability in medicinal products or which are less likely to be successfully abused as doping agents."

A doping violation involving such substances may result in a reduced sanction provided that the "*...Athlete can establish that the Use of such a specfied substance was not intended to enhance sport performance...*"

Preparations

Multi-ingredient: ***Chile:*** Cheracol; ***Hong Kong:*** Asmeton; ***Irl.:*** Casacol; ***Venez.:*** Metoxifilin.

Methyclothiazide

Other names: Méthyclothiazide; Methyclothiazidum; Meticlotiazida; Metyklotiatsidi; Metyklotiazid; NSC-110431.

Метиклотиазид

Clinical profile: Methyclothiazide is a thiazide diuretic used for oedema, including that associated with heart failure, and for hypertension.

WADA Status: Banned in and out of competition

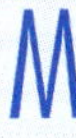

WADA Class: Diuretics and Other Masking Agents

Includes diuretics or substances with a similar chemical structure or similar biological effect(s).

Preparations
Single ingredient: ***USA:*** Enduron.
Multi-ingredient: ***Fr.:*** Isobar.

Methylenedioxymethamfetamine

Other names: MDMA; Methylenedioxymethamphetamine; 3,4-Methylenedioxymethamphetamine; Metilendioximetanfetamina.

Clinical profile: Methylenedioxymethamfetamine (also known as Adam, E, Ecstasy, M & M, MDM, and XTC) is a phenylethylamine compound structurally related to amfetamine and mescaline and is an analogue of tenamfetamine. It is subject to abuse.

WADA Status: Banned in competition

WADA Class: Stimulants

Includes methylenedioxymethamfetamine and any optical isomers.

Methylephedrine Hydrochloride

Other names: *dl*-Methylephedrine Hydrochloride; *dl*-*N*-Methylephedrine Hydrochloride; Metilefedrina, hidrocloruro de.

Метилэфедрина Гидрохлорид

Clinical profile: Methylephedrine hydrochloride is a sympathomimetic that has been used as a bronchodilator and in combination preparations for the relief of cough and nasal congestion.

WADA Status: Banned in competition

WADA Class: Stimulants

Methylephedrine is prohibited when its concentration in urine is greater than 10 micrograms per milliliter.

WADA Class: Specified Substances

Also listed as a specified substance.

"The prohibited List may identify specified substances which are particularly susceptible to unintentional anti-doping rule violations because of their general availability in medicinal products or which are less likely to be successfully abused as doping agents."

A doping violation involving such substances may result in a reduced sanction provided that the "*...Athlete can establish that the Use of such a specfied substance was not intended to enhance sport performance...*"

Preparations
Multi-ingredient: ***Austria:*** Tussoretardin; ***Hong Kong:*** Codaewon; ***Jpn:*** Colgen Kowa IB Toumei; Sin Colgen Kowa Kaze; ***S.Afr.:*** Ilvico; ***Switz.:*** Tossamine plus; ***Thai.:*** Methorcon; ***Venez.:*** Ilvico.

Methylphenidate Hydrochloride

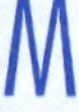

Other names: Hidrocloruro de metilfenidato; Methyl Phenidate Hydrochloride; Méthylphénidate, chlorhydrate de; Methylphenidati hydrochloridum; Metilfenidat

Hidroklorür.

Метилфенидата Гидрохлорид

Clinical profile: Methylphenidate hydrochloride is a central stimulant and indirect-acting sympathomimetic used in the treatment of narcolepsy and in the treatment of hyperactivity disorders in children.

WADA Status: Banned in competition

WADA Class: Stimulants

Includes methylphenidate and any optical isomers.

Preparations
Single ingredient: ***Arg.:*** Concerta; Methylin; Ritalina; Rubifen; ***Austral.:*** Attenta; Concerta; Ritalin; ***Austria:*** Concerta; Ritalin; ***Belg.:*** Concerta; Rilatine; ***Braz.:*** Concerta; Ritalina; ***Canad.:*** Concerta; Ritalin; ***Chile:*** Aradix; Concerta; Nebapul; Ritalin; Ritrocel; ***Cz.:*** Ritalin; ***Denm.:*** Equasym; Motiron; Ritalin; ***Fin.:*** Concerta; ***Fr.:*** Concerta; Ritaline; ***Ger.:*** Concerta; Equasym; Medikinet; Ritalin; ***Gr.:*** Concerta; Ritaline; ***Hong Kong:*** Concerta; Ritalin; ***Hung.:*** Ritalin; ***Indon.:*** Concerta; Ritalin; ***Irl.:*** Concerta; Equasym; Ritalin; ***Israel:*** Concerta; Metadate; Ritalin; ***Malaysia:*** Ritalin; ***Mex.:*** Concerta; Ritalin; Tradea; ***Neth.:*** Concerta; Equasym; Ritalin; Tifinidat; ***Norw.:*** Concerta; Equasym; Ritalin; ***NZ:*** Concerta; Ritalin; Rubifen; ***Philipp.:*** Concerta; ***Pol.:*** Concerta; ***Port.:*** Concerta; Ritalina; ***S.Afr.:*** Adaphen; Concerta; Ritalin; ***Singapore:*** Concerta; Ritalin; Rubifen; ***Spain:*** Concerta; Rubifen; ***Swed.:*** Concerta; Ritalin; ***Switz.:*** Concerta; Ritaline; ***Thai.:*** Concerta; ***Turk.:*** Concerta; Ritalin; ***UK:*** Concerta; Equasym; Medikinet; Ritalin; ***USA:*** Concerta; Daytrana; Metadate; Methylin; Ritalin; ***Venez.:*** Concerta; Ritalin.

Methylprednisolone

Other names: Meilprednizolon; Methylprednisolon; Méthylprednisolone; 6α-Methylprednisolone; Methylprednisolonum; Metilprednisolona; Metilprednizolon; Metilprednizolonas; Metylprednisolon; Metyyliprednisoloni; NSC-19987.

Метилпреднизолон

Methylprednisolone Acetate

Other names: Acetato de metilprednisolona; Methylprednisolon-acetát; Méthylprednisolone, acétate de; Methylprednisoloni acetas; Metilprednizolon Asetat; Metilprednizolon-acetát; Metilprednizolono acetatas; Metylprednisolonacetat; Metyyliprednisoloniasetaatti.

Метилпреднизолона Ацетат

Methylprednisolone Hydrogen Succinate

Other names: Hidrogenosuccinato de metilprednisolona; Methylprednisolone Hemisuccinate; Méthylprednisolone, Hémisuccinate de; Méthylprednisolone, Hydrogénosuccinate de; Methylprednisolon-hydrogen-sukcinát; Methylprednisoloni Hemisuccinas; Methylprednisoloni hydrogenosuccinas; Metilprednizolon-hidrogénszukcinát; Metilprednizolono-vandenilio sukcinatas; Metylprednisolonvätesuccinat; Metyyliprednisolonivetysuksinaatti.

Метилпреднизолона Гемисукцинат

Methylprednisolone Sodium Succinate

Other names: Methylprednisolone Sodium Hemisuccinate; Méthylprednisolone, Succinate Sodique de; Methylprednisoloni Natrii Succinas; Metilprednizolon Sodyum Süksinat; Succinato sódico de metilprednisolona.

Метилпреднизолона Натрия Сукцинат

Clinical profile: Methylprednisolone is a glucocorticoid corticosteroid. It has been used, either in the form of the free alcohol or in one of the esterified forms, in the treatment of

a wide range of conditions that respond to the anti-inflammatory and immunosuppressant effects of corticosteroid therapy.

WADA Status: Banned in competition

WADA Class: Glucocorticosteroids

All glucocorticosteroids are prohibited when administered orally, rectally, intravenously or intramuscularly. Their use requires a Therapeutic Use Exemption approval. Other routes of administration (intraarticular / periarticular / peritendinous / epidural / intradermal injections and inhalation) require an Abbreviated Therapeutic Use Exemption except as noted below.

Topical preparations when used for dermatological (including iontophoresis / phonophoresis), auricular, nasal, ophthalmic, buccal, gingival and perianal disorders are not prohibited and do not require any form of Therapeutic Use Exemption.

WADA Class: Specified Substances

Also listed as a specified substance.

"The prohibited List may identify specified substances which are particularly susceptible to unintentional anti-doping rule violations because of their general availability in medicinal products or which are less likely to be successfully abused as doping agents."

A doping violation involving such substances may result in a reduced sanction provided that the "*...Athlete can establish that the Use of such a specfied substance was not intended to enhance sport performance...*"

Preparations

Single ingredient: ***Arg.:*** Advantan; Cipridanol; Solu-Medrol; ***Austral.:*** Advantan; Depo-Medrol; Depo-Nisolone; Medrol; Solu-Medrol; ***Austria:*** Advantan; Depo-Medrol; Solu-Medrol; Urbason; ***Belg.:*** Advantan; Depo-Medrol; Medrol; Solu-Medrol; ***Braz.:*** Advantan; Alergolon; Depo-Medrol; Predmetil; Solu-Medrol; Solu-Pred; Solupren; ***Canad.:*** Depo-Medrol; Medrol; Solu-Medrol; ***Chile:*** Depo-Medrol; Medrol; Solu-Medrol; ***Cz.:*** Advantan; Depo-Medrol; Medrol; Metypred; Solu-Medrol; Urbason; ***Denm.:*** Depo-Medrol; Medrol; Solu-Medrol; ***Fin.:*** Advantan; Depo-Medrol; Medrol; Solomet; Solu-Medrol; ***Fr.:*** Depo-Medrol; Medrol; Solu-Medrol; ***Ger.:*** Advantan; M-PredniHexal; Medrate; Metypred; Metysolon; Predni M; Urbason; ***Gr.:*** Advantan; Depo-Medrol; Medrol; Solu-Medrol; ***Hong Kong:*** Advantan; Depo-Medrol; Medrol; Solu-Medrol; ***Hung.:*** Depo-Medrol; Medrol; Metypred; Solu-Medrol; ***India:*** Depo-Medrol; Solu-Medrol; ***Indon.:*** Advantan; Depo-Medrol; Flason; Hexilon; Intidrol; Lameson; Lexcomet; Medixon; Medrol; Meprilon; Meproson; Mesol; Methylon; Metidrol; Metisol; Nichomedson; Prednicort; Prednox; Pretilon; Sanexon; Solu-Medrol; Somerol; Sonicor; Stenirol; Thimelon; Tison; Tropidrol; Urbason; Yalone; ***Irl.:*** Depo-Medrone; Solu-Medrone; ***Israel:*** Depo-Medrol; Medrol; Solu-Medrol; ***Ital.:*** Advantan; Asmacortone; Avancort; Depo-Medrol; Medrol; Metilbetasone Solubile; Solu-Medrol; Supresol; Urbason; ***Malaysia:*** Depo-Medrol; Solu-Medrol; ***Mex.:*** Advantan; Cryosolona; Depo-Medrol; Metisona; Prednilem; Radilem; Solipred; Solu-Medrol; ***Neth.:*** Depo-Medrol; Solu-Medrol; ***Norw.:*** Depo-Medrol; Medrol; Solu-Medrol; ***NZ:*** Advantan; Depo-Medrol; Medrol; Solu-Medrol; ***Philipp.:*** Adrena; Advantan; Depo-Medrol; Medixon; Medrol; Solu-Medrol; ***Pol.:*** Advantan; Depo-Medrol; Medrol; Metypred; Solu-Medrol; ***Port.:*** Advantan; Depo-Medrol; Medrol; Metilpren; Solu-Medrol; ***Rus.:*** Advantan (Адвантан); Medrol (Медрол); Metypred (Метипред); Solu-Medrol (Солу-медрол); ***S.Afr.:*** Advantan; Depo-Medrol; Medrol; Metypresol; Solu-Medrol; ***Singapore:*** Solu-Medrol; ***Spain:*** Adventan; Lexxema; Solu-Moderin; Urbason; ***Swed.:*** Depo-Medrol; Medrol; Solu-Medrol; ***Switz.:*** Advantan; Depo-Medrol; Medrol; Solu-Medrol; ***Thai.:*** Depo-Medrol; Solu-Medrol; ***Turk.:*** Advantan; Depo-Medrol; Prednol; ***UK:*** Depo-Medrone; Medrone; Solu-Medrone; ***USA:*** A-Methapred; depMedalone; Depo-Medrol; Medrol; Solu-Medrol; ***Venez.:*** Advantan; Depo-Medrol; Medrol; Prednicort; Solu-Medrol.

Multi-ingredient: ***Austral.:*** Neo-Medrol; ***Austria:*** Depo-Medrol mit Lidocain; ***Belg.:*** Depo-Medrol + Lidocaine; ***Canad.:*** Depo-Medrol with Lidocaine; Medrol Acne Lotion; Neo-Medrol Acne; ***Fin.:*** Depo-Medrol cum Lidocain; Solomet c bupivacain hydrochlorid; ***Hong Kong:*** Depo-Medrol with Lidocaine; Neo-Medrol Acne; ***Irl.:*** Depo-Medrone with Lidocaine; ***Israel:*** Depo-Medrol with Lidocaine; Neo-Medrol; ***Ital.:*** Depo-Medrol + Lidocaina; ***Malaysia:*** Neo-Medrol; ***Neth.:*** Depo-Medrol + Lidocaine; ***Norw.:*** Depo-Medrol cum Lidocain; ***NZ:*** Depo-Medrol with Lidocaine; ***Pol.:*** Depo-Medrol z Lidokaina; ***Port.:*** Depo-Medrol com Lidocaina; ***S.Afr.:*** Depo-Medrol with Lidocaine; Neo-Medrol; ***Singapore:*** Neo-Medrol; ***Swed.:*** Depo-Medrol cum Lidocain; ***Switz.:*** Depo-Medrol Lidocaine; ***Thai.:*** Neo-Medrol; ***UK:*** Depo-Medrone with Lidocaine.

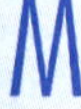

Methyltestosterone

Other names: Methyltestosteron; Méthyltestostérone; Methyltestosteronum;

Metiltestosterona; Metiltestosteronas; Metiltesztoszteron; Metylotestosteron; Metyl-testosteron; Metyylitestosteroni; NSC-9701.
Метилтестостерон

Clinical profile: Methyltestosterone has androgenic and anabolic properties and is used for androgen replacement therapy in male hypogonadism. It has also been given for metastatic breast carcinoma in postmenopausal women, and with oestrogens for the short-term treatment of menopausal vasomotor symptoms unresponsive to oestrogens alone.

WADA Status: Banned in and out of competition

WADA Class: Anabolic; Androgenic Steroids (exogenous)

Includes exogenous anabolic androgenic steroids or other substances with a similar chemical structure or similar biological effect(s).

Preparations
Single ingredient: ***USA:*** Android; Testred; Virilon.
Multi-ingredient: ***Austria:*** Pasuma-Dragees; ***Braz.:*** Gabecon M; Testonus; ***Chile:*** Delitan; Feminova-T; ***Hong Kong:*** Wari-Procomil; ***India:*** Mixogen; ***Mex.:*** Bigenol; ***Thai.:*** Men Hormone; ***UK:*** Prowess; ***USA:*** Covaryx; Estratest; Syntest.

Methyl-1-testosterone

Other names: 17β-Hydroxy-17α-methyl-5α-androst-1-en-3-one; M1T.
Метил-1-тестостерон

Clinical profile: Methyl-1-testosterone is an anabolic steroid that appears to be widely abused by body-builders.

WADA Status: Banned in and out of competition

WADA Class: Anabolic; Androgenic Steroids (exogenous)

Includes exogenous anabolic androgenic steroids or other substances with a similar chemical structure or similar biological effect(s).

Meticrane

Other names: Méticrane; Meticrano; Meticranum; SD-17102.
Метикран

Clinical profile: Meticrane is a thiazide diuretic that has been used in the treatment of hypertension.

WADA Status: Banned in and out of competition

WADA Class: Diuretics and Other Masking Agents

Includes diuretics or substances with a similar chemical structure or similar biological effect(s).

Metipamide

Other names: Metipamid; Metipamidum; VÚFB-14429.

Clinical profile: Metipamide is a diuretic structurally related to indapamide; it is used as an antihypertensive.

WADA Status: Banned in and out of competition

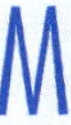

Metipranolol

WADA Class: Diuretics and Other Masking Agents

Includes diuretics or substances with a similar chemical structure or similar biological effect(s).

Preparations
Single ingredient: ***Cz.:*** Hypotylin.

Metipranolol

Other names: BMOI-004; Methypranolol; Métipranolol; Metipranololum; VUAB-6453 (SPOFA); VUFB-6453.

Метипранолол

Clinical profile: Metipranolol is a non-cardioselective beta blocker used in the management of open-angle glaucoma and ocular hypertension. It has also been used in the management of cardiovascular disorders.

WADA Status: Banned in and out of competition as specified below

WADA Class: Beta-Blockers

Unless otherwise specified, beta-blockers are prohibited *In-Competition* only in the following sports.

- Aeronautics (FAI)
- Archery (FITA, IPC) (also prohibited *Out-of-Competition*)
- Automobile (FIA)
- Billiards (WCBS)
- Bobsleigh (FIBT)
- Boules (CMSB, IPC bowls)
- Bridge (FMB)
- Curling (WCF)
- Gymnastics (FIG)
- Motorcycling (FIM)
- Modern Pentathlon (UIPM) for disciplines involving shooting
- Nine-pin bowling (FIQ)
- Powerboating (UIM)
- Sailing (ISAF) for match race helms only
- Shooting (ISSF, IPC) (also prohibited *Out-of-Competition*)
- Skiing/Snowboarding (FIS) in ski jumping, freestyle aerials/halfpipe and snowboard halfpipe/big air
- Wrestling (FILA)

WADA Class: Specified Substances

Also listed as a specified substance.

"*The prohibited List may identify specified substances which are particularly susceptible to unintentional anti-doping rule violations because of their general availability in medicinal products or which are less likely to be successfully abused as doping agents.*"

A doping violation involving such substances may result in a reduced sanction provided that the "*...Athlete can establish that the Use of such a specfied substance was not intended to enhance sport performance...*"

Preparations
Single ingredient: ***Austria:*** Beta-Ophtiole; ***Belg.:*** Beta-Ophtiole; ***Cz.:*** Trimepranol; ***Ger.:***

Betamann; ***Ital.:*** Turoptin; ***Neth.:*** Beta-Ophtiole; ***Philipp.:*** Beta-Ophtiole; ***Pol.:*** Betamann; ***Port.:*** Beta-Ophtiole; ***S.Afr.:*** Beta-Ophtiole; ***Turk.:*** Turoptin; ***USA:*** OptiPranolol.
Multi-ingredient: ***Austria:*** Betacarpin; ***Belg.:*** Normoglaucon; ***Cz.:*** Trimecryton; ***Ger.:*** Normoglaucon; ***Gr.:*** Beta Opthiole; ***Ital.:*** Ripix; ***Neth.:*** Normoglaucon; ***Pol.:*** Normoglaucon; ***Port.:*** Normoglaucon; ***Switz.:*** Ripix.

Metizoline Hydrochloride

Other names: EX-10-781; Hidrocloruro de metizolina; Métizoline, Chlorhydrate de; Metizolini Hydrochloridum; Metyzoline Hydrochloride; RMI-10482A.
Метизолина Гидрохлорид

Clinical profile: Metizoline hydrochloride is a sympathomimetic with vasoconstrictor activity that has been given for the relief of nasal congestion.

WADA Status: Banned in competition

WADA Class: Stimulants

Includes stimulants or substances with a similar chemical structure or similar biological effect(s). Metizoline is an imidazole derivative. Imidazole derivatives for topical use are exempt.

Metolazone

Other names: Metolatsoni; Metolazon; Metolazona; Métolazone; Metolazonum; SR-720-22.
Метолазон

Clinical profile: Metolazone is a diuretic similar to the thiazide diuretics. It is used for oedema, including that associated with heart failure, and for hypertension.

WADA Status: Banned in and out of competition

WADA Class: Diuretics and Other Masking Agents

Includes diuretics or substances with a similar chemical structure or similar biological effect(s).

Preparations
Single ingredient: ***Canad.:*** Zaroxolyn; ***Chile:*** Pavedal; ***Gr.:*** Metenix; ***Hong Kong:*** Zaroxolyn; ***India:*** Metoz; ***Israel:*** Zaroxolyn; ***Ital.:*** Zaroxolyn; ***Port.:*** Diulo; ***UK:*** Metenix; ***USA:*** Mykrox; Zaroxolyn.

Metoprolol

Other names: Métoprolol; Metoprololi; Metoprololum.
Метопролол

Metoprolol Fumarate

Other names: CGP-2175C; Fumarato de metoprolol; Métoprolol, Fumarate de; Metoprololi Fumaras.
Метопролола Фумарат

Metoprolol Succinate

Other names: Métoprolol, succinate de; Metoprolol Suksinat; Metoprololi succi-

nas; Metoprololio sukcinatas; Metoprololisuksinaatti; Metoprololsuccinat; Metoprolol-sukcinát; Metoprolol-szukcinát; Succinato de metoprolol.
Метопролола Суксинат

Metoprolol Tartrate

Other names: CGP-2175E; H-93/26; Metoprolol tartarát; Metoprolol Tartarat; Métoprolol, tartrate de; Metoprololi tartras; Metoprololio tartratas; Metoprololitartraatti; Metoprolol-tartarát; Metoprololtartrat; Tartrato de metoprolol.
Метопролола Тартрат

Clinical profile: Metoprolol is a cardioselective beta blocker used in the management of hypertension, angina pectoris, cardiac arrhythmias, myocardial infarction, and heart failure. It is also used in the management of hyperthyroidism and migraine.

WADA Status: Banned in and out of competition as specified below

WADA Class: Beta-Blockers

Unless otherwise specified, beta-blockers are prohibited *In-Competition* only in the following sports.

- Aeronautics (FAI)
- Archery (FITA, IPC) (also prohibited *Out-of-Competition*)
- Automobile (FIA)
- Billiards (WCBS)
- Bobsleigh (FIBT)
- Boules (CMSB, IPC bowls)
- Bridge (FMB)
- Curling (WCF)
- Gymnastics (FIG)
- Motorcycling (FIM)
- Modern Pentathlon (UIPM) for disciplines involving shooting
- Nine-pin bowling (FIQ)
- Powerboating (UIM)
- Sailing (ISAF) for match race helms only
- Shooting (ISSF, IPC) (also prohibited *Out-of-Competition*)
- Skiing/Snowboarding (FIS) in ski jumping, freestyle aerials/halfpipe and snowboard halfpipe/big air
- Wrestling (FILA)

WADA Class: Specified Substances

Also listed as a specified substance.

"*The prohibited List may identify specified substances which are particularly susceptible to unintentional anti-doping rule violations because of their general availability in medicinal products or which are less likely to be successfully abused as doping agents.*"

A doping violation involving such substances may result in a reduced sanction provided that the "...*Athlete can establish that the Use of such a specfied substance was not intended to enhance sport performance...*"

Preparations

Single ingredient: ***Arg.:*** Belozok; Lopresor; ***Austral.:*** Betaloc; Lopresor; Metohexal; Metrol; Minax; Toprol; ***Austria:*** Beloc; Lanoc; Metohexal; MetoMed; Metostadol; Seloken; ***Belg.:*** Lopresor; Selo-Zok; Seloken; Slow-Lopresor; ***Braz.:*** Lopressor; Selo-Zok; Seloken; ***Canad.:*** Betaloc; Lopresor; Novo-Metoprol; Nu-Metop; ***Cz.:*** Betaloc; Corvitol; Egilok; Metohexal; Vasocardin; ***Denm.:*** Mepronet; Metocar; Selo-Zok; Seloken; ***Fin.:*** Metoprolin; Seloken ZOC; Seloken; Selopral; Spesicor; ***Fr.:*** Lopressor; Seloken; Selozok; ***Ger.:*** Beloc-Zok; Beloc; Jeprolol; Jutabloc; Lopresor; Meprolol; Meto-Succinat; Meto-Tablinen; Meto; Metobeta; Metodoc; Metodura; Metohexal; Metoprogamma; Prelis; ***Gr.:*** Lopresor; ***Hong Kong:*** Betaloc; CP-Metolol; Minax; Novo-Metoprol; Sefloc; ***Hung.:*** Betaloc; Egilok; ***India:*** Betaloc; Metolar; Revelol; Selopres; ***Indon.:*** Cardiosel; Lopresor; Loprolol; Seloken; ***Irl.:*** Betaloc; Lopresor; Metocor; Metop; ***Israel:*** Lopresor; Neobloc; ***Ital.:*** Lopresor; Seloken; ***Jpn:*** Seloken; ***Malaysia:*** Beatrolol; Betaloc; Denex; ***Mex.:*** Bioprol; Eurolol; Futaline; Kenaprol; Lopresor; Metopresol; Prolaken; Promiced; Prontol; Ritmolol; Seloken; Sermetrol; ***Neth.:*** Lopresor; Selokeen; ***Norw.:*** Selo-Zok; Seloken; ***NZ:*** Betaloc; Lopresor; Slow-Lopresor; ***Philipp.:*** Betaloc; Betaryx; Betazok; Cardiosel; Cardiostat; Cardiotab; Metocare; Metoprim; Metospec; Metostad; Montebloc; Neobloc; Prolohex; Valvexin; ***Pol.:*** Betaloc; Beto; Metocard; Metohexal; ***Port.:*** Lopresor; ***Rus.:*** Betaloc ZOK (Беталок ЗОК); Corvitol (Корвадил); Egilok (Эгилок); Emzok (Эмзок); Metocard (Метокард); Serdol (Сердол); Vasocardin (Вазокардин); ***S.Afr.:*** Lopresor; ***Singapore:*** Betaloc; Denex; ***Spain:*** Beloken; Lopresor; ***Swed.:*** Seloken ZOC; Seloken; ***Switz.:*** Beloc-Zok; Beloc; Lopresor; Metopress; ***Thai.:*** Betaloc;

M

Cardeloc; Cardoxone; Melol; Metoblock; Metolol; Minax; Sefloc; ***Turk.:*** Beloc; Lopresor; Problok; ***UK:*** Betaloc; Lopresor; ***USA:*** Lopressor; Toprol; ***Venez.:*** Lopresor.

Multi-ingredient: ***Austria:*** Beloc comp; Metoprolol compositum; Seloken retard Plus; Triloc; ***Belg.:*** Logimat; Logroton; Selozide; Zok-Zid; ***Braz.:*** Selopress; ***Cz.:*** Logimax; ***Denm.:*** Logimax; Zok-Zid; ***Fin.:*** Logimax; Selocomp ZOC; ***Fr.:*** Logimax; Logroton; ***Ger.:*** Belnif; Beloc-Zok comp; Meprolol Comp; Metobeta comp; Metodura comp; Metohexal comp; Metoprolol comp; Metostad Comp; Mobloc; Prelis comp; Treloc; ***Gr.:*** Logimax; ***Hong Kong:*** Betaloc Comp; CP-Metolol Co; Logimax; ***Hung.:*** Logimax; ***India:*** Metolar-H; ***Irl.:*** Co-Betaloc; ***Israel:*** Logimax; ***Ital.:*** Igroton-Lopresor; ***Malaysia:*** Logroton; ***Mex.:*** Logimax; Selopres; ***Neth.:*** Logimax; Selokomb; ***Philipp.:*** Betazide; Logimax; ***Rus.:*** Logimax (Логимакс); ***Spain:*** Higrotensin; Logimax; ***Swed.:*** Logimax; ***Switz.:*** Logimax; Logroton; ***USA:*** Lopressor HCT.

Mibolerone

Other names: Mibolerona; Mibolérone; Miboleronum; NSC-72260; U-10997.

Миболерон

Clinical profile: Mibolerone is an androgen that is used in veterinary practice as a contraceptive for female dogs. It also has anabolic properties.

WADA Status: Banned in and out of competition

WADA Class: Anabolic; Androgenic Steroids (exogenous)

Includes exogenous anabolic androgenic steroids or other substances with a similar chemical structure or similar biological effect(s).

Midodrine Hydrochloride

Other names: Hidrocloruro de midodrina; Midodrine, Chlorhydrate de; Midodrini Hydrochloridum; ST-1085 (midodrine or midodrine hydrochloride).

Мидодрина Гидрохлорид

Clinical profile: Midodrine hydrochloride is a direct-acting sympathomimetic with selective alpha-agonist activity; the active moiety is stated to be its major metabolite deglymidodrine (ST-1059). It is used in the treatment of hypotensive states and may also be used as an adjunct in the management of urinary incontinence.

WADA Status: Banned in competition

WADA Class: Stimulants

Includes stimulants or substances with a similar chemical structure or similar biological effect(s).

WADA Class: Specified Substances

Also listed as a specified substance.

"The prohibited List may identify specified substances which are particularly susceptible to unintentional anti-doping rule violations because of their general availability in medicinal products or which are less likely to be successfully abused as doping agents."

A doping violation involving such substances may result in a reduced sanction provided that the *"...Athlete can establish that the Use of such a specfied substance was not intended to enhance sport performance..."*

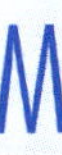

Preparations

Single Ingredient: ***Austria:*** Gutron; ***Canad.:*** Amatine; ***Chile:*** Gutron; ***Cz.:*** Gutron; ***Fr.:*** Gutron; ***Ger.:*** Gutron; ***Hong Kong:*** Gutron; ***Hung.:*** Gutron; ***Irl.:*** Midon; ***Israel:*** Gutron; ***Ital.:***

Gutron; Xerotil; ***Jpn:*** Metligine; ***Neth.:*** Gutron; ***NZ:*** Gutron; ***Pol.:*** Gutron; ***Port.:*** Gutron; ***Rus.:*** Gutron (Гутрон); ***Singapore:*** Gutron; ***Switz.:*** Gutron; ***USA:*** ProAmatine.

Modafinil

Other names: CEP-1538; CRL-40476; Modafinilo; Modafinilum.

Модафинил

Clinical profile: Modafinil is a central stimulant used in the treatment of excessive daytime sleepiness associated with the narcoleptic syndrome, obstructive sleep apnoea, and shift-work sleep disorder.

WADA Status: Banned in competition

WADA Class: Stimulants

Includes modafinil and any optical isomers.

Preparations
Single ingredient: ***Arg.:*** Forcilin; Vigicer; ***Austral.:*** Modavigil; ***Austria:*** Modasomil; ***Belg.:*** Provigil; ***Canad.:*** Alertec; ***Chile:*** Mentix; Naxelan; Resotyl; ***Cz.:*** Vigil; ***Denm.:*** Modiodal; ***Fr.:*** Modiodal; ***Ger.:*** Vigil; ***Gr.:*** Modiodal; ***Irl.:*** Provigil; ***Israel:*** Provigil; ***Ital.:*** Provigil; ***Mex.:*** Modiodal; ***Neth.:*** Modiodal; ***Norw.:*** Modiodal; ***NZ:*** Modavigil; ***Pol.:*** Vigil; ***Port.:*** Modiodal; ***S.Afr.:*** Provigil; ***Spain:*** Modiodal; ***Swed.:*** Modiodal; ***Switz.:*** Modasomil; ***Turk.:*** Modiodal; ***UK:*** Provigil; ***USA:*** Provigil.

Mometasone Furoate

Other names: Furoato de mometasona; Mométasone, furoate de; Mometasonfuroat; Mometason-furoát; Mometasoni furoas; Mometasonifuroaatti; Mometazon Furoat; Mometazon-furoát; Mometazono furoatas; Mometazonu furoinian; Sch-32088.

Мометазона Фуроат

Clinical profile: Mometasone furoate is a corticosteroid used topically in the treatment of various skin disorders, as a nasal spray for allergic rhinitis and for nasal polyps, and by inhalation for the management of asthma.

WADA Status: Banned in competition

WADA Class: Glucocorticosteroids

All glucocorticosteroids are prohibited when administered orally, rectally, intravenously or intramuscularly. Their use requires a Therapeutic Use Exemption approval. Other routes of administration (intraarticular / periarticular / peritendinous / epidural / intradermal injections and inhalation) require an Abbreviated Therapeutic Use Exemption except as noted below.

Topical preparations when used for dermatological (including iontophoresis / phonophoresis), auricular, nasal, ophthalmic, buccal, gingival and perianal disorders are not prohibited and do not require any form of Therapeutic Use Exemption.

WADA Class: Specified Substances

Also listed as a specified substance.

"The prohibited List may identify specified substances which are particularly susceptible to unintentional anti-doping rule violations because of their general availability in medicinal products or which are less likely to be successfully abused as doping agents."

A doping violation involving such substances may result in a reduced sanction provided that the "*...Athlete can establish that the Use of such a specfied substance was not intended to enhance sport performance...*"

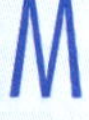

Preparations

Single ingredient: ***Arg.:*** Elocon; Fenisona; Metason; Momeplus; Nasonex; Novasone; Uniclar; ***Austral.:*** Elocon; Nasonex; Novasone; ***Austria:*** Asmanex; Elocon; Elovent; Nasonex; ***Belg.:*** Elocom; Nasonex; ***Braz.:*** Asmanex; Elocom; Nasonex; ***Canad.:*** Elocom; Nasonex; ***Chile:*** Dermosona; Elocom; Flogocort; Lisoder; Momelab; Nasonex; Uniclar; ***Cz.:*** Asmanex; Elocom; Nasonex; ***Denm.:*** Asmanex; Elocon; Nasonex; ***Fin.:*** Elocon; Nasonex; ***Fr.:*** Nasonex; ***Ger.:*** Asmanex; Ecural; Nasonex; ***Gr.:*** Asmanex; Bioelementa; Ecelecort; Elocon; Esine; F-Din; Fremomet; Makiren; Metason; Mofur; Molken; Momecort; Movesan; Mozeton; Nasamet; Nasonex; Pharmecort; Yperod; ***Hong Kong:*** Elomet; Nasonex; Topcort; ***Hung.:*** Elocom; Nasonex; ***India:*** Elocon; Metaspray; Momate; Topcort; ***Indon.:*** Dermovel; Elocon; Eloskin; Elox; Intercon; Mefurosan; Mesone; Mofacort; Mofulex; Momet; Motaderm; Moteson; Nasonex; ***Irl.:*** Asmanex; Elocon; Nasonex; ***Israel:*** Elocom; Nasonex; ***Ital.:*** Altosone; Elocon; Nasonex; Rinelon; ***Malaysia:*** Elomet; Nasonex; ***Mex.:*** Elica; Elomet; Elovent; Rinelon; Uniclar; ***Neth.:*** Asmanex; Elocon; Elovent; Nasonex; ***Norw.:*** Elocon; Nasonex; ***NZ:*** Asmanex; Bronconex; Elocon; ***Philipp.:*** Elica; Elocon; Momate; Nasonex; Rinelon; ***Pol.:*** Elocom; Elosone; Nasonex; ***Port.:*** Elocom; Nasomet; ***Rus.:*** Elocom (Элоком); Nasonex (Назонекс); ***S.Afr.:*** Elocon; Nasonex; ***Singapore:*** Elomet; Nasonex; ***Spain:*** Elica; Elocom; Nasonex; Rinelon; ***Swed.:*** Asmanex; Elocon; Nasonex; ***Switz.:*** Asmanex; Elocom; Nasonex; ***Thai.:*** Elomet; Nasonex; ***Turk.:*** Elocon; M-Furo; Nasonex; ***UK:*** Asmanex; Elocon; Nasonex; ***USA:*** Asmanex; Elocon; Nasonex; ***Venez.:*** Asmanex; Cortynase; Dergentil; Elocon; Elomet; Nasonex.

Multi-ingredient: ***Austria:*** Elosalic; ***Chile:*** Velosalic; ***Cz.:*** Monsalic; ***Ger.:*** Elosalic; ***Hong Kong:*** Elosalic; ***India:*** Momate-S; ***Indon.:*** Elosalic; ***Pol.:*** Elosalic; ***Rus.:*** Elocom-S (Элоком-С); ***S.Afr.:*** Elosalic; ***Swed.:*** Elosalic; ***Turk.:*** Elosalic; ***Venez.:*** Elosalic.

Morphine

Other names: Morfiini; Morfin; Morfina; Morphinum.

Morphine Hydrochloride

Other names: Morfiinihydrokloridi; Morfin Hidroklorür; Morfina, hidrocloruro de; Morfin-hidroklorid; Morfin-hydrochlorid trihydrát; Morfinhydroklorid; Morfino hidrochloridas; Morfiny chlorowodorek; Morphine, chlorhydrate de; Morphini hydrochloridum; Morphini Hydrochloridum Trihydricum; Morphinii Chloridum; Morphinum Chloratum.

Morphine Sulfate

Other names: Morfiinisulfaatti; Morfin Sülfat; Morfina, sulfato de; Morfino sulfatas; Morfinsulfat; Morfin-sulfát pentahydrát; Morfin-szulfát; Morfiny siarczan; Morphine, sulfate de; Morphine Sulphate; Morphini sulfas; Morphini Sulfas Pentahydricus.

Morphine Tartrate

Other names: Morfina, tartrato de.

Clinical profile: Morphine, a phenanthrene derivative and the principal alkaloid of opium, is an opioid analgesic with agonist activity at μ opioid receptors and perhaps at κ and δ receptors. It is used for the relief of moderate to severe pain, especially that associated with cancer, myocardial infarction, and surgery. Morphine reduces intestinal motility and has been used in the symptomatic treatment of diarrhoea. It relieves the dyspnoea of pulmonary oedema and of left ventricular failure. Morphine is sometimes used for the suppression of cough as for example in the control of intractable cough associated with terminal lung cancer.

WADA Status: Banned in competition

WADA Class: Narcotics

Includes specified narcotics.

Preparations

Single ingredient: ***Arg.:*** Algedol; Amidiaz; Analmorph; Duramorph; GNO; MST Continus; Neocalmans; ***Austral.:*** Anamorph; Kapanol; MS Contin; MS Mono; Ordine; ***Austria:*** Compensan; Kapabloc; Kapanol; M-Dolor; Morapid; Mundidol; Substitol; Vendal; ***Belg.:*** Docmorfine; Kapanol; MS Contin; MS Direct; Oramorph; Stellorphinad; Stellorphine; ***Braz.:*** Dimorf; ***Canad.:***

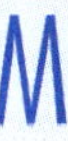

Kadian; M-Eslon; MOS; MS Contin; MSIR; ***Chile:*** M-Eslon; ***Cz.:*** Doltard; M-Eslon; MST Continus; MST Uno; Oramorph; Sevredol; Skenan; Slovalgin; Vendal; ***Denm.:*** Contalgin; Depolan; Doltard; ***Fin.:*** Depolan; Dolcontin; ***Fr.:*** Actiskenan; Kapanol; Moscontin; Oramorph; Sevredol; Skenan; ***Ger.:*** Capros; Kapanol; M-beta; M-long; M-Stada; Morph; Morphanton; MSI; MSR; MST; Oramorph; Painbreak; Sevredol; ***Hong Kong:*** M-Eslon; MST Continus; ***Hung.:*** M-Eslon; Moretal; MST Continus; Sevredol; ***India:*** Morcontin; ***Indon.:*** MST; ***Irl.:*** MST Continus; MXL; Oramorph; Sevredol; ***Israel:*** MCR; MIR; Morphex; MSP; ***Ital.:*** MS Contin; Oramorph; Ticinan; Twice; ***Jpn:*** MS Contin; ***Mex.:*** Analfin; Graten; ***Neth.:*** Kapanol; MS Contin; Oramorph; Sevredol; Skenan; ***Norw.:*** Dolcontin; ***NZ:*** Kapanol; LA Morph; M-Eslon; RA Morph; Sevredol; ***Philipp.:*** M-Dolor; MST Continus; Relimal; ***Pol.:*** MST Continus; Sevredol; Vendal; ***Port.:*** MST; MXL; Sevredol; Skenan; ***S.Afr.:*** MST Continus; SRM-Rhotard; ***Singapore:*** MST Continus; Statex; ***Spain:*** MST Continus; MST Unicontinus; Oramorph; Sevredol; Skenan; ***Swed.:*** Depolan; Dolcontin; ***Switz.:*** Kapanol; M-retard; MST Continus; Sevre-Long; Sevredol; ***Turk.:*** M-Eslon; Vendal; ***UK:*** Filnarine; Morphgesic; MST Continus; MXL; Oramorph; Rhotard; Sevredol; Zomorph; ***USA:*** Astramorph; Avinza; DepoDur; Duramorph; Infumorph; Kadian; MS Contin; MSIR; Oramorph; RMS; Roxanol; ***Venez.:*** MS Contin.

Multi-ingredient: ***Austral.:*** Morphalgin; ***Austria:*** Modiscop; ***Irl.:*** Cyclimorph; ***Ital.:*** Cardiostenol; ***Pol.:*** Doltard; ***S.Afr.:*** Chloropect; Cyclimorph; Enterodyne; Pectrolyte; ***Swed.:*** Spasmofen; ***Switz.:*** Spasmosol; ***UK:*** Collis Browne's; Collis Browne's; Cyclimorph; Diocalm Dual Action; Opazimes.

Muzolimine

Other names: Bay-g-2821; Mutsolimiini; Muzolimin; Muzolimina; Muzoliminum.

Музолимин

Clinical profile: Although chemically unrelated, muzolimine is a diuretic similar to the loop diuretics. Severe neurological symptoms were associated with the administration of high doses of muzolimine in patients with renal impairment and led to its withdrawal worldwide.

WADA Status: Banned in and out of competition

WADA Class: Diuretics and Other Masking Agents

Includes diuretics or substances with a similar chemical structure or similar biological effect(s).

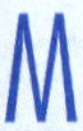

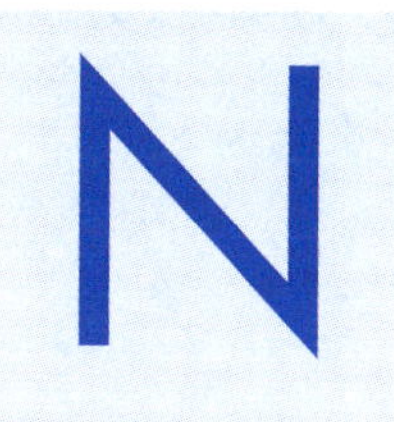

Nabilone

Other names: Compound 109514; Lilly-109514; Nabilon; Nabilona; Nabiloni; Nabilonum.

Набилон

Clinical profile: Nabilone, a synthetic cannabinoid with antiemetic and anxiolytic properties, is used for the control of nausea and vomiting associated with cancer chemotherapy in patients who have failed to respond adequately to conventional antiemetics.

WADA Status: Banned in competition

WADA Class: Cannabinoids

E.g. hashish, marijuana

WADA Class: Specified Substances

Also listed as a specified substance.

"The prohibited List may identify specified substances which are particularly susceptible to unintentional anti-doping rule violations because of their general availability in medicinal products or which are less likely to be successfully abused as doping agents."

A doping violation involving such substances may result in a reduced sanction provided that the *"...Athlete can establish that the Use of such a specfied substance was not intended to enhance sport performance..."*

Preparations
Single ingredient: ***Arg.:*** Cesamet; ***Canad.:*** Cesamet; ***USA:*** Cesamet.

Nadolol

Other names: Nadololi; Nadololis; Nadololum; SQ-11725.

Надолол

Clinical profile: Nadolol is a non-cardioselective beta blocker used in the management of hypertension, angina pectoris, and cardiac arrhythmias. It is also used in the management of hyperthyroidism and migraine.

WADA Status: Banned in and out of competition as specified below

WADA Class: Beta-Blockers

Unless otherwise specified, beta-blockers are prohibited *In-Competition* only in the following sports.

- Aeronautics (FAI)

- Archery (FITA, IPC) (also prohibited *Out-of-Competition*)
- Automobile (FIA)
- Billiards (WCBS)
- Bobsleigh (FIBT)
- Boules (CMSB, IPC bowls)
- Bridge (FMB)
- Curling (WCF)
- Gymnastics (FIG)
- Motorcycling (FIM)
- Modern Pentathlon (UIPM) for disciplines involving shooting
- Nine-pin bowling (FIQ)
- Powerboating (UIM)
- Sailing (ISAF) for match race helms only
- Shooting (ISSF, IPC) (also prohibited *Out-of-Competition*)
- Skiing/Snowboarding (FIS) in ski jumping, freestyle aerials/halfpipe and snowboard halfpipe/big air
- Wrestling (FILA)

WADA Class: Specified Substances

Also listed as a specified substance.

"The prohibited List may identify specified substances which are particularly susceptible to unintentional anti-doping rule violations because of their general availability in medicinal products or which are less likely to be successfully abused as doping agents."

A doping violation involving such substances may result in a reduced sanction provided that the "*...Athlete can establish that the Use of such a specfied substance was not intended to enhance sport performance...*"

Preparations
Single ingredient: ***Arg.:*** Corgard; ***Belg.:*** Corgard; ***Braz.:*** Corgard; ***Canad.:*** Apo-Nadol; Corgard; ***Chile:*** Corgard; ***Fr.:*** Corgard; ***Ger.:*** Solgol; ***Hong Kong:*** Apo-Nadol; ***Ital.:*** Corgard; ***Mex.:*** Corgard; ***NZ:*** Corgard; ***Port.:*** Anabet; ***S.Afr.:*** Corgard; ***Spain:*** Corgard; Solgol; ***Switz.:*** Corgard; ***UK:*** Corgard; ***USA:*** Corgard; ***Venez.:*** Corgard.
Multi-ingredient: ***Ger.:*** Sotaziden N; ***Mex.:*** Corgaretic; ***S.Afr.:*** Corgaretic; ***USA:*** Corzide.

Nafarelin Acetate

Other names: Acetato de nafarelina; Nafareliiniasetaatti; Nafarelin Asetat; Nafarelinacetat; Nafaréline, Acétate de; Nafarelini Acetas; D-Nal(2)^6-LHRH acetate hydrate; RS-94991298.

Нафарелина Ацетат

Clinical profile: Nafarelin acetate is an analogue of gonadorelin used for the treatment of endometriosis. It is also used in the treatment of precocious puberty, and as an adjunct to ovulation induction with gonadotrophins in the treatment of infertility.

WADA Status: Banned in and out of competition

WADA Class: Hormones and Related Substances: Gonadotrophins

Includes gonadotrophin or a substance with a similar chemical structure or similar biological effect(s), or one of their releasing factors. Prohibited in males only.

Preparations
Single ingredient: ***Arg.:*** Synrelin; ***Austral.:*** Synarel; ***Braz.:*** Synarel; ***Canad.:*** Synarel; ***Cz.:*** Synarel; ***Denm.:*** Synarela; ***Fin.:*** Synarela; ***Fr.:*** Synarel; ***Ger.:*** Synarela; ***India:*** Nasarel; ***Irl.:*** Synarel; ***Israel:*** Synarel; ***Neth.:*** Synarel; ***Norw.:*** Synarela; ***Pol.:*** Synarel; ***S.Afr.:*** Synarel; ***Spain:*** Synarel; ***Swed.:*** Synarela; ***Switz.:*** Synrelina; ***Turk.:*** Synarel; ***UK:*** Synarel; ***USA:*** Synarel.

Nandrolone

Other names: Estrenolona; Hidroxiestrenona; Nandrolon; Nandrolona; Nandroloni; Nandrolonum; Norandrostenolona; 19-Nortestosterone; Nortestrionato.

Нандролон

N

Nandrolone Cyclohexylpropionate

Other names: Ciclohexilpropionato de nandrolona; Nandrolone Cyclohexane-propionate; Nandrolone, Cyclohexylpropionate de; Nandroloni Cyclohexylpropionas; Nortestosterone Cyclohexylpropionate.

Нандролона Циклогексилпропионат

Nandrolone Decanoate

Other names: Decanoato de nandrolona; Nandrolon-dekanoát; Nandrolone, décanoate de; Nandroloni decanoas; Nandrolonu dekanonian; Nortestosterone Decanoate; Nortestosterone Decylate.

Нандролона Деканоат

Nandrolone Laurate

Other names: Dodecanoato de nandrolona; Laurato de nandrolona; Nandrolone Dodecanoate; Nandrolone, Laurate de; Nandroloni Lauras; Nortestosterone Laurate.

Нандролона Лаурат

Nandrolone Phenylpropionate

Other names: Fenilpropionato de nandrolona; Nandrolone Hydrocinnamate; Nandrolone Phenpropionate; Nandrolone, Phénylpropionate de; Nandroloni Phenylpropionas; Nandrolonu fenylopropionian; 19-Norandrostenolone Phenylpropionate; Nortestosterone Phenylpropionate; NSC-23162.

Нандролона Фенилпропионат

Nandrolone Sodium Sulfate

Other names: Nandrolone Sodium Sulphate; Nandrolone, Sulfate Sodique de; Nandroloni Natrii Sulfas; Nortestosterone Sodium Sulphate; Sulfato sódico de nandrolona.

Нандролона Натрия Сульфат

Nandrolone Undecylate

Other names: Nandrolone Undecanoate; Nandrolone, Undécylate de; Nandroloni Undecylas; Nortestosterone Undecanoate; Undecilato de nandrolona.

Нандролона Ундесилат

Clinical profile: Nandrolone is an anabolic steroid. Nandrolone decanoate, nandrolone phenylpropionate, and nandrolone undecylate have been used for their anabolic effects after debilitating illness. The cyclohexylpropionate, the decanoate, the phenylpropionate, and the undecylate have been used in osteoporosis. Nandrolone decanoate and nandrolone phenylpropionate have also been given in postmenopausal metastatic breast carcinoma, and nandrolone decanoate has also been given for the treatment of anaemias. Nandrolone sodium sulfate is used in the treatment of corneal damage. The cyclohexylpropionate, the laurate, and the phenylpropionate have been used in veterinary medicine.

WADA Status: Banned in and out of competition

WADA Class: Anabolic; Androgenic Steroids (exogenous)

Includes exogenous anabolic androgenic steroids or other substances with a similar chemical structure or similar biological effect(s).

N

Preparations
Single ingredient: ***Arg.:*** Deca-Durabolin; ***Austral.:*** Deca-Durabolin; ***Austria:*** Deca-Durabolin; ***Belg.:*** Deca-Durabolin; ***Braz.:*** Deca-Durabolin; ***Canad.:*** Deca-Durabolin; ***Chile:*** Anaprolina; Deca-Durabolin; Nandrosande; ***Cz.:*** Keratyl; Superanabolon; ***Fin.:*** Deca-Durabolin; ***Ger.:*** Deca-Durabolin; ***Gr.:*** Anaboline Depot; Deca-Durabolin; Extraboline; ***Hong Kong:*** Deca-Durabolin; ***Hung.:*** Retabolil; ***India:*** Deca-Durabolin; Durabolin; Metabol; Metadec; Neurabol; ***Indon.:*** Deca-Durabolin; ***Ital.:*** Deca-Durabolin; ***Malaysia:*** Deca-Durabolin; ***Mex.:*** Deca-Durabolin; ***Neth.:*** Deca-Durabolin; Durabolin; ***Norw.:*** Deca-Durabolin; ***NZ:*** Deca-Durabolin; ***Pol.:*** Deca-Durabolin; ***Port.:*** Deca-Durabolin; Nandain; ***Rus.:*** Retabolil (Ретаболил); ***S.Afr.:*** Deca-Durabolin; ***Singapore:*** Deca-Durabolin; ***Spain:*** Deca-Durabolin; ***Swed.:*** Deca-Durabol; ***Switz.:*** Deca-Durabolin; Keratyl; ***Thai.:*** Deca-Durabolin; Keratyl; ***UK:*** Deca-Durabolin; ***USA:*** Androlone-D; Deca-Durabolin; Durabolin; Hybolin; Neo-Durabolic; ***Venez.:*** Deca-Durabolin.
Multi-ingredient: ***Indon.:*** Dexatopic.

Naphazoline

Other names: Nafatsoliini; Nafazolin; Nafazolina; Naphazolinum.

Нафазолин

Naphazoline Hydrochloride

Other names: Hidrocloruro de nafazolina; Nafatsoliinihydrokloridi; Nafazolin Hidroklorür; Nafazolin-hidroklorid; Nafazolin-hydrochlorid; Nafazolinhydroklorid; Nafazolino hidrochloridas; Naphazoline, chlorhydrate de; Naphazolini hydrochloridum.

Нафазолина Гидрохлорид

Naphazoline Nitrate

Other names: Nafatsoliininitraatti; Nafazolin Nitrat; Nafazolinnitrat; Nafazolinnitrát; Nafazolino nitratas; Nafazoliny azotan; Naphazoline, nitrate de; Naphazolini nitras; Naphazolinium Nitricum; Naphthizinum; Nitrato de nafazolina.

Нафазолина Нитрат

Clinical profile: Naphazoline is a sympathomimetic with marked alpha-adrenergic activity. It is a vasoconstrictor with a rapid and prolonged action in reducing swelling and congestion when applied to mucous membranes. It has also sometimes been added to solutions of local anaesthetics as an adjunct to diminish absorption and localise the effect. It is used for the symptomatic relief of nasal congestion and has been instilled into the eye as a conjunctival decongestant.

WADA Status: Banned in competition

WADA Class: Stimulants

Includes stimulants or substances with a similar chemical structure or similar biological effect(s). Naphazoline is an imidazole derivative. Imidazole derivatives for topical use are exempt.

Preparations
Single ingredient: ***Arg.:*** Actifedrin Nasal; Bactio Rhin; Bano Ocular Agrand; Dazolin; Disel; Gotabiotic D; Gotinal; Let-Nasal; Mirasan; Mirus-S; Nafazolex; Nasalex; Privina; Rhinal; ***Austral.:*** Albalon; Naphcon; Optazine; ***Austria:*** Aconex; Coldan; Isoftal; Mertan; Privin; Rhinon; Rhinoperd; ***Belg.:*** Deltarhinol-Mono; Naphcon; Neusinol; Priciasol; Vasocedine; ***Braz.:*** Clarivit; Claroft; Multisoro; Narial; Narix; Nazicol; Neosoro; Privina; Rino Resfenol; Rinos-A; ***Canad.:*** Ak-Con; Albalon; Allergy Drops; Clear Eyes; Diopticon; Naphcon Forte; ***Chile:*** Clarimir; Red Off; ***Cz.:*** Proculin; Sanorin; ***Ger.:*** Privin; Proculin; Rhinex mit Naphazolin; Tele-Stulln; ***Gr.:*** Coldan; Naphcon; ***Hong Kong:*** Albalon; All Clear; ***India:*** Clearine; Ocustress; ***Indon.:*** Optrine; ***Israel:*** Naphasal; Naphcon Forte; ***Ital.:*** Collirio Alfa; Desamin Same; Imidazyl; Iridina Due; Naftazolina; Pupilla; Rinazina; Rino Naftazolina; Video-Mill; ***Malaysia:*** Albalon; ***Mex.:*** Afazol; Alphadinal; Celunaf; Fazolin; Gotinal; Nazil; ***Neth.:*** Albalon; ***NZ:*** Clear Eyes; Naphcon; ***Philipp.:*** Cosooth; ***Pol.:*** Rhinazin; ***Rus.:*** Sanorin (Санорин); ***S.Afr.:*** Safyr Bleu; ***Spain:*** Alfa; Euboral; Miraclar; Vasoconstrictor Pensa; ***Switz.:*** Albalon; ***Thai.:*** Albalon; Naphcon; ***Turk.:*** Deltarhinol; Enflucide; ***UK:*** Murine; ***USA:*** Ak-Con; Albalon; All Clear; Clear Eyes Plus Redness Relief; Clear Eyes; Napha

Forte; Naphcon; Privine; ***Venez.:*** Clarasol; Clearize; Fazolan; Gotinal; Naphcon; Nas; Niazol; Ninazo.

Multi-ingredient: ***Arg.:*** Bactio Rhin Prednisolona; Bideon; Biotaer Nasal; Dexalergin; Disel Hidrocortisona; Drynisan; Factioneye; Fadanasal; Hyalcrom; Mira Klonal; Mirus; Nasomicina; Neo-Currino; Neodexa Plus; Neosona; Nexadron Compuesto; Nexadron Plus; Panoptic; Provacsin Nasal; Refenax Colirio; Refenax Gotas Nasales; Rinofilax AG M; Rinogel; Suavithiol; ***Austral.:*** Albalon-A; Antistine-Privine; In A Wink; Naphcon-A; Optrex; ***Austria:*** Coldistan; Coldophthal; Histophtal; Luuf-Nasenspray; Ophtaguttal; Rhinodrin; Rhinon; Rhinoperd comp; ***Belg.:*** Minhavez; Naphcon-A; Neofenox; Sofraline; Sofrasolone; ***Braz.:*** Alergotox Nasal; Claril; Colirio Legrand; Colirio Teuto; Conidrin; Fluo-Vaso; Hemodotti; Hidrocin; Inhadrina; Lerin; Maxibell; Mentodrin; Naridrin; Nariflux; Naso-Josp; Nazobel; Nazobio; Neo Quimica Colirio; Nitrileno; Novo Rino; Rhinosept; Rinisone; Rinocito; Sinustrat Vasoconstritor; Sorine Adulto; Stilux; Visiplex; Visual; Zincolok; ***Canad.:*** Albalon-A; Clear Eyes Allergy; Diopticon A; Naphcon-A; Onrectal; Opcon-A; Visine Advance Allergy; Zincfrin-A; ***Chile:*** Clarimir F; Dessolets; Miral; Naphcon-A; Naphtears; Nico Drops; Novo-Tears; Oculosan; Oftalirio; Red Off Aqua; Red Off Plus; ***Cz.:*** Sanorin-Analergin; ***Denm.:*** Ansal; Antistina-Privin; Sesal; ***Fr.:*** Collyre Bleu; Derinox; ***Ger.:*** Antistin-Privin; duraultra; Oculosan N; Siozwo; ***Gr.:*** Neo-Priphen; Oculosan; Septobore; Zabysept; ***Hong Kong:*** Clear Blue; Frazoline; Naphcon-A; Nazin; Oculosan; Opcon-A; ***India:*** Andre-I-Kul; Andre; Betnesol-N Nasal; Efcorlin; Fenox; Ocurest-AH; Ocurest-Z; Ocurest; Proto-Boric; ***Indon.:*** Flamergi; Indofrin-A; Isotic Azora; Naphcon-A; Oculosan; Zincopto; ***Israel:*** Alnase; Optryl; Proaf; ***Ital.:*** Alfaflor; Antisettico Astringente Sedativo; Antistin-Privina; Collirio Alfa Antistaminico; Deltarinolo; Fotofil; Genalfa; Imidazyl Antistaminico; Indaco; Iristamina; Oftalmil; Pupilla Antistaminico; Rinocidina; Zinc-Imizol; ***Malaysia:*** Alergoftal; Naphcon-A; Oculosan; ***Mex.:*** Afazol Z; Biofrin; Biotarson O; Eyrasil; Istasol; Midazol Ofteno; Mirus; Naphacel; Naphtears; Opcon-A; Soltrictor con Lagrifilm; Solutina; Sulvi; Zincfrin-A; ***NZ:*** Betnesol Aqueous; Naphcon-A; Optrex Red-Eye Relief; Visine Allergy; ***Philipp.:*** Decocon A; Moisturizing All Clear; Naphcon-A; Oculosan; Optaphen; ***Pol.:*** Betadrin; Cincol; Dermophenazol; Mibalin; Oculosan; Oftophenazol; Rhinophenazol; Sulfarinol; ***Port.:*** Alergiftalmina; Colircusi Anestesico; Naso-Prieulina; ***Rus.:*** Betadrin (Бетадрин); Polynadim (Полинадим); Sanorin (Санорин); Sanorin-Analergin (Санорин-аналергин); ***S.Afr.:*** Antistin-Privin; Covomycin; Covosan; ENT; Nasdro; Oculosan; Universal Nasal Drops; Zincfrin-A; ***Singapore:*** Antistin-Privin; Naphcon-A; ***Spain:*** Alergoftal; Centilux; Cloram Zinc; Coliriocilina Adren Astr; Epistaxol; Kanafosal Predni; Kanafosal; Oftalmol Ocular; Ojosbel; Rinovel; Zolina; ***Swed.:*** Antasten-Privin; ***Switz.:*** Antistin-Privin; Collyre Bleu Laiter; Oculosan; Spray nasal comp pour adultes; ***Thai.:*** Levoptin; Naphcon-A; Oculosan; ***Turk.:*** Alergoftal; Sulfarhin; ***UK:*** Eye Dew; Optrex Red Eyes; ***USA:*** 4-Way Fast Acting; Antazoline-V; Clear Eyes Seasonal Relief; Maximum Strength Allergy Drops; Naphazoline Plus; Naphcon-A; Naphoptic-A; Ocuhist; Opcon-A; Vaso-Clear A; Vasocon-A; Visine-A; ***Venez.:*** Camolyn Plus; Pinazo; Soltin; Soluclear.

Adjunct-ingredient: ***Fr.:*** Xylocaine; ***Spain:*** Anestesico.

Natriuretic Peptides

Other names: Péptidos natriuréticos.

Clinical profile: Atrial natriuretic peptide (ANP) is an endogenous substance secreted by the heart that possesses diuretic and natriuretic properties. Synthetic forms include anaritide and carperitide. Natriuretic peptides related structurally to atrial natriuretic peptide include brain natriuretic peptide and ularitide. Atrial natriuretic peptide and brain natriuretic peptide are closely involved in fluid and electrolyte homoeostasis and in the regulation of blood pressure, together with other complex systems such as the renin-angiotensin-aldosterone cascade. Their physiological and pathological role and potential clinical applications are under investigation. Carperitide and nesiritide (recombinant brain natriuretic peptide) are used in acute heart failure.

WADA Status: Banned in and out of competition

N

WADA Class: Diuretics and Other Masking Agents

Includes diuretics or substances with a similar chemical structure or similar biological effect(s).

Nebivolol

Other names: Narbivolol; Nébivolol; Nebivololi, Nebivololum; R-65824.

Небиволол

Nebivolol Hydrochloride

Other names: Hidrocloruro de nebivolol; Nébivolol, Chlorhydrate de; Nebivololi Hydrochloridum; R-67555; R-067555.

Небиволола Гидрохлорид

Clinical profile: Nebivolol is a cardioselective beta blocker also reported to have vasodilating activity. It is given by mouth as the hydrochloride in the management of hypertension and heart failure.

WADA Status: Banned in and out of competition as specified below

WADA Class: Beta-Blockers

Unless otherwise specified, beta-blockers are prohibited *In-Competition* only in the following sports.

- Aeronautics (FAI)
- Archery (FITA, IPC) (also prohibited *Out-of-Competition*)
- Automobile (FIA)
- Billiards (WCBS)
- Bobsleigh (FIBT)
- Boules (CMSB, IPC bowls)
- Bridge (FMB)
- Curling (WCF)
- Gymnastics (FIG)
- Motorcycling (FIM)
- Modern Pentathlon (UIPM) for disciplines involving shooting
- Nine-pin bowling (FIQ)
- Powerboating (UIM)
- Sailing (ISAF) for match race helms only
- Shooting (ISSF, IPC) (also prohibited *Out-of-Competition*)
- Skiing/Snowboarding (FIS) in ski jumping, freestyle aerials/halfpipe and snowboard halfpipe/big air
- Wrestling (FILA)

WADA Class: Specified Substances

Also listed as a specified substance.

"*The prohibited List may identify specified substances which are particularly susceptible to unintentional anti-doping rule violations because of their general availability in medicinal products or which are less likely to be successfully abused as doping agents.*"

A doping violation involving such substances may result in a reduced sanction provided that the "*...Athlete can establish that the Use of such a specfied substance was not intended to enhance sport performance...*"

Preparations

Single ingredient: ***Arg.:*** Nebilet; ***Austria:*** Nomexor; ***Belg.:*** Nobiten; ***Chile:*** Nebilet; ***Cz.:*** Nebilet; ***Fr.:*** Nebilox; Temerit; ***Ger.:*** Nebilet; ***Gr.:*** Lobivon; ***Hung.:*** Nebilet; ***India:*** Nodon; ***Irl.:*** Nebilet; ***Ital.:*** Lobivon; Nebilox; ***Neth.:*** Hypoloc; Lobivon; Nebilet; Nebiloc; ***Pol.:*** Nebilet; ***Port.:*** Nebilet; ***Rus.:*** Nebilet (Небилет); ***S.Afr.:*** Nebilet; ***Singapore:*** Nebilet; ***Spain:*** Lobivon;

Nebilet; Nebilox; Silostar; ***Switz.:*** Nebilet; ***Thai.:*** Nebilet; ***Turk.:*** Vasoxen; ***UK:*** Nebilet; ***Venez.:*** Nebilet.

Nesiritide Citrate

Other names: Citrato de nesiritida; Nésiritide, Citrate de; Nesiritidi Citras.

Незиритида Цитрат

Clinical profile: Nesiritide is a recombinant brain natriuretic peptide used in acutely decompensated heart failure.

WADA Status: Banned in and out of competition

WADA Class: Diuretics and Other Masking Agents

Includes diuretics or substances with a similar chemical structure or similar biological effect(s).

Preparations
Single ingredient: ***Arg.:*** Natrecor; ***Indon.:*** Natrecor; ***Israel:*** Noratak; ***Switz.:*** Noratak; ***USA:*** Natrecor; ***Venez.:*** Natrecor.

Nifenalol

Other names: Nifénalol; Nifenalolum.

Нифеналол

Clinical profile: Nifenalol is a beta blocker.

WADA Status: Banned in and out of competition as specified below

WADA Class: Beta-Blockers

Unless otherwise specified, beta-blockers are prohibited *In-Competition* only in the following sports.

- Aeronautics (FAI)
- Archery (FITA, IPC) (also prohibited *Out-of-Competition*)
- Automobile (FIA)
- Billiards (WCBS)
- Bobsleigh (FIBT)
- Boules (CMSB, IPC bowls)
- Bridge (FMB)
- Curling (WCF)
- Gymnastics (FIG)
- Motorcycling (FIM)
- Modern Pentathlon (UIPM) for disciplines involving shooting
- Nine-pin bowling (FIQ)
- Powerboating (UIM)
- Sailing (ISAF) for match race helms only
- Shooting (ISSF, IPC) (also prohibited *Out-of-Competition*)
- Skiing/Snowboarding (FIS) in ski jumping, freestyle aerials/halfpipe and snowboard halfpipe/big air
- Wrestling (FILA)

WADA Class: Specified Substances

Also listed as a specified substance.

"The prohibited List may identify specified substances which are particularly susceptible to unintentional anti-doping rule violations because of their general availability in medicinal products or which are less likely to be successfully abused as doping agents."

A doping violation involving such substances may result in a reduced sanction pro-

vided that the "*...Athlete can establish that the Use of such a specfied substance was not intended to enhance sport performance...*"

N

Nikethamide

Other names: Cordiaminum; Nicetamid; Nicéthamide; Nicethamidum; Nicotinic Acid Diethylamide; Nicotinoyldiaethylamidum; Niketamid; Niketamidas; Niketamidi; Nikethamid; Nikethylamide; Niquetamida.

Никетамид

Clinical profile: Nikethamide was formerly used as a respiratory stimulant, but such use has largely been abandoned because of toxicity. It has also been used as a central stimulant and in preparations for hypotensive disorders.

WADA Status: Banned in competition

WADA Class: Stimulants

Includes nikethamide and any optical isomers.

WADA Class: Specified Substances

Also listed as a specified substance.

"*The prohibited List may identify specified substances which are particularly susceptible to unintentional anti-doping rule violations because of their general availability in medicinal products or which are less likely to be successfully abused as doping agents.*"

A doping violation involving such substances may result in a reduced sanction provided that the "*...Athlete can establish that the Use of such a specfied substance was not intended to enhance sport performance...*"

Preparations

Single ingredient: ***Pol.:*** Cardiamidum.

Multi-ingredient: ***Fr.:*** Coramine Glucose; ***Pol.:*** Cardiamid-Coffein; Glucardiamid; ***Switz.:*** Gly-Coramin.

Nipradilol

Other names: K-351; Nipradilolum; Nipradolol.

Нипрадилол

Clinical profile: Nipradilol is a non-cardioselective beta blocker also reported to have direct vasodilating activity. It is used in the management of glaucoma and ocular hypertension.

WADA Status: Banned in and out of competition as specified below

WADA Class: Beta-Blockers

Unless otherwise specified, beta-blockers are prohibited *In-Competition* only in the following sports.

- Aeronautics (FAI)
- Archery (FITA, IPC) (also prohibited *Out-of-Competition*)
- Automobile (FIA)
- Billiards (WCBS)
- Bobsleigh (FIBT)
- Boules (CMSB, IPC bowls)
- Bridge (FMB)
- Curling (WCF)
- Gymnastics (FIG)
- Motorcycling (FIM)
- Modern Pentathlon (UIPM) for disciplines involving shooting
- Nine-pin bowling (FIQ)

- Powerboating (UIM)
- Sailing (ISAF) for match race helms only
- Shooting (ISSF, IPC) (also prohibited *Out-of-Competition*)
- Skiing/Snowboarding (FIS) in ski jumping, freestyle aerials/halfpipe and snowboard halfpipe/big air
- Wrestling (FILA)

WADA Class: Specified Substances

Also listed as a specified substance.

"The prohibited List may identify specified substances which are particularly susceptible to unintentional anti-doping rule violations because of their general availability in medicinal products or which are less likely to be successfully abused as doping agents."

A doping violation involving such substances may result in a reduced sanction provided that the "*...Athlete can establish that the Use of such a specfied substance was not intended to enhance sport performance...*"

Preparations
Single ingredient: ***Jpn:*** Hypadil.

Noradrenaline

Other names: Norepinephrine; Levarterenol; Noradrenaliini; Noradrenalin; Noradrenalinum; Norepinefriini; Norepinefrin; Norepinefrina; Norépinéphrine; Norepinephrinum; Norepirenamine.

Норэпинефрин

Noradrenaline Acid Tartrate

Other names: Norepinephrine Bitartrate; Arterenol Acid Tartrate; *l*-Arterenol Bitartrate; Bitartrato de norepinefrina; Levarterenol Acid Tartrate; Levarterenol Bitartrate; Levarterenoli Bitartras; Noradrenaliinitartraatti; Noradrenaline Bitartrate; Noradrenaline Tartrate; Noradrénaline, tartrate de; Noradrenalini tartras; Noradrenalino tartratas; Noradrenalin-tartarát; Noradrenalintartrat; Norepinefrin tartarát monohydrát; Norepinefryny wodorowinian; Norepinephrine Acid Tartrate; *l*-Norepinephrine Bitartrate; Norépinéphrine, Bitartrate de; Norepinephrini Bitartras; Norepinephrini Tartras Monohydricus.

Норэпинефрина Битартрат

Noradrenaline Hydrochloride

Other names: Norepinephrine Hydrochloride; Hidrocloruro de norepinefrina; Noradrenaliinihydrokloridi; Noradrénaline, chlorhydrate de; Noradrenalin-hidroklorid; Noradrenalinhydroklorid; Noradrenalini hydrochloridum; Noradrenalino hidrochloridas; Norepinefrin hydrochlorid; Norépinéphrine, Chlorhydrate de; Norepinephrini Hydrochloridum.

Норэпинефрина Гидрохлорид

Clinical profile: The catecholamine, noradrenaline, is a direct-acting sympathomimetic with pronounced effects on alpha-adrenergic receptors and less marked effects on beta-adrenergic receptors. It is a neurotransmitter. Noradrenaline may be used for the emergency restoration of blood pressure in acute hypotensive states. It has also sometimes been added to solutions of local anaesthetics as an adjunct to diminish absorption and localise the effect. Locally applied noradrenaline solutions have also been used to control bleeding in upper gastrointestinal haemorrhage and similar disorders.

WADA Status: Banned in competition

N

WADA Class: Stimulants

Includes stimulants or substances with a similar chemical structure or similar biological effect(s).

WADA Class: Specified Substances

Also listed as a specified substance.

"*The prohibited List may identify specified substances which are particularly susceptible to unintentional anti-doping rule violations because of their general availability in medicinal products or which are less likely to be successfully abused as doping agents.*"

A doping violation involving such substances may result in a reduced sanction provided that the "*...Athlete can establish that the Use of such a specfied substance was not intended to enhance sport performance...*"

Preparations

Single ingredient: ***Arg.:*** Fioritina; ***Austral.:*** Levophed; ***Belg.:*** Levophed; ***Braz.:*** Levophed; Norephed; ***Canad.:*** Levophed; ***Chile:*** Adine; ***Ger.:*** Arterenol; ***Gr.:*** Levophed; Noradren; ***India:*** Adrenor; ***Indon.:*** Levophed; N-Epi; Raivas; Vascon; ***Irl.:*** Levophed; ***Israel:*** Levophed; ***Malaysia:*** Levophed; ***Mex.:*** Pridam; ***NZ:*** Levophed; ***Philipp.:*** Inotrop; Levophed; ***Pol.:*** Levonor; ***Spain:*** Norages; ***Thai.:*** Levophed; ***USA:*** Levophed.

Adjunct-ingredient: ***Austria:*** Neo-Xylestesin forte; Scandonest; ***Braz.:*** Xylestesin; Xylocaina; ***Ital.:*** Xylonor; ***Port.:*** Xilonibsa; ***S.Afr.:*** Xylotox; ***Spain:*** Xylonor Especial; ***Switz.:*** Scandonest.

Norclostebol Acetate

Other names: Acetato de norclostebol; Norclostébol, Acétate de; Norclosteboli Acetas.

Норклостебола Ацетат

Clinical profile: Norclostebol acetate has been used as an anabolic agent.

WADA Status: Banned in and out of competition

WADA Class: Anabolic; Androgenic Steroids (exogenous)

Includes exogenous anabolic androgenic steroids or other substances with a similar chemical structure or similar biological effect(s).

Norethandrolone

Other names: 17α-Ethyl-17β-hydroxyestr-4-en-3-one; 17β-Hydroxy-19-nor-17α-pregn-4-en-3-one; Noretandrolona; Noréthandrolone; Norethandrolonum.

Норэтандролон

Clinical profile: Norethandrolone is an anabolic steroid used in the treatment of aplastic anaemia.

WADA Status: Banned in and out of competition

WADA Class: Anabolic; Androgenic Steroids (exogenous)

Includes exogenous anabolic androgenic steroids or other substances with a similar chemical structure or similar biological effect(s).

Preparations
Single ingredient: ***Fr.:*** Nilevar.

Norfenefrine Hydrochloride

Other names: Hidrocloruro de norfenefrina; Norfenefrin Hidroklorür; Norfénéfrine, Chlorhydrate de; Norfenefrini Hydrochloridum; Norphenylephrine Hydrochloride; *m*-Norsynephrine Hydrochloride; WV-569.

Норфенефрина Гидрохлорид

Clinical profile: Norfenefrine hydrochloride is a sympathomimetic with predominantly alpha-adrenergic activity used in the treatment of hypotensive states.

WADA Status: Banned in competition

WADA Class: Stimulants
Includes norfenefrine and any optical isomers.

WADA Class: Specified Substances
Also listed as a specified substance.
"The prohibited List may identify specified substances which are particularly susceptible to unintentional anti-doping rule violations because of their general availability in medicinal products or which are less likely to be successfully abused as doping agents."
A doping violation involving such substances may result in a reduced sanction provided that the "*...Athlete can establish that the Use of such a specfied substance was not intended to enhance sport performance...*"

Preparations
Single ingredient: ***Austria:*** Novadral; ***Mex.:*** AS Cor; ***Switz.:*** Novadral; ***Turk.:*** Novadral.
Multi-ingredient: ***Switz.:*** Ortho-Maren retard.

Normethandrone

Other names: Methylestrenolone; Methylestrenolonum; Methylnortestosterone; 17α-Methyl-19-nortestosterone; Metylöstrenolon; Metyyliestrenoloni; Normethandrolone; NSC-10039.

Норметандрон

Clinical profile: Normethandrone has androgenic, anabolic, and progestogenic properties and has been given orally with an oestrogen for the treatment of amenorrhoea and menopausal disorders.

WADA Status: Banned in and out of competition

WADA Class: Anabolic; Androgenic Steroids (exogenous)
Includes exogenous anabolic androgenic steroids or other substances with a similar chemical structure or similar biological effect(s).

Preparations
Multi-ingredient: ***Indon.:*** Mediol; Renodiol; ***Venez.:*** Ginecosid.

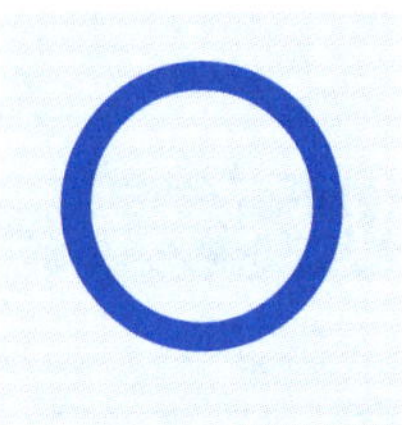

Octodrine

Other names: Octodrina; Octodrinum; SKF-51.
Октодрин

Clinical profile: Octodrine is a sympathomimetic with predominantly alpha-adrenergic activity. It has been used in the treatment of hypotensive states and in obstructive airways disease.

WADA Status: Banned in competition

WADA Class: Stimulants

Includes stimulants or substances with a similar chemical structure or similar biological effect(s).

WADA Class: Specified Substances

Also listed as a specified substance.
"The prohibited List may identify specified substances which are particularly susceptible to unintentional anti-doping rule violations because of their general availability in medicinal products or which are less likely to be successfully abused as doping agents."
A doping violation involving such substances may result in a reduced sanction provided that the "*...Athlete can establish that the Use of such a specfied substance was not intended to enhance sport performance...*"

Preparations
Multi-ingredient: ***Austria:*** Ambredin.

Octopamine

Other names: β,4-Dihydroxyphenethylamine; *p*-Hydroxymandelamine; ND-50; Noroxedrine; *p*-Norsynephrine; Octopamina; *p*-Octopamine; Octopaminum.
Октопамин

Clinical profile: Octopamine is a sympathomimetic with predominantly alpha-adrenergic activity. It has been given in the treatment of hypotensive states.

WADA Status: Banned in competition

WADA Class: Stimulants

Includes octopamine and any optical isomers.

WADA Class: Specified Substances

Also listed as a specified substance.

"The prohibited List may identify specified substances which are particularly susceptible to unintentional anti-doping rule violations because of their general availability in medicinal products or which are less likely to be successfully abused as doping agents."
A doping violation involving such substances may result in a reduced sanction provided that the "*...Athlete can establish that the Use of such a specfied substance was not intended to enhance sport performance...*"

Orciprenaline Sulfate

Other names: Metaproterenol Sulfate; Metaproterenol Sulphate; Orciprenalin sulfát; Orciprénaline, sulfate d'; Orciprenaline Sulphate; Orciprenalini sulfas; Orciprenalino sulfatas; Orciprenalinsulfat; Orciprenalin-szulfát; Orcyprenaliny siarczan; Orsiprenaliinisulfaatti; Orsiprenalin Sülfat; Sulfato de orciprenalina; Th-152.

Орципреналина Сульфат

Clinical profile: Orciprenaline sulfate is a direct-acting sympathomimetic with beta-adrenoceptor stimulant activity. It is used for its bronchodilator properties in the management of respiratory disorders such as asthma and chronic obstructive pulmonary disease.

WADA Status: Banned in and out of competition

WADA Class: Beta-2 Agonists
Includes beta-2 agonists or their isomers.

WADA Class: Specified Substances
Also listed as a specified substance.
"The prohibited List may identify specified substances which are particularly susceptible to unintentional anti-doping rule violations because of their general availability in medicinal products or which are less likely to be successfully abused as doping agents."
A doping violation involving such substances may result in a reduced sanction provided that the "*...Athlete can establish that the Use of such a specfied substance was not intended to enhance sport performance...*"

Preparations
Single ingredient: ***Austral.:*** Alupent; ***Austria:*** Alupent; ***Ger.:*** Alupent; ***Gr.:*** Alupent; ***India:*** Alupent; ***Indon.:*** Alupent; ***Irl.:*** Alupent; ***Ital.:*** Alupent; ***Jpn:*** Alotec; ***Mex.:*** Alupent; ***Pol.:*** Astmopent; ***Rus.:*** Astmopent (Астмопент); ***UK:*** Alupent; ***USA:*** Alupent.

Multi-ingredient: ***Chile:*** Broncodual Compuesto; Cloval Compuesto; Pulbronc; Solvanol; Tusabron; Vapoflu; ***Indon.:*** Silomat Compositum; ***Irl.:*** Alupent Expectorant; ***Mex.:*** Bisolpent Ex; ***Philipp.:*** Bisolpent; ***S.Afr.:*** Adco-Linctopent; Benylin Chesty; Bisolvon Linctus DA; Bronkese Compound; Flemeze; ***UAE:*** Orcinol.

Ormeloxifene

Other names: Centchroman; Orméloxifène; Ormeloxifeno; Ormeloxifenum.

Ормелоксифен

Clinical profile: Ormeloxifene is a nonsteroidal benzopyran derivative with anti-oestrogenic and antiprogestogenic actions that has been used as an oral contraceptive and investigated in the management of osteoporosis.

WADA Status: Banned in and out of competition

WADA Class: Hormone Antagonists and Modulators
Includes selective estrogen receptor modulators.

Preparations
Single ingredient: ***India:*** Centron.

Oxabolone Cipionate

Other names: Cipionato de oxabolona; FI-5852; Oxabolone, Cipionate d'; Oxabolone Cypionate; Oxaboloni Cipionas.

Оксаболона Ципионат

Clinical profile: Oxabolone cipionate has been used for its anabolic properties.

WADA Status: Banned in and out of competition

WADA Class: Anabolic; Androgenic Steroids (exogenous)
Includes exogenous anabolic androgenic steroids or other substances with a similar chemical structure or similar biological effect(s).

Oxandrolone

Other names: NSC-67068; Oxandrolona; Oxandrolonum; SC-11585.

Оксандролон

Clinical profile: Oxandrolone is an anabolic steroid that is used to promote weight gain in various catabolic states. It may also be given to promote growth in the treatment of constitutional delay of growth and puberty in boys and Turner's syndrome in girls.

WADA Status: Banned in and out of competition

WADA Class: Anabolic; Androgenic Steroids (exogenous)
Includes exogenous anabolic androgenic steroids or other substances with a similar chemical structure or similar biological effect(s).

Preparations
Single ingredient: ***Austral.:*** Oxandrin; ***Israel:*** Lonavar; ***Mex.:*** Xtendrol; ***USA:*** Oxandrin.

Oxedrine

Other names: Oksedriini; Oxedrin; Oxedrinum; Sinefrina; Sympaethaminum; Synephrine; *p*-Synephrine.

Oxedrine Hydrochloride

Other names: Sinefrina, hidrocloruro de.

Oxedrine Tartrate

Other names: Aetaphen. Tartrat.; Aethaphenum Tartaricum; Oksedriinitartraatti; Oxedrini Tartras; Oxedrintartrat; Oxyphenylmethylaminoethanol Tartrate; Sinefrina Tartrato; Sinefrina, tartrato de; Synephrine Tartrate.

Clinical profile: Oxedrine is a sympathomimetic used in hypotensive states. It has also been used as an ocular decongestant.

WADA Status: Banned in competition

WADA Class: Stimulants

Includes stimulants or substances with a similar chemical structure or similar biological effect(s).

WADA Class: Specified Substances

Also listed as a specified substance.

"The prohibited List may identify specified substances which are particularly susceptible to unintentional anti-doping rule violations because of their general availability in medicinal products or which are less likely to be successfully abused as doping agents."

A doping violation involving such substances may result in a reduced sanction provided that the "*...Athlete can establish that the Use of such a specfied substance was not intended to enhance sport performance...*"

Preparations
Single ingredient: ***Austria:*** Sympatol; ***Hong Kong:*** Ocuton; ***Hung.:*** Sympathomim; ***Ital.:*** Sympatol; ***Switz.:*** Sympalept.
Multi-ingredient: ***Austria:*** Dacrin; Pasuma-Dragees; ***Fr.:*** Dacryne; Dacryoboraline; Polyfra; Sedacollyre; Uvicol.

O

Oxilofrine Hydrochloride

Other names: Hidrocloruro de oxilofrina; *p*-Hydroxyephedrine Hydrochloride; Methylsynephrine Hydrochloride; Oxilofrine, Chlorhydrate d'; Oxilofrini Hydrochloridum; Oxyephedrine Hydrochloride.

Оксилофрина Гидрохлорид

Clinical profile: Oxilofrine is a sympathomimetic used in the treatment of hypotensive states. It has also been used in antitussive preparations.

WADA Status: Banned in competition

WADA Class: Stimulants

Includes oxilofrine and any optical isomers.

WADA Class: Specified Substances

Also listed as a specified substance.

"The prohibited List may identify specified substances which are particularly susceptible to unintentional anti-doping rule violations because of their general availability in medicinal products or which are less likely to be successfully abused as doping agents."

A doping violation involving such substances may result in a reduced sanction provided that the "*...Athlete can establish that the Use of such a specfied substance was not intended to enhance sport performance...*"

Preparations
Single ingredient: ***Austria:*** Carnigen; ***Ger.:*** Carnigen.
Multi-ingredient: ***Canad.:*** Cophylac.

Oxprenolol Hydrochloride

Other names: Ba-39089; Hidrocloruro de oxiprenolol; Hidrocloruro de oxprenolol; Oksprenolol Hidroklorür; Oksprenololihydrokloridi; Oksprenololio hidrochloridas; Oksprenololu chlorowodorek; Oxprénolol, chlorhydrate d'; Oxprenolol hydrochlorid; Oxprenolol-hidroklorid; Oxprenololhydroklorid; Oxprenololi hydrochloridum; Oxyprenolol Hydrochloride.

Окспренолола Гидрохлорид

Clinical profile: Oxprenolol is a non-cardioselective beta blocker used in the management of hypertension, angina pectoris, cardiac arrhythmias, and in anxiety.

WADA Status: Banned in and out of competition as specified below

WADA Class: Beta-Blockers

Unless otherwise specified, beta-blockers are prohibited *In-Competition* only in the following sports.

- Aeronautics (FAI)
- Archery (FITA, IPC) (also prohibited *Out-of-Competition*)
- Automobile (FIA)
- Billiards (WCBS)
- Bobsleigh (FIBT)
- Boules (CMSB, IPC bowls)
- Bridge (FMB)
- Curling (WCF)
- Gymnastics (FIG)
- Motorcycling (FIM)
- Modern Pentathlon (UIPM) for disciplines involving shooting
- Nine-pin bowling (FIQ)
- Powerboating (UIM)
- Sailing (ISAF) for match race helms only
- Shooting (ISSF, IPC) (also prohibited *Out-of-Competition*)
- Skiing/Snowboarding (FIS) in ski jumping, freestyle aerials/halfpipe and snowboard halfpipe/big air
- Wrestling (FILA)

WADA Class: Specified Substances

Also listed as a specified substance.

"The prohibited List may identify specified substances which are particularly susceptible to unintentional anti-doping rule violations because of their general availability in medicinal products or which are less likely to be successfully abused as doping agents."

A doping violation involving such substances may result in a reduced sanction provided that the "*...Athlete can establish that the Use of such a specfied substance was not intended to enhance sport performance...*"

Preparations

Single ingredient: ***Austral.:*** Corbeton; ***Austria:*** Trasicor; ***Canad.:*** Trasicor; ***Fr.:*** Trasicor; ***Ger.:*** Trasicor; ***Gr.:*** Trasicor; ***Neth.:*** Trasicor; ***Spain:*** Trasicor; ***Switz.:*** Slow-Trasicor; Trasicor; ***Turk.:*** Trasicor; ***UK:*** Slow-Trasicor; Trasicor.

Multi-ingredient: ***Austria:*** Trasitensin; Trepress; ***Fr.:*** Trasitensine; ***Ger.:*** Trepress; ***Gr.:*** Trasitensin; ***Ital.:*** Trasitensin; ***Spain:*** Trasitensin; ***Switz.:*** Slow-Trasitensine; ***UK:*** Trasidrex.

Oxycodone

Other names: Dihydrone; 14-Hydroxydihydrocodeinone; NSC-19043; Oksikodoni; Oxicodona; Oxikodon; Oxycodonum.
Оксикодон

Oxycodone Hydrochloride

Other names: 7,8-Dihydro-14-hydroxycodeinone hydrochloride; Dihydrone Hydrochloride; Hidrocloruro de oxicodona; Oksikodonihydrokloridi; Oksikodono hidrochloridas; Oxikodonhydroklorid; Oxycodone, chlorhydrate d'; Oxycodoni hydrochloridum; Oxycone Hydrochloride; Oxykodon-hydrochlorid; Thecodine.
Оксикодона Гидрохлорид

Oxycodone Terephthalate

Other names: Oxicodona, tereftalato de.

Clinical profile: Oxycodone, a phenanthrene derivative, is an opioid analgesic used for the relief of moderate to severe pain.

WADA Status: Banned in competition

WADA Class: Narcotics

Includes specified narcotics.

Preparations

Single ingredient: ***Arg.:*** Oxicalmans; Oxinovag; Oxycontin; ***Austral.:*** Endone; Oxycontin; Oxynorm; Proladone; ***Austria:*** Oxycontin; Oxynorm; ***Belg.:*** Oxycontin; ***Braz.:*** Oxycontin; ***Canad.:*** Oxy IR; Oxycontin; Supeudol; ***Chile:*** Oxycontin; ***Cz.:*** Oxycontin; ***Denm.:*** Oxycontin; Oxynorm; ***Fin.:*** Oxanest; Oxycontin; Oxynorm; ***Fr.:*** Oxycontin; Oxynorm; ***Ger.:*** Oxygesic; ***Hung.:*** Oxycontin; ***Irl.:*** Oxycontin; Oxynorm; ***Israel:*** Oxycod; Oxycontin; ***Ital.:*** Oxycontin; ***Jpn:*** Oxycontin; ***Neth.:*** Oxycontin; Oxynorm; ***Norw.:*** Oxycontin; Oxynorm; ***NZ:*** Oxycontin; Oxynorm; ***Philipp.:*** Oxycontin; ***Singapore:*** Oxycontin; Oxynorm; ***Spain:*** Oxycontin; Oxynorm; ***Swed.:*** Oxycontin; Oxynorm; ***Switz.:*** Oxycontin; Oxynorm; ***UK:*** Oxycontin; Oxynorm; ***USA:*** ETH-Oxydose; Oxycontin; Oxyfast; OxyIR; Roxicodone; ***Venez.:*** Oxycontin.

Multi-ingredient: ***Arg.:*** Oxinovag Complex; ***Canad.:*** Endocet; Endodan; Percocet; Percodan; ratio-Oxycocet; ratio-Oxycodan; ***Israel:*** Percocet; Percodan; ***Ital.:*** Depalgos; ***USA:*** Combunox; Endocet; Magnacet; Narvox; Percocet; Percodan; Perloxx; Roxicet; Roxilox; Roxiprin; Tylox.

O

Oxymetazoline Hydrochloride

Other names: H-990; Hidrocloruro de oximetazolina; Oksimetatsoliinihydrokloridi; Oksimetazolin Hidroklorür; Oksimetazolino hidrochloridas; Oximetazolin-hidroklorid; Oximetazolinhydroklorid; Oxymetazolin hydrochlorid; Oxymétazoline, chlorhydrate d'; Oxymetazolini hydrochloridum; Sch-9384.

Оксиметазолина Гидрохлорид

Clinical profile: Oxymetazoline is a direct-acting sympathomimetic used as a vasoconstrictor to relieve nasal and conjunctival congestion.

WADA Status: Banned in competition

WADA Class: Stimulants

Includes stimulants or substances with a similar chemical structure or similar biological effect(s). Oxymetazoline is an imidazole derivative. Imidazole derivatives for topical use are exempt.

Preparations

Single ingredient: ***Arg.:*** Apracur Nasal; Lidil; Newclar; Rinox VX; Visine D; Yusin; ***Austral.:*** Dimetapp 12 Hour Nasal; Drixine Nasal; Logicin Rapid Relief; Ordov Sinudec; ***Austria:*** Nasivin; ***Belg.:*** Nesivine; Rhino Humex; Vicks Sinex; ***Braz.:*** Afrin; Desfrin; Freenal; Nasivin; ***Canad.:*** Claritin Allergic Congestion Relief; Claritin Eye Allergy Relief; Decongestant Nasal Mist; Dristan; Drixoral; Long Lasting Nasal Mist; Vicks Sinex; Visine Workplace; ***Chile:*** Facimin; Iliadin; Oxilin; ***Cz.:*** Iversal; Nasivin; ***Denm.:*** Drixin; Iliadin; ***Fin.:*** Vicks Sinex; ***Fr.:*** Aturgyl; ***Ger.:*** Nasivin Sanft; Nasivin; Vistoxyn; Wick Sinex; ***Gr.:*** Narol; Ronal; ***Hong Kong:*** Afrin; Duration; Iliadin; Logicin Rapid Relief; Long Lasting Decongestant Nasal Mist; ***Hung.:*** Afrin; Nasivin; ***India:*** Naselin; Nasivion; Sinarest-PD; Sinarest; ***Indon.:*** Afrin; Iliadin; Visine LR; ***Israel:*** Af-Tipa; Alrin; Rhinoclir; Sinulen; ***Ital.:*** Actifed Nasale; Oxilin; Rino Calyptol; ***Jpn:*** Nasivin; ***Malaysia:*** Afrin; Iliadin; Oxynase; ***Mex.:*** Afrin; Iliadin; Naztril; Oxylin; Sinex; Visine AD; ***Neth.:*** Nasivin; Oxylin; Vicks Sinex; ***Norw.:*** Iliadin; Rhinox; ***NZ:*** At-Eze; Dimetapp 12 Hour Nasal; ***Philipp.:*** Drixine; Nasivin; ***Pol.:*** Acatar; Afrin; Nasivin; Nosox; Oxalin; Resoxym; ***Port.:*** Alerjon; Bisolspray; Nasex; Nasorhinathiol; Rinerge; ***Rus.:*** Nasivin (Називин); Nazol (Назол); Sanorinchik (Саноринчик); ***S.Afr.:*** Dristan; Drixine; Iliadin; Oxylin; Sparkling White Eye Drops; Vicks Decongestant; ***Singapore:*** Afrin; Iliadin; Nazolin; Oxy-Nase; Utabon; ***Spain:*** Alerfrin; Antirrinum; Corilisina; Couldespir; Ilvinax; Nasolina; Nebulicina; Oftinal; Respibien; Respir; Serranasal; Utabon; ***Swed.:*** Iliadin; Nasin; Nezeril; ***Switz.:*** Nasivine; ***Thai.:*** Iliadin; Oxymet; ***Turk.:*** Iliadin; Oksinazal; ***UAE:*** Nasivin; ***UK:*** Afrazine; Nasivin; Vicks Sinex; ***USA:*** 4-Way Long Lasting; Afrin; Allerest 12 Hour Nasal; Chlorphed-LA; Dristan 12-hr Nasal Decongestant Spray; Dristan Long Lasting; Duramist Plus; Duration; Genasal; Nasal Relief; Nasal Spray; Neo-Synephrine 12 Hour; Nostrilla; NTZ Long Acting Nasal; Twice-A-Day; Vicks Sinex 12-Hour; Visine LR; ***Venez.:*** Afrin; Airfen; Clarix; Drixine; Nasin.

Multi-ingredient: ***Arg.:*** Panoxi; ***Austral.:*** Nasex; Vasylox; Vicks Sinex; ***Austria:*** Wick Sinex; ***Fr.:*** Deturgylone; ***Hong Kong:*** Bonjedex; ***Hung.:*** Nasopax; ***Israel:*** Sinaf; ***Ital.:*** Triaminic; Vicks

Sinex; ***Mex.:*** Grimal; Hyalox; ***NZ:*** Vicks Sinex; ***Rus.:*** Nazol Advance (Назол Адванс); ***S.Afr.:*** Nazene Z; ***Spain:*** Seniospray; Vicks Spray; ***Switz.:*** Vicks Sinex.

Oxymetholone

Other names: CI-406; HMD; Oksimetolon; Oksimetoloni; Oximetolon; Oximetolona; Oxymétholone; Oxymetholonum.

Оксиметолон

Clinical profile: Oxymetholone is an anabolic steroid that has been used in the treatment of anaemias such as aplastic anaemia.

WADA Status: Banned in and out of competition

WADA Class: Anabolic; Androgenic Steroids (exogenous)

Includes exogenous anabolic androgenic steroids or other substances with a similar chemical structure or similar biological effect(s).

Preparations
Single ingredient: ***Braz.:*** Hemogenin; ***India:*** Adroyd; ***Thai.:*** Androlic; ***Turk.:*** Anapolon; ***USA:*** Anadrol.

Oxymorphone Hydrochloride

Other names: 7,8-Dihydro-14-hydroxymorphinone hydrochloride; Hidrocloruro de oximorfona; Oximorphone Hydrochloride; Oxymorphone, Chlorhydrate d'; Oxymorphoni Hydrochloridum.

Оксиморфона Гидрохлорид

Clinical profile: Oxymorphone hydrochloride, a phenanthrene derivative, is an opioid analgesic used in the treatment of moderate to severe pain. It is also used for premedication, as an adjunct to anaesthesia, and to relieve dyspnoea due to pulmonary oedema resulting from left ventricular failure.

WADA Status: Banned in competition

WADA Class: Narcotics

Includes specified narcotics.

Preparations
Single ingredient: ***USA:*** Numorphan; Opana.

Oxypolygelatin

Other names: Oxipoligelatina.

Clinical profile: Oxypolygelatin is a polymer derived from gelatin and is used as a plasma volume expander.

WADA Status: Banned in and out of competition

WADA Class: Diuretics and Other Masking Agents

Masking agents including alpha-reductase inhibitors or plasma expanders or substances with similar biological effect(s).

Preparations
Single ingredient: ***Austria:*** Gelifundol; ***Thai.:*** Gelifundol.

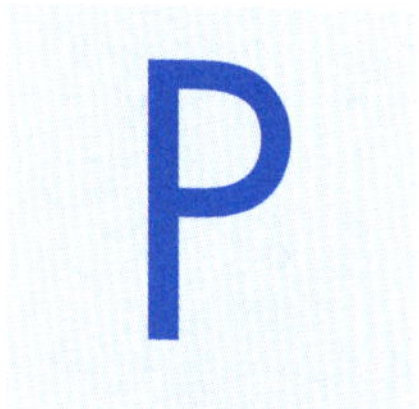

Pamabrom

Other names: Pamabromo.

Clinical profile: Pamabrom is a weak diuretic used for symptomatic relief of the premenstrual syndrome.

WADA Status: Banned in and out of competition

WADA Class: Diuretics and Other Masking Agents
Includes diuretics or substances with a similar chemical structure or similar biological effect(s).

Preparations
Single ingredient: ***USA:*** Maximum Strength Aqua-Ban.
Multi-ingredient: ***Arg.:*** Everfem; ***Canad.:*** Midol PMS Extra Strength; Painaid PMF; Pamprin; Relievol PMS; Tylenol Menstrual; ***Chile:*** Kitadol Periodo Menstrual; Minfaden; Predual; Tapsin Periodo Menstrual; ***Malaysia:*** Panadol Menstrual; ***Mex.:*** Femsedin Kutz; ***Singapore:*** Panadol Menstrual; ***USA:*** Lurline PMS; Midol Pre-Menstrual Syndrome; Midol Teen Formula; Painaid PMF Premenstrual Formula; Pamprin; Premsyn PMS; Womens Tylenol Multi-Symptom Menstrual Relief.

Paraflutizide

Other names: LD-3612; Parafluthiazide; Paraflutizida; Paraflutizidum.
Парафлутизид

Clinical profile: Paraflutizide is a thiazide diuretic that has been used in the treatment of hypertension.

WADA Status: Banned in and out of competition

WADA Class: Diuretics and Other Masking Agents
Includes diuretics or substances with a similar chemical structure or similar biological effect(s).

Paramethasone Acetate

Other names: Acetato de parametasona; 6α-Fluoro-16α-methylprednisolone 21-

Acetate; Parametazon Asetat; Paraméthasone, Acétate de; Paramethasoni Acetas.
Параметазона Ацетат

Clinical profile: Paramethasone acetate is a glucocorticoid corticosteroid that has been used systemically.

WADA Status: Banned in competition

WADA Class: Glucocorticosteroids

All glucocorticosteroids are prohibited when administered orally, rectally, intravenously or intramuscularly. Their use requires a Therapeutic Use Exemption approval. Other routes of administration (intraarticular / periarticular / peritendinous / epidural / intradermal injections and inhalation) require an Abbreviated Therapeutic Use Exemption except as noted below.

Topical preparations when used for dermatological (including iontophoresis / phonophoresis), auricular, nasal, ophthalmic, buccal, gingival and perianal disorders are not prohibited and do not require any form of Therapeutic Use Exemption.

WADA Class: Specified Substances

Also listed as a specified substance.

"The prohibited List may identify specified substances which are particularly susceptible to unintentional anti-doping rule violations because of their general availability in medicinal products or which are less likely to be successfully abused as doping agents."

A doping violation involving such substances may result in a reduced sanction provided that the "*...Athlete can establish that the Use of such a specfied substance was not intended to enhance sport performance...*"

Preparations
Single ingredient: ***Mex.:*** Dilar; ***Spain:*** Cortidene; ***Turk.:*** Depo-Dilar.
Multi-ingredient: ***Mex.:*** Dilarmine.

Pegzerepoetin Alfa

Other names: Methoxy Polyethylene Glycol-Epoetin Beta; Pegserepoetin Alfa; R-744; Ro-50-3821.

Clinical profile: Pegzerepoetin alfa is described as a continuous erythropoietin receptor activator, and has similar properties to the epoetins. It is used in the treatment of anaemia associated with chronic renal failure.

WADA Status: Banned in and out of competition

WADA Class: Hormones and Related Substances: Erythropoietin

Includes erythropoietin or a substance with a similar chemical structure or similar biological effect(s), or one of their releasing factors.

Preparations
Single ingredient: ***UK:*** Mircera.

Pemoline

Other names: LA-956; NSC-25159; Pemoliini; Pemolin; Pemolina; Pémoline; Pemolinum; Phenoxazole; Phenylisohydantoin; Phenylpseudohydantoin.
Пемолин

Clinical profile: Pemoline is a central stimulant that has been used in the management of hyperactivity disorders in children.

WADA Status: Banned in competition

WADA Class: Stimulants

Includes pemoline and any optical isomers.

Preparations
Single ingredient: ***Chile:*** Ceractiv; Cylert; ***Ger.:*** Tradon; ***Israel:*** Cylert; Nitan.
Multi-ingredient: ***UK:*** Prowess.

Penbutolol Sulfate

P

Other names: Hoe-39-893d; Hoe-893d; Levopenbutolol Sulfate; Penbutolol Hemisulfate; Penbutolol sulfát; Penbutolol, sulfate de; Penbutolol Sulphate; Penbutololi sulfas; Penbutololio sulfatas; Penbutololisulfaatti; Penbutololsulfat; Penbutololszulfát; Sulfato de penbutolol.

Пенбутолола Сульфат

Clinical profile: Penbutolol is a non-cardioselective beta blocker used in the management of hypertension and angina.

WADA Status: Banned in and out of competition as specified below

WADA Class: Beta-Blockers

Unless otherwise specified, beta-blockers are prohibited *In-Competition* only in the following sports.

- Aeronautics (FAI)
- Archery (FITA, IPC) (also prohibited *Out-of-Competition*)
- Automobile (FIA)
- Billiards (WCBS)
- Bobsleigh (FIBT)
- Boules (CMSB, IPC bowls)
- Bridge (FMB)
- Curling (WCF)
- Gymnastics (FIG)
- Motorcycling (FIM)
- Modern Pentathlon (UIPM) for disciplines involving shooting
- Nine-pin bowling (FIQ)
- Powerboating (UIM)
- Sailing (ISAF) for match race helms only
- Shooting (ISSF, IPC) (also prohibited *Out-of-Competition*)
- Skiing/Snowboarding (FIS) in ski jumping, freestyle aerials/halfpipe and snowboard halfpipe/big air
- Wrestling (FILA)

WADA Class: Specified Substances

Also listed as a specified substance.

"*The prohibited List may identify specified substances which are particularly susceptible to unintentional anti-doping rule violations because of their general availability in medicinal products or which are less likely to be successfully abused as doping agents.*"

A doping violation involving such substances may result in a reduced sanction provided that the "...*Athlete can establish that the Use of such a specfied substance was not intended to enhance sport performance*..."

Preparations
Single ingredient: ***Ger.:*** Betapressin; ***USA:*** Levatol.
Multi-ingredient: ***Ger.:*** Betarelix; Betasemid.

Penflutizide

Other names: Penflutizida; Penflutizidum; Penfluzide; Pentylhydroflumethiazide.

Пенфлутизид

Clinical profile: Penflutizide is a thiazide diuretic that has been used in the treatment of oedema.

WADA Status: Banned in and out of competition

WADA Class: Diuretics and Other Masking Agents

Includes diuretics or substances with a similar chemical structure or similar biological effect(s).

P

Pentazocine

Other names: NIH-7958; NSC-107430; Pentatsosiini; Pentazocin; Pentazocina; Pentazocinas; Pentazocinum; Win-20228.

Пентазоцин

Pentazocine Hydrochloride

Other names: Hidrocloruro de pentazocina; Pentatsosiinihydrokloridi; Pentazocine, chlorhydrate de; Pentazocin-hidroklorid; Pentazocin-hydrochlorid; Pentazocin-hydroklorid; Pentazocini hydrochloridum; Pentazocino hidrochloridas.

Пентазоцина Гидрохлорид

Pentazocine Lactate

Other names: Lactato de pentazocina; Pentatsosiinilaktaatti; Pentazocine, lactate de; Pentazocini lactas; Pentazocinlaktat; Pentazocin-laktát; Pentazocino laktatas.

Пентазоцина Лактат

Clinical profile: Pentazocine, a benzomorphan derivative, is an opioid analgesic with mixed opioid agonist and antagonist actions used for the relief of moderate to severe pain, for pre-operative sedation, and as an adjunct to anaesthesia.

WADA Status: Banned in competition

WADA Class: Narcotics

Includes specified narcotics.

Preparations

Single ingredient: ***Austral.:*** Fortral; ***Austria:*** Fortral; ***Belg.:*** Fortal; ***Canad.:*** Talwin; ***Cz.:*** Fortral; ***Ger.:*** Fortral; ***Gr.:*** Fortal; ***India:*** Fortwin; Pentawin; ***Ital.:*** Talwin; ***Neth.:*** Fortral; ***Port.:*** Sosegon; ***S.Afr.:*** Ospronim; Sosenol; ***Spain:*** Sosegon; ***Thai.:*** Pangon; ***UK:*** Fortral; ***USA:*** Talwin NX; Talwin.

Multi-ingredient: ***India:*** Expergesic; Foracet; ***USA:*** Emergent-Ez; Talacen; Talwin Compound.

Pentetrazol

Other names: Corazol; Leptazol; Pentamethazol; 1,5-Pentamethylenetetrazole; Pentazol; Pentetratsoli; Pentétrazol, Pentetrazolum; Pentylenetetrazol.

Пентетразол

Clinical profile: Pentetrazol is a central and respiratory stimulant that has been used in respiratory depression. It has also been included in multi-ingredient preparations intended for the treatment of respiratory-tract disorders including cough, cardiovascular disorders including hypotension, and for the treatment of pruritus.

WADA Status: Banned in competition

WADA Class: Stimulants

Includes pentetrazol and any optical isomers.

Preparations
Multi-ingredient: ***Braz.:*** Belacodid; Belacodid; Revulsan; ***Ital.:*** Cardiazol-Paracodina; ***Port.:*** Broncodiazina.

Perflubron

Other names: Perflubrón; Perflubronum; Perfluorooctylbromide; PFOB.

Перфлуброн

Clinical profile: Perflubron is a perfluorocarbon tried as an alternative to red blood cell preparations to improve gaseous transport, in particular oxygen supply, to the tissues. It may also be instilled directly to the lungs for use in partial liquid ventilation as an adjunct to mechanical ventilation in patients with respiratory failure. Perflubron is being studied as an intravenous contrast medium in computed tomography and ultrasound. It has also been given by mouth to enhance delineation of the bowel during magnetic resonance imaging. Other perfluorocarbons have also been used to prevent myocardial ischaemia during percutaneous transluminal coronary angioplasty, and used in eye surgery.

WADA Status: Banned in and out of competition

WADA Class: Enhancement of Oxygen Transfer: Artificial Enhancers

Includes products that may be used to artificially enhance the uptake, transport, or delivery of oxygen.

Preparations
Single ingredient: ***USA:*** Imagent GI; LiquiVent.

Perflunafene

Other names: Perflunafène; Perflunafeno; Perflunafenum; Perfluorodecahydronaphthalene; Perfluorodecalin; Perfluorodekalin.

Перфлунафен

Clinical profile: Intra-ocular injection of perflunafene is used to provide temporary tamponade in ophthalmic procedures such as retinal re-attachment. Perflunafene and perfluamine have been used together for their oxygen-carrying properties in blood substitute preparations and to prevent myocardial ischaemia during percutaneous transluminal coronary angioplasty.

WADA Status: Banned in and out of competition

WADA Class: Enhancement of Oxygen Transfer: Artificial Enhancers

Includes products that may be used to artificially enhance the uptake, transport, or delivery of oxygen.

Preparations
Single ingredient: ***Neth.:*** Eftiar Decalin; ***Turk.:*** DK-Line.

Pethidine Hydrochloride

Other names: Hidrocloruro de petidina; Meperidine Hydrochloride; Péthidine, chlorhydrate de; Pethidin-hydrochlorid; Pethidini hydrochloridum; Petidiinihydrokloridi; Petidin Hidroklorür; Petidin-hidroklorid; Petidinhydroklorid; Petidino hidrochloridas; Petydyny chlorowodorek.

Петидина Гидрохлорид

Clinical profile: Pethidine hydrochloride, a phenylpiperidine derivative, is an opioid analgesic that acts mainly as a μ opioid agonist. It is used for the relief of most types of moderate to severe acute pain including the pain of labour and that associated with biliary colic and pancreatitis. It is not suitable for the management of chronic pain. It is also used as pre-operative medication and as an adjunct to anaesthesia.

WADA Status: Banned in competition

WADA Class: Narcotics

Includes specified narcotics.

Preparations
Single ingredient: ***Arg.:*** Cluyer; Meperol; ***Austria:*** Alodan; ***Belg.:*** Dolantine; ***Braz.:*** Dolantina; Dolosal; ***Canad.:*** Demerol; ***Cz.:*** Dolsin; ***Ger.:*** Dolantin; ***Hung.:*** Dolargan; ***Israel:*** Dolestine; ***Philipp.:*** Demerol; ***Pol.:*** Dolargan; Dolcontral; ***Spain:*** Dolantina; ***Turk.:*** Aldolan; ***USA:*** Demerol.
Multi-ingredient: ***UK:*** Pamergan P100.

P

Phendimetrazine Tartrate

Other names: Phendimetrazine Acid Tartrate; Phendimetrazine Bitartrate; Phendimétrazine, Tartrate de; Phendimetrazini Tartras; Tartrato de fendimetrazina.

Фендиметразина Тартрат

Clinical profile: Phendimetrazine is a central stimulant and indirect-acting sympathomimetic that has been used as an anorectic in the short-term treatment of obesity.

WADA Status: Banned in competition

WADA Class: Stimulants

Includes phendimetrazine and any optical isomers.

Preparations
Single ingredient: ***S.Afr.:*** Obesan-X; Obex-LA; ***USA:*** Bontril; Melfiat; Prelu-2.

Phenmetrazine Hydrochloride

Other names: Hidrocloruro de fenmetrazina; Oxazimédrine; Phenmétrazine, Chlorhydrate de; Phenmetrazini Hydrochloridum.

Фенметразина Гидрохлорид

Clinical profile: Phenmetrazine hydrochloride is a central stimulant and indirect-acting sympathomimetic that has been used as an anorectic in the treatment of obesity.

WADA Status: Banned in competition

WADA Class: Stimulants

Includes phenmetrazine and any optical isomers.

Phentermine

Other names: Fentermiini; Fentermin; Fentermina; Phenterminum.

Фентермин

Phentermine Hydrochloride

Other names: Hidrocloruro de fentermina; Phentermine, Chlorhydrate de; Phentermini Hydrochloridum.

Фентермина Гидрохлорид

Clinical profile: Phentermine is a central stimulant and indirect-acting sympathomimetic used as an anorectic in the treatment of obesity.

WADA Status: Banned in competition

WADA Class: Stimulants

Includes phentermine and any optical isomers.

Preparations
Single ingredient: ***Austral.:*** Duromine; ***Canad.:*** Ionamin; ***Cz.:*** Adipex; ***Hong Kong:*** Duromine; Panbesy; Redusa; ***Israel:*** Razin; ***Malaysia:*** Adipex; Duromine; Ionamin; ***Mex.:*** Acxion; Ifa Acxion; Ifa Reduccing; Sinpet; Terfamex; ***NZ:*** Duromine; ***Philipp.:*** Duromine; ***S.Afr.:*** Duromine, ***Singapore:*** Duromine; Panbesy; ***Switz.:*** Adipex; ***Thai.:*** Panbesy; ***USA:*** Adipex-P; Ionamin; ***Venez.:*** Mirubal.

4-Phenylpiracetam

Other names: BRN-5030440; Carphedon; Karfedon.

Clinical profile: 4-Phenylpiracetam is a nootropic that has been abused in sport.

WADA Status: Banned in competition

WADA Class: Stimulants

Includes 4-phenylpiracetam and any optical isomers.

Preparations
Single ingredient: ***Rus.:*** Phenotropil (Фенотропил).

Pholedrine Sulfate

Other names: Isodrine Sulphate; Pholédrine, Sulfate de; Pholedrine Sulphate; Pholedrini Sulfas; Sulfato de foledrina; Sympropaminum (pholedrine).

Фоледрина Сульфат

Clinical profile: Pholedrine sulfate is a sympathomimetic used in the treatment of hypotensive states. It has also been used in preparations promoted for vascular disorders.

WADA Status: Banned in competition

WADA Class: Stimulants

Includes stimulants or substances with a similar chemical structure or similar biological effect(s).

WADA Class: Specified Substances

Also listed as a specified substance.

"The prohibited List may identify specified substances which are particularly susceptible to unintentional anti-doping rule violations because of their general availability in medicinal products or which are less likely to be successfully abused as doping agents."

A doping violation involving such substances may result in a reduced sanction provided that the *"...Athlete can establish that the Use of such a specfied substance was not intended to enhance sport performance..."*

Preparations
Multi-ingredient: ***Switz.:*** Ortho-Maren retard.

Pindolol

Other names: LB-46; Pindololi; Pindololis; Pindololum; Prindolol; Prinodolol.

Пиндолол

Clinical profile: Pindolol is a non-cardioselective beta blocker used in the management of hypertension, angina pectoris, and other cardiovascular disorders. It is also used in glaucoma.

WADA Status: Banned in and out of competition as specified below

WADA Class: Beta-Blockers

Unless otherwise specified, beta-blockers are prohibited *In-Competition* only in the following sports.

- Aeronautics (FAI)
- Archery (FITA, IPC) (also prohibited *Out-of-Competition*)
- Automobile (FIA)
- Billiards (WCBS)
- Bobsleigh (FIBT)
- Boules (CMSB, IPC bowls)
- Bridge (FMB)
- Curling (WCF)
- Gymnastics (FIG)
- Motorcycling (FIM)
- Modern Pentathlon (UIPM) for disciplines involving shooting
- Nine-pin bowling (FIQ)
- Powerboating (UIM)
- Sailing (ISAF) for match race helms only
- Shooting (ISSF, IPC) (also prohibited *Out-of-Competition*)
- Skiing/Snowboarding (FIS) in ski jumping, freestyle aerials/halfpipe and snowboard halfpipe/big air
- Wrestling (FILA)

WADA Class: Specified Substances

Also listed as a specified substance.
"The prohibited List may identify specified substances which are particularly susceptible to unintentional anti-doping rule violations because of their general availability in medicinal products or which are less likely to be successfully abused as doping agents."
A doping violation involving such substances may result in a reduced sanction provided that the "*...Athlete can establish that the Use of such a specfied substance was not intended to enhance sport performance...*"

Preparations
Single ingredient: ***Austral.:*** Barbloc; Visken; ***Austria:*** Visken; ***Belg.:*** Visken; ***Braz.:*** Visken; ***Canad.:*** Apo-Pindol; Novo-Pindol; Nu-Pindol; Visken; ***Cz.:*** Apo-Pindol; Visken; ***Denm.:*** Hexapindol; Visken; ***Fin.:*** Pindocor; Pinloc; Visken; ***Fr.:*** Visken; ***Ger.:*** Glauco-Stulln; Visken; ***Gr.:*** Visken; ***Hong Kong:*** Visken; ***Hung.:*** Visken; ***India:*** Visken; ***Irl.:*** Visken; ***Israel:*** Pinden; ***Ital.:*** Visken; ***Mex.:*** Visken; ***Neth.:*** Visken; ***NZ:*** Pindol; ***Philipp.:*** Pyndale; Visken; ***Pol.:*** Visken; ***Rus.:*** Visken (Вискен); ***Swed.:*** Visken; ***Switz.:*** Viskene; ***Turk.:*** Visken; ***UK:*** Visken; ***USA:*** Visken.

Multi-ingredient: ***Austria:*** Viskenit; ***Belg.:*** Viskaldix; ***Braz.:*** Viskaldix; ***Canad.:*** Viskazide; ***Chile:*** Viskaldix; ***Fr.:*** Viskaldix; ***Ger.:*** Viskaldix; ***Gr.:*** Viskaldix; ***Hung.:*** Viskaldix; ***Irl.:*** Viskaldix;

Malaysia: Viskaldix; ***Neth.:*** Viskaldix; ***Philipp.:*** Viskaldix; ***Rus.:*** Viskaldix (Вискалдикс); ***Switz.:*** Viskaldix; ***UK:*** Viskaldix.

Pirbuterol

Other names: Pirbuterol; Pirbutérol; Pirbuteroli; Pirbuterolum; Pyrbuterol.

Пирбутерол

P

Pirbuterol Acetate

Other names: Acetato de pirbuterol; CP-24314-14; Pirbutérol, Acétate de; Pirbuteroli Acetas; Pyrbuterol Acetate.

Пирбутерола Ацетат

Pirbuterol Hydrochloride

Other names: CP-24314-1; Hidrocloruro de pirbuterol; Pirbutérol, Chlorhydrate de; Pirbuteroli Hydrochloridum; Pyrbuterol Hydrochloride.

Пирбутерола Гидрохлорид

Clinical profile: Pirbuterol is a direct-acting sympathomimetic with a selective action on beta$_2$ adrenoceptors. It is used as a bronchodilator in the management of respiratory disorders such as asthma and chronic obstructive pulmonary disease.

WADA Status: Banned in and out of competition

WADA Class: Beta-2 Agonists

Includes beta-2 agonists or their isomers.

WADA Class: Specified Substances

Also listed as a specified substance.

"The prohibited List may identify specified substances which are particularly susceptible to unintentional anti-doping rule violations because of their general availability in medicinal products or which are less likely to be successfully abused as doping agents."

A doping violation involving such substances may result in a reduced sanction provided that the "*...Athlete can establish that the Use of such a specfied substance was not intended to enhance sport performance...*"

Preparations
Single ingredient: ***Fr.:*** Maxair; ***USA:*** Maxair.

Piretanide

Other names: Hoe-118; Piretanid; Piretanida; Piretanidas; Pirétanide; Piretanidi; Piretanidum; S73-4118.

Пиретанид

Clinical profile: Piretanide is a loop diuretic used in the treatment of oedema and hypertension.

WADA Status: Banned in and out of competition

WADA Class: Diuretics and Other Masking Agents

Includes diuretics or substances with a similar chemical structure or similar biological effect(s).

Preparations
Single ingredient: ***Austria:*** Arelix; ***Braz.:*** Arelix; ***Fr.:*** Eurelix; ***Ger.:*** Arelix; ***Irl.:*** Arelix; ***Ital.:*** Tauliz; ***Mex.:*** Diural; ***S.Afr.:*** Arelix; ***Spain:*** Perbilen; ***Switz.:*** Arelix.
Multi-ingredient: ***Austria:*** Trialix; ***Ger.:*** Arelix ACE; Aretensin; Betarelix; ***Irl.:*** Trialix; ***Ital.:*** Prilace; ***Switz.:*** Trialix.

Plasma Protein Fraction

Other names: Fracción proteica del plasma.

P

Clinical profile: Plasma protein fraction consists mainly of albumin with a small proportion of globulins. It is used for plasma volume replacement and to restore colloid osmotic pressure in acute hypovolaemic shock, burns, and severe albumin loss.

WADA Status: Banned in and out of competition

WADA Class: Diuretics and Other Masking Agents

Masking agents including alpha-reductase inhibitors or plasma expanders or substances with similar biological effect(s).

Preparations
Single ingredient: ***Austria:*** Biseko; ***Ger.:*** Biseko; ***Gr.:*** Alburex; ***Hung.:*** Biseko; ***Indon.:*** Plasmanate; ***Israel:*** Plasmanate; ***Ital.:*** PPS; Uman-Serum; ***Philipp.:*** Plasmanate; ***S.Afr.:*** Bioplasma FDP; ***Thai.:*** Biseko; ***USA:*** Plasma-Plex; Plasmanate; Protenate.
Multi-ingredient: ***Fin.:*** Tisseel Duo Quick; ***Ger.:*** Tissucol Duo S; Tissucol-Kit; ***Hung.:*** Tissucol-Kit; ***Ital.:*** Tissucol; ***Swed.:*** Tisseel Duo Quick; ***Switz.:*** Tissucol Duo S.

Polygeline

Other names: Poligelina; Polygéline; Polygelinum.

Полигелин

Clinical profile: Polygeline is a polymer prepared by cross-linking polypeptides derived from denatured gelatin and is used as a plasma volume expander. It is also used in patients undergoing extracorporeal circulation, as a perfusion fluid for isolated organs, as fluid replacement in plasma exchange, and as a carrier solution for insulin.

WADA Status: Banned in and out of competition

WADA Class: Diuretics and Other Masking Agents

Masking agents including alpha-reductase inhibitors or plasma expanders or substances with similar biological effect(s).

Preparations
Single ingredient: ***Austral.:*** Haemaccel; ***Austria:*** Haemaccel; ***Braz.:*** Haemaccel; ***Cz.:*** Haemaccel; ***Ger.:*** Haemaccel; ***India:*** Haemaccel; ***Indon.:*** Haemaccel; ***Ital.:*** Emagel; Gelplex; ***Mex.:*** Haemaccel; Phygelin; ***Neth.:*** Haemaccel; ***NZ:*** Haemaccel; ***S.Afr.:*** Haemaccel; ***Singapore:*** Haemaccel; ***Thai.:*** Haemaccel; Plasmax; ***UK:*** Haemaccel.

Polythiazide

Other names: NSC-108161; P-2525; Politiazida; Polythiazidum; Polytiatsidi; Polytiazid.

Политиазид

Clinical profile: Polythiazide is a thiazide diuretic used for hypertension, and for oedema, including that associated with heart failure.

WADA Status: Banned in and out of competition

WADA Class: Diuretics and Other Masking Agents

Includes diuretics or substances with a similar chemical structure or similar biological effect(s).

Potassium Canrenoate

P

Other names: Aldadiene Potassium; Canrénoate de Potassium; Canrenoate Potassium; Canrenoato de potasio; Kalii Canrenoas; Kaliumkanrenoaatti; Kaliumkanrenoat; MF-465a; SC-14266.

Калия Канреноат

Clinical profile: Potassium canrenoate is a potassium-sparing diuretic and aldosterone antagonist used in oedema.

WADA Status: Banned in and out of competition

WADA Class: Diuretics and Other Masking Agents

Includes diuretics or substances with a similar chemical structure or similar biological effect(s).

Preparations

Single ingredient: ***Austria:*** Aldactone; ***Belg.:*** Canrenol; Soldactone; ***Cz.:*** Aldactone; Canrenol; ***Fr.:*** Soludactone; ***Ger.:*** Aldactone; Kalium-Can; ***Ital.:*** Dikantal; Diurek; Kanrenol; Luvion; ***Neth.:*** Soldactone; ***Pol.:*** Aldactone; ***Switz.:*** Soldactone.

Multi-ingredient: ***Ital.:*** Kadiur.

Potassium Nitrate

Other names: Dusičnan draselný; E252; Kalii nitras; Kalio nitratas; Kalium Nitricum; Kaliumnitraatti; Kaliumnitrat; Kálium-nitrát; Nitrato potásico; Nitre; Potassium, nitrate de; Potasu azotan; Saltpetre.

Clinical profile: Potassium nitrate is used as a preservative in foods. It was formerly used as a diuretic.

WADA Status: Banned in and out of competition

WADA Class: Diuretics and Other Masking Agents

Includes diuretics or substances with a similar chemical structure or similar biological effect(s).

Preparations

Single ingredient: ***Chile:*** Crowne; ***USA:*** Denquel; Original Sensodyne.

Multi-ingredient: ***Arg.:*** Esmedent Dientes Sens Blanq + Ctrol Sarro; Esmedent Dientes Sensibles; Fluorogel 2001 para Dientes Sensibles; Hyper Sensitive; Sebulex; Sensigel; Sensodyne Antisarro; Sensodyne Bicarbonato de Sodio; Sensodyne Proteccion Total; Sensodyne-F; ***Austral.:*** Oral-B Sensitive; ***Braz.:*** Malvatricin Dentes Sensiveis; Pilulas De Witt's; Sensodyne Antitartaro; Sensodyne C/Bicarbonato de Sodio; Sensodyne Cool; Sensodyne Fresh Mint; Sensodyne Protecao Total; Sensodyne-F; ***Canad.:*** Sensodyne-F; ***Chile:*** Sensaid; ***Fr.:*** Emoform Dents Sensibles; Emoform Gencives; Fluocaril dents sensibles; Sensigel; ***Ital.:*** Dentosan Sensibile; Fluocaril; Oral-B Sensitive; ***Mex.:*** Dentsiblen; Dentsiblen; ***Port.:*** Biofluor Sensitive; ***Rus.:*** Sensigel (Сенсигель);

Singapore: Sensigel; ***Turk.:*** Sensodyne-F Gel; ***UK:*** Avoca; ***USA:*** Sensitivity Protection Crest; Sensodyne-F; ***Venez.:*** Sensodyne.

Practolol

Other names: AY-21011; ICI-50172; Practololum; Praktolol; Praktololi.

Практолол

Clinical profile: Practolol is a cardioselective beta blocker. It is no longer used clinically due to serious adverse effects, in particular the potentially fatal oculomucocutaneous syndrome comprising serious adverse effects on the skin, eyes, and mucous membranes, deafness, systemic lupus erythematosus, and sclerosing peritonitis.

WADA Status: Banned in and out of competition as specified below

WADA Class: Beta-Blockers

Unless otherwise specified, beta-blockers are prohibited *In-Competition* only in the following sports.

- Aeronautics (FAI)
- Archery (FITA, IPC) (also prohibited *Out-of-Competition*)
- Automobile (FIA)
- Billiards (WCBS)
- Bobsleigh (FIBT)
- Boules (CMSB, IPC bowls)
- Bridge (FMB)
- Curling (WCF)
- Gymnastics (FIG)
- Motorcycling (FIM)
- Modern Pentathlon (UIPM) for disciplines involving shooting
- Nine-pin bowling (FIQ)
- Powerboating (UIM)
- Sailing (ISAF) for match race helms only
- Shooting (ISSF, IPC) (also prohibited *Out-of-Competition*)
- Skiing/Snowboarding (FIS) in ski jumping, freestyle aerials/halfpipe and snowboard halfpipe/big air
- Wrestling (FILA)

WADA Class: Specified Substances

Also listed as a specified substance.

"The prohibited List may identify specified substances which are particularly susceptible to unintentional anti-doping rule violations because of their general availability in medicinal products or which are less likely to be successfully abused as doping agents."

A doping violation involving such substances may result in a reduced sanction provided that the "*...Athlete can establish that the Use of such a specfied substance was not intended to enhance sport performance...*"

Pralmorelin Dihydrochloride

Other names: Dihidrocloruro de pralmorelina; GHRP-2 (pralmorelin); Growth Hormone-releasing Peptide-2 (pralmorelin); KP-102 (pralmorelin); Pralmoréline, Dichlorhydrate de; Pralmorelini Dihydrochloridum; WAY-GPA-748.

Пральморелина Дигидрохлорид

Clinical profile: Pralmorelin is a small synthetic peptide that stimulates the release of growth hormone. It is under investigation in the diagnosis of growth hormone deficiency and for the treatment of growth retardation.

WADA Status: Banned in and out of competition

WADA Class: Hormones and Related Substances: Growth Hormone, Insulin-like Growth Factors, Mechano Growth Factors
Includes growth hormone or insulin-like growth factors or mechano growth factor or substances with a similar chemical structure or similar biological effect(s), or one of their releasing factors.

Prasterone

Other names: Dehydroandrosterone; Dehydroepiandrosteron; Dehydroepiandrosterone; Dehydroepiandrosteroni; Dehydroepiandrosteronum; Dehydroisoandrosterone; DHEA; GL-701; Prasterona; Prastérone; Prasteronum.

Прастерон

Prasterone Enantate

Other names: Dehydroepiandrosterone Enanthate; EDHEA; Enantato de prasterona; Prastérone, Enantate de; Prasterone Enanthate; Prasteroni Enantas.

Прастерона Энантат

Prasterone Sodium Sulfate

Other names: Dehydroepiandrosterone Sulphate Sodium; DHA-S (prasterone sulfate); DHEAS (prasterone sulfate); PB-005; Prasterone Sodium Sulphate; Prastérone, Sulfate Sodique de; Prasteroni Natrii Sulfas; Sulfato sódico de prasterona.

Прастерона Натрия Сульфат

Clinical profile: Prasterone is a naturally occurring but relatively weak androgen that is under investigation for a variety of disorders including adrenal insufficiency and SLE. The enantate is used in menopausal disorders and the sodium sulfate has been investigated for burns and acute asthma.

WADA Status: Banned in and out of competition

WADA Class: Anabolic; Androgenic Steroids (endogenous)
Includes endogenous anabolic androgenic steroids or specified metabolites or isomers.

Preparations
Single ingredient: ***Mex.:*** Biolaif; ***Pol.:*** Biosteron; ***Port.:*** Dinistenile.
Multi-ingredient: ***Arg.:*** Dastonil; Gynodian Depot; Supligol NF; ***Austria:*** Gynodian Depot; ***Chile:*** Gynodian Depot; ***Cz.:*** Gynodian Depot; ***Ger.:*** Gynodian Depot; ***Ital.:*** Gynodian Depot; ***Mex.:*** Binodian; Sten; ***Pol.:*** Gynodian Depot; ***Rus.:*** Gynodian Depot (Гинодиан Депо); ***Switz.:*** Gynodian Depot; ***Venez.:*** Gynodian Depot.

Prednazoline

Other names: Prednazolina; Prednazolinum; Prednisolone-Fenoxazoline Compound.

Предназолин

Clinical profile: Prednazoline is a compound of the corticosteroid prednisolone with the sympathomimetic fenoxazoline and has been used locally in the treatment of pharyngitis, rhinitis, and sinusitis.

WADA Status: Banned in competition

WADA Class: Glucocorticosteroids

All glucocorticosteroids are prohibited when administered orally, rectally, intravenously or intramuscularly. Their use requires a Therapeutic Use Exemption approval. Other routes of administration (intraarticular / periarticular / peritendinous / epidural / intradermal injections and inhalation) require an Abbreviated Therapeutic Use Exemption except as noted below.

Topical preparations when used for dermatological (including iontophoresis / phonophoresis), auricular, nasal, ophthalmic, buccal, gingival and perianal disorders are not prohibited and do not require any form of Therapeutic Use Exemption.

WADA Class: Specified Substances

Also listed as a specified substance.

"The prohibited List may identify specified substances which are particularly susceptible to unintentional anti-doping rule violations because of their general availability in medicinal products or which are less likely to be successfully abused as doping agents."

A doping violation involving such substances may result in a reduced sanction provided that the "*...Athlete can establish that the Use of such a specfied substance was not intended to enhance sport performance...*"

Prednicarbate

Other names: Hoe-777; Prednicarbato; Prednicarbatum; Prednikarbaatti; Prednikarbát; Prednikarbat; Prednikarbatas; S-77-0777.

Предникарбат

Clinical profile: Prednicarbate is a corticosteroid used topically in the treatment of various skin disorders.

WADA Status: Banned in competition

WADA Class: Glucocorticosteroids

All glucocorticosteroids are prohibited when administered orally, rectally, intravenously or intramuscularly. Their use requires a Therapeutic Use Exemption approval. Other routes of administration (intraarticular / periarticular / peritendinous / epidural / intradermal injections and inhalation) require an Abbreviated Therapeutic Use Exemption except as noted below.

Topical preparations when used for dermatological (including iontophoresis / phonophoresis), auricular, nasal, ophthalmic, buccal, gingival and perianal disorders are not prohibited and do not require any form of Therapeutic Use Exemption.

WADA Class: Specified Substances

Also listed as a specified substance.

"The prohibited List may identify specified substances which are particularly susceptible to unintentional anti-doping rule violations because of their general availability in medicinal products or which are less likely to be successfully abused as doping agents."

A doping violation involving such substances may result in a reduced sanction provided that the "*.. Athlete can establish that the Use of such a specfied substance was not intended to enhance sport performance...*"

Preparations

Single ingredient: ***Austria:*** Prednitop; ***Braz.:*** Dermatop; Invex; ***Canad.:*** Dermatop; ***Chile:*** Dermatop; ***Cz.:*** Dermatop; ***Ger.:*** Dermatop; Prednitop; ***Indon.:*** Dermatop; ***Ital.:*** Dermatop;

Mex.: Alisyd; ***Spain:*** Batmen; Peitel; ***Switz.:*** Prednitop; ***Thai.:*** Dermatop; ***Turk.:*** Dermatop; ***USA:*** Dermatop.

Prednisolamate Hydrochloride

Other names: Hidrocloruro de prednisolamato; Prednisolamate, Chlorhydrate de; Prednisolamati Hydrochloridum; Prednisolone 21-Diethylaminoacetate Hydrochloride.

Преднизоламата Гидрохлорид

Clinical profile: Prednisolamate hydrochloride is a water-soluble form of the corticosteroid prednisolone.

WADA Status: Banned in competition

WADA Class: Glucocorticosteroids

All glucocorticosteroids are prohibited when administered orally, rectally, intravenously or intramuscularly. Their use requires a Therapeutic Use Exemption approval. Other routes of administration (intraarticular / periarticular / peritendinous / epidural / intradermal injections and inhalation) require an Abbreviated Therapeutic Use Exemption except as noted below.

Topical preparations when used for dermatological (including iontophoresis / phonophoresis), auricular, nasal, ophthalmic, buccal, gingival and perianal disorders are not prohibited and do not require any form of Therapeutic Use Exemption.

WADA Class: Specified Substances

Also listed as a specified substance.

"*The prohibited List may identify specified substances which are particularly susceptible to unintentional anti-doping rule violations because of their general availability in medicinal products or which are less likely to be successfully abused as doping agents.*"

A doping violation involving such substances may result in a reduced sanction provided that the "*...Athlete can establish that the Use of such a specfied substance was not intended to enhance sport performance...*"

Prednisolone

Other names: 1,2-Dehydrohydrocortisone; Deltahydrocortisone; Δ^1-Hydrocortisone; Metacortandralone; NSC-9120; Prednisolon; Prednisolona; Prednisoloni; Prednisolonum; Prednizolon; Prednizolonas.

Преднизолон

Prednisolone Acetate

Other names: Acetato de prednisolona; Prednisolonacetat; Prednisolon-acetát; Prednisolone, acétate de; Prednisoloni acetas; Prednisoloniasetaatti; Prednizolon Asetat; Prednizolon-acetát; Prednizolono acetatas; Prednizolonu octan.

Преднизолона Ацетат

Prednisolone Caproate

Other names: Caproato de prednisolona; Prednisolone, Caproate de; Prednisolone Hexanoate; Prednisoloni Caproas.

Преднизолона Капроат

Prednisolone Hydrogen Succinate

Other names: Hidrogenosuccinato de prednisolona; Prednisolone Hemisuccinate; Prednisolone, Hémisuccinate de; Prednisoloni Hemisuccinas.

Преднизолона Гемисукцинат

Prednisolone Metasulfobenzoate Sodium

Other names: Metasulfobenzoato sódico de prednisolona; Natrii Prednisoloni Metasulfobenzoas; Prednisolone Métasulfobenzoate Sodique; Prednisolone Metasulphobenzoate Sodium; Prednisolone Sodium Metasulphobenzoate; R-812.

Натрий Метасульфобензоат Преднизолон

P

Prednisolone Pivalate

Other names: Pivalato de prednisolona; Prednisolone, pivalate de; Prednisolone Trimethylacetate; Prednisoloni pivalas; Prednisolonipivalaatti; Prednisolonpivalat; Prednisolon-pivalát; Prednizolono pivalatas; Prednizolon-pivalát; Prednizolonu piwalan.

Преднизолона Пивалат

Prednisolone Sodium Phosphate

Other names: Fosfato sódico de prednisolona; Natrii Prednisoloni Phosphas; Prednisolone, phosphate sodique de; Prednisolonfosfát sodná sůl; Prednisoloni natrii phosphas; Prednisoloninatriumfosfaatti; Prednisolonnatriumfosfat; Prednizolon Sodyum Fosfat; Prednizolon-nárium-foszfát; Prednizolono natrio fosfatas.

Натрия Преднизолона Фосфат

Prednisolone Sodium Succinate

Other names: Prednisolone Sodium Hemisuccinate; Prednisolone, Succinate Sodique de; Prednisoloni Natrii Succinas; Succinato sódico de prednisolona.

Преднизолона Натрия Сукцинат

Prednisolone Steaglate

Other names: Esteaglato de prednisolona; Prednisolone, Stéaglate de; Prednisoloni Steaglas.

Преднизолона Стеаглат

Prednisolone Tebutate

Other names: Prednisolone Butylacetate; Prednisolone 21-*tert*-Butylacetate; Prednisolone, Tébutate de; Prednisolone Tertiary-butylacetate; Prednisoloni Tebutas; Tebutato de prednisolona.

Преднизолона Тебутат

Clinical profile: Prednisolone is a glucocorticoid corticosteroid. It has been used, either in the form of the free alcohol or in one of the esterified forms, in the treatment of a wide range of conditions that respond to the anti-inflammatory and immunosuppressant effects of corticosteroid therapy.

WADA Status: Banned in competition

WADA Class: Glucocorticosteroids

All glucocorticosteroids are prohibited when administered orally, rectally, intravenously or intramuscularly. Their use requires a Therapeutic Use Exemption approval. Other routes of administration (intraarticular / periarticular / peritendinous / epidural / intradermal injections and inhalation) require an Abbreviated Therapeutic Use Exemption except as noted below.

Topical preparations when used for dermatological (including iontophoresis / pho-

nophoresis), auricular, nasal, ophthalmic, buccal, gingival and perianal disorders are not prohibited and do not require any form of Therapeutic Use Exemption.

WADA Class: Specified Substances

Also listed as a specified substance.

"The prohibited List may identify specified substances which are particularly susceptible to unintentional anti-doping rule violations because of their general availability in medicinal products or which are less likely to be successfully abused as doping agents."

A doping violation involving such substances may result in a reduced sanction provided that the *"...Athlete can establish that the Use of such a specfied substance was not intended to enhance sport performance..."*

Preparations

Single ingredient: ***Arg.:*** Cortizul; Ultracortenol; ***Austral.:*** Panafcortelone; Predmix; Predsol; Predsolone; Redipred; Solone; Sterofrin; ***Austria:*** Aprednislon; Kuhlprednon; Prednihexal; Rectopred; Solu-Dacortin; Ultracortenol; ***Belg.:*** Pred Forte; Ultracortenol; ***Braz.:*** Oftpred; Pred Fort; Pred Mild; Predsim; Prelone; ***Canad.:*** Ak-Tate; Pediapred; Pred Forte; Pred Mild; ***Chile:*** Pred Forte; Predsolets; ***Cz.:*** Inflanefran; Linola-H N; Linola-H-Fett N; Predni-POS; Solu-Decortin H; Ultracortenol; ***Denm.:*** Pred-Clysma; Ultracortenol; ***Fin.:*** Di-Adreson-F; Pred Forte; Ultracortenol; ***Fr.:*** Hydrocortancyl; Solupred; ***Ger.:*** Decortin H; Dermosolon; Dontisolon D; duraprednisolon; hefasolon; Infectocortikrupp; Inflanefran; Klismacort; Linola-H N; Linola-H-Fett N; Lygal Kopftinktur N; Prednabene; Predni H; Predni-Ophtal; Predni-POS; Predni; Prednigalen; Prednihexal; Prednisolut; Solu-Decortin H; Ultracortenol; ***Gr.:*** Adelcort; Adelone; Deltacortril; Prezolon; ***Hong Kong:*** Dhasolone; Di-Adreson-F; Panafcortelone; Pred Forte; Pred Mild; Predenema; Predfoam; Redipred; Ultracortenol; ***Hung.:*** Di-Adreson-F; Linola-H N; Linola-H-Fett N; Ultracortenol; ***India:*** Predone; Wysolone; ***Irl.:*** Deltacortril; Pred Mild; Predenema; Predfoam; Prednesol; Predsol; ***Israel:*** Pred Forte; Ultracortenol; ***Jpn:*** Farnerate; Farnezone; ***Malaysia:*** Dhasolone; Pred Forte; Pred Mild; ***Mex.:*** Cetapred; Delta-Diona; Fisopred; Meticortelone; Pred-NF; Pred; Prednefrin SF; Sophipren; ***Neth.:*** Di-Adreson-F; Pred Forte; Ultracortenol; ***Norw.:*** Pred-Clysma; Ultracortenol; ***NZ:*** Pred Forte; Pred Mild; Redipred; ***Philipp.:*** Histacort; Inflastat; Liquipred; Optipred; Pred Forte; Predisyr; Prednecort; Syrupred; ***Pol.:*** Encortolon; Fenicort; Mecortolon; ***Port.:*** Frisolona; Lepicortinolo; Predniocil; Sintisone; Solu-Dacortina; ***Rus.:*** Medopred (Медопред); ***S.Afr.:*** Capsoid; Lenisolone; Pred Mild; Preflam; Prelone; ***Singapore:*** Dhasolone; Econopred; Pred; Walesolone; ***Spain:*** Estilsona; Pred Forte; ***Swed.:*** Precortalon aquosum; Pred-Clysma; Ultracortenol; ***Switz.:*** Hexacortone; Pred Forte; Pred Mild; Spiricort; Ultracortenol; ***Thai.:*** Di-Adreson-F; Inf-Oph; Opredsone; Polypred; Pred Forte; Pred Mild; Prednersone; Prednisil; ***Turk.:*** Codelsol; Codelton; Deltacortril; Hexacorton; Neocorten; Norsol; Pred Forte; Prednol; ***UAE:*** Gupisone; ***UK:*** Deltacortril; Deltastab; Precortisyl; Pred Forte; Predenema; Predfoam; Predsol; ***USA:*** Key-Pred-SP; Orapred; Pediapred; Pred Forte; Pred Mild; Pred-Phosphate; Pred; Predcor; Prednisol; Prelone; ***Venez.:*** Meticortelone; Ocupred; Sintisone; Sophipren.

Multi-ingredient: ***Arg.:*** Bactio Rhin Prednisolona; Blefamide; Cortizul; Delta Tomanil B12; Deltar; Efecoryl Forte; Esodar; Fenipred; Neocortizul; Otidrops; Prednefrin; Prednifarma; Procto Venart; Relefrina; Rucaten Prednisolona; Scheriproct; Solupred; ***Austral.:*** Prednefrin; Scheriproct; ***Austria:*** Alpicort; Delta-Hadensa; Phoscortil; Scheriproct; ***Belg.:*** Hemosedan; Predmycin P; Scheriproct; Sofrasolone; ***Braz.:*** Colutoide; Isopto Cetapred; Polipred; Predmicin; Reumazine; Rifocort; Rinisone; ***Canad.:*** Blephamide; ***Chile:*** Banedif Oftalmico con Prednisolona; Blefamide; Blefamide; Deltamid; Gemitin con Prednisolona; Scheriproct; Sintoftona; ***Cz.:*** Alpicort F; Alpicort; Imacort; Isopto Cetapred; Linola-H-compositum N; Linoladiol-H N; Prednisolon J; ***Fin.:*** Scheriproct; Septison; ***Fr.:*** Cortisal; Deliproct; Derinox; Deturgylone; ***Ger.:*** Alpicort F; Alpicort; Aquapred; Berlicetin; Bismolan H Corti; Blephamide; Imazol comp; Inflanegent; Leioderm P; Linoladiol-H N; ***Gr.:*** Dermol; Isopto Cetapred; Scheriproct Neo; ***Hong Kong:*** Blephamide; Pilelife; ***Hung.:*** Alpicort F; Alpicort; Aurobin; Prednisolon J; Rheosolon; ***India:*** Atrisolon; Perfocyn; ***Indon.:*** Borraginol-S; Chloramphecort-H; Klorfeson; ***Irl.:*** Scheriproct; ***Israel:*** Aflumycin; Blephamide; Blephamide; Threolone; ***Ital.:*** Bio-Delta Cortilen; Deltamidrina; Solprene; ***Malaysia:*** Blephamide; ***Mex.:*** Artrilan; Blefamide-F; Blefamide; Dartrizon; Deltamid; Deltron; Isopto Cetapred; Obrypre; Otalgan; Premid; Scheriproct; ***Norw.:*** Scheriproct; ***NZ:*** Blephamide; ***Philipp.:*** Cetapred; Histacort; Isopto Cetapred; Predmycin-P; ***Pol.:*** Alpicort E; Alpicort; Mecortolon N; ***Port.:*** Anacal; Ciclobiotico; Meocil; Mobilat; Predniderma; Predniftalmina; Scheriproct; ***Rus.:*** Aurobin (Ауробин); Dermosolon (Дермозолон); Hepatrombin H (Гепатромбин Г); Terginan (Тержинан); ***S.Afr.:*** Scheriproct; ***Singapore:*** Blephamide; ***Spain:*** Alergical; Alergical; Antigrietun; Kanapomada; Nasopomada; Poly Pred; Predni Azuleno; Proctium; Rinobanedif; Rinovel; Ruscus; Scheriproct; Teolixir Compositum; ***Swed.:*** Scheriproct N; ***Switz.:*** Alpicort F; Blephamide; Calpred; Imacort; Locaseptil-Neo; Mycinopred; Premandol; Scheriproct; ***Thai.:*** Denson; Farakil; Levoptin; Mysolone-N; Neozolone; Pred Oph; Prednisil-N; Unipred; ***Turk.:*** Blephamid;

Otimisin; Prednol-A; Suprenil; ***UK:*** Predsol-N; Scheriproct; ***USA:*** Blephamide; Metimyd; Poly-Pred; Pred G; Sulfamide; Vasocidin; Vasocine; ***Venez.:*** Clorasona; Permucal; Scheriproct; Sulfacort.

Prednisone

P

Other names: Δ^1-Cortisone; 1,2-Dehydrocortisone; Deltacortisone; Deltadehydrocortisone; Metacortandracin; NSC-10023; Prednison; Prednisona; Prednisoni; Prednisonum; Prednizon; Prednizonas.

Преднизон

Prednisone Acetate

Other names: Acetato de prednisona; Prednisone, Acétate de; Prednisoni Acetas; Prednizonu octan.

Преднизона Ацетат

Clinical profile: Prednisone is a biologically inert glucocorticoid corticosteroid which is converted to prednisolone in the liver. It has been used, either in the form of the free alcohol or in one of the esterified forms, in the treatment of a wide range of conditions that respond to the anti-inflammatory and immunosuppressant effects of corticosteroid therapy.

WADA Status: Banned in competition

WADA Class: Glucocorticosteroids

All glucocorticosteroids are prohibited when administered orally, rectally, intravenously or intramuscularly. Their use requires a Therapeutic Use Exemption approval. Other routes of administration (intraarticular / periarticular / peritendinous / epidural / intradermal injections and inhalation) require an Abbreviated Therapeutic Use Exemption except as noted below.

Topical preparations when used for dermatological (including iontophoresis / phonophoresis), auricular, nasal, ophthalmic, buccal, gingival and perianal disorders are not prohibited and do not require any form of Therapeutic Use Exemption.

WADA Class: Specified Substances

Also listed as a specified substance.

"The prohibited List may identify specified substances which are particularly susceptible to unintentional anti-doping rule violations because of their general availability in medicinal products or which are less likely to be successfully abused as doping agents."

A doping violation involving such substances may result in a reduced sanction provided that the "*...Athlete can establish that the Use of such a specfied substance was not intended to enhance sport performance...*"

Preparations

Single ingredient: ***Arg.:*** Meticorten; Metilpres; Prednipirine; ***Austral.:*** Panafcort; Predsone; Sone; ***Braz.:*** Artinizona; Becortem; Corticorten; Meticorten; Metilen; Precortil; Predicorten; Predval; ***Canad.:*** Winpred; ***Chile:*** Berseri; Cortiprex; Meticorten; Procion; ***Cz.:*** Rectodelt; ***Fr.:*** Cortancyl; ***Ger.:*** Decortin; Predni Tablinen; Rectodelt; ***Hung.:*** Rectodelt; ***Indon.:*** Inflason; ***Ital.:*** Deltacortene; ***Mex.:*** Ednapron; Meprosona-F; Meticorten; Norapred; Prednidib; ***Philipp.:*** Bi-oster; Oracort; Orasone; Pred; Prolix; Steerometz; ***Pol.:*** Encorton; ***Port.:*** Meticorten; ***S.Afr.:***

Meticorten; Panafcort; Predeltin; Pulmison; ***Spain:*** Dacortin; ***Swed.:*** Deltison; ***USA:*** Deltasone; Liquid Pred; Meticorten; Panasol-S; Sterapred; ***Venez.:*** Meticorten.
Multi-ingredient: ***Arg.:*** Peganix; ***Austria:*** Fluorex Plus; Oleomycetin-Prednison; ***Chile:*** Alerzona; ***Mex.:*** Barigesic; Pre Clor; ***Spain:*** Coliriocilina Prednisona; Fiacin; Kanafosal Predni; Prednisona Neomicina.

Prednylidene

P

Other names: 16-Methyleneprednisolone; Prednilideeni; Prednilideno; Prednyliden; Prednylidène; Prednylidenum.

Преднилиден

Clinical profile: Prednylidene is a glucocorticoid corticosteroid related to prednisolone.

WADA Status: Banned in competition

WADA Class: Glucocorticosteroids

All glucocorticosteroids are prohibited when administered orally, rectally, intravenously or intramuscularly. Their use requires a Therapeutic Use Exemption approval. Other routes of administration (intraarticular / periarticular / peritendinous / epidural / intradermal injections and inhalation) require an Abbreviated Therapeutic Use Exemption except as noted below.

Topical preparations when used for dermatological (including iontophoresis / phonophoresis), auricular, nasal, ophthalmic, buccal, gingival and perianal disorders are not prohibited and do not require any form of Therapeutic Use Exemption.

WADA Class: Specified Substances

Also listed as a specified substance.

"*The prohibited List may identify specified substances which are particularly susceptible to unintentional anti-doping rule violations because of their general availability in medicinal products or which are less likely to be successfully abused as doping agents.*"

A doping violation involving such substances may result in a reduced sanction provided that the "...*Athlete can establish that the Use of such a specfied substance was not intended to enhance sport performance...*"

Prethcamide

Other names: G-5668; Pretcamida.

Cropropamide

Other names: Cropropamida; Cropropamidum; Kropropamid; Kropropamidi.

Кропропамид

Crotetamide

Other names: Crotetamida; Crotétamide; Crotetamidum; Crotethamide.

Кротетамид

Clinical profile: Prethcamide is a mixture of equal parts by weight of cropropamide and crotetamide; it has been used as a respiratory stimulant.

WADA Status: Banned in competition

WADA Class: Stimulants

Includes cropropamide, crotetamide and any optical isomers.

WADA Class: Specified Substances

Also listed as a specified substance.

"The prohibited List may identify specified substances which are particularly susceptible to unintentional anti-doping rule violations because of their general availability in medicinal products or which are less likely to be successfully abused as doping agents."

A doping violation involving such substances may result in a reduced sanction provided that the "*...Athlete can establish that the Use of such a specfied substance was not intended to enhance sport performance...*"

Preparations
Single ingredient: ***Ital.:*** Micoren.

P

Prizidilol Hydrochloride

Other names: Hidrocloruro de prizidilol; Prizidilol, Chlorhydrate de; Prizidiloli Hydrochloridum; SKF-92657-A[2].

Призидилола Гидрохлорид

Clinical profile: Prizidilol hydrochloride was investigated as an antihypertensive because of its vasodilator and beta blocking properties.

WADA Status: Banned in and out of competition as specified below

WADA Class: Beta-Blockers

Unless otherwise specified, beta-blockers are prohibited *In-Competition* only in the following sports.

- Aeronautics (FAI)
- Archery (FITA, IPC) (also prohibited *Out-of-Competition*)
- Automobile (FIA)
- Billiards (WCBS)
- Bobsleigh (FIBT)
- Boules (CMSB, IPC bowls)
- Bridge (FMB)
- Curling (WCF)
- Gymnastics (FIG)
- Motorcycling (FIM)
- Modern Pentathlon (UIPM) for disciplines involving shooting
- Nine-pin bowling (FIQ)
- Powerboating (UIM)
- Sailing (ISAF) for match race helms only
- Shooting (ISSF, IPC) (also prohibited *Out-of-Competition*)
- Skiing/Snowboarding (FIS) in ski jumping, freestyle aerials/halfpipe and snowboard halfpipe/big air
- Wrestling (FILA)

WADA Class: Specified Substances

Also listed as a specified substance.

"The prohibited List may identify specified substances which are particularly susceptible to unintentional anti-doping rule violations because of their general availability in medicinal products or which are less likely to be successfully abused as doping agents."

A doping violation involving such substances may result in a reduced sanction provided that the "*...Athlete can establish that the Use of such a specfied substance was not intended to enhance sport performance...*"

Probenecid

Other names: Probenecidas; Probénécide; Probenecidum; Probenesid; Probenesidi.

Пробенецид

Clinical profile: Probenecid is a uricosuric used in chronic gout to reduce the incidence and severity of attacks. It is of no value in acute gout. Probenecid also reduces the renal tubular excretion of many other drugs, thereby increasing their plasma concentrations, and has therefore been used as an adjunct to antibacterial therapy.

WADA Status: Banned in and out of competition

P

WADA Class: Diuretics and Other Masking Agents

Masking agents including alpha-reductase inhibitors or plasma expanders or substances with similar biological effect(s).

WADA Class: Specified Substances

Also listed as a specified substance.

"The prohibited List may identify specified substances which are particularly susceptible to unintentional anti-doping rule violations because of their general availability in medicinal products or which are less likely to be successfully abused as doping agents."

A doping violation involving such substances may result in a reduced sanction provided that the "*...Athlete can establish that the Use of such a specfied substance was not intended to enhance sport performance...*"

Preparations

Single ingredient: ***Austral.:*** Pro-Cid; ***Canad.:*** Benuryl; ***Fr.:*** Benemide; ***Gr.:*** Benemid; ***India:*** Bencid; ***Mex.:*** Benecid; ***Norw.:*** Probecid; ***S.Afr.:*** Proben; ***Swed.:*** Probecid; ***Thai.:*** Benacid; Bencid; ***USA:*** Benemid.

Multi-ingredient: ***USA:*** ColBenemid.

Adjunct-ingredient: ***Braz.:*** Emicilin; Gonol; ***Spain:*** Blenox.

Procaterol Hydrochloride

Other names: CI-888; Hidrocloruro de procaterol; OPC-2009; Procatérol, Chlorhydrate de; Procateroli Hydrochloridum; Prokaterolhydroklorid; Prokaterolihydrokloridi.

Прокатерола Гидрохлорид

Clinical profile: Procaterol hydrochloride is a direct-acting sympathomimetic with beta$_2$-adrenoceptor stimulant activity. It is used as a bronchodilator in the treatment of respiratory disorders such as asthma and chronic obstructive pulmonary disease.

WADA Status: Banned in and out of competition

WADA Class: Beta-2 Agonists

Includes beta-2 agonists or their isomers.

WADA Class: Specified Substances

Also listed as a specified substance.

"The prohibited List may identify specified substances which are particularly susceptible to unintentional anti-doping rule violations because of their general availability in medicinal products or which are less likely to be successfully abused as doping agents."

A doping violation involving such substances may result in a reduced sanction provided that the "*...Athlete can establish that the Use of such a specfied substance was not intended to enhance sport performance...*"

Preparations

Single ingredient: ***Cz.:*** Lontermin; ***Hong Kong:*** Meptin; ***Indon.:*** Ataroc; Meptin; ***Ital.***

Procadil; Propulm; ***Jpn:*** Meptin; ***Malaysia:*** Meptin; ***Philipp.:*** Meptin; ***Port.:*** Onsudil; ***Singapore:*** Meptin; ***Thai.:*** Caterol; Meptin.

Procinonide

Other names: Procinonida; Procinonidum; RS-2362.

Процинонид

Clinical profile: Procinonide is a derivative of the corticosteroid fluocinolone acetonide that has been applied topically with fluocinonide and ciprocinonide in the management of various skin disorders.

WADA Status: Banned in competition

WADA Class: Glucocorticosteroids

All glucocorticosteroids are prohibited when administered orally, rectally, intravenously or intramuscularly. Their use requires a Therapeutic Use Exemption approval. Other routes of administration (intraarticular / periarticular / peritendinous / epidural / intradermal injections and inhalation) require an Abbreviated Therapeutic Use Exemption except as noted below.

Topical preparations when used for dermatological (including iontophoresis / phonophoresis), auricular, nasal, ophthalmic, buccal, gingival and perianal disorders are not prohibited and do not require any form of Therapeutic Use Exemption.

WADA Class: Specified Substances

Also listed as a specified substance.

"*The prohibited List may identify specified substances which are particularly susceptible to unintentional anti-doping rule violations because of their general availability in medicinal products or which are less likely to be successfully abused as doping agents.*"

A doping violation involving such substances may result in a reduced sanction provided that the "*...Athlete can establish that the Use of such a specfied substance was not intended to enhance sport performance...*"

Prolintane Hydrochloride

Other names: Hidrocloruro de prolintano; Prolintane, Chlorhydrate de; Prolintani Hydrochloridum; SP-732.

Пролинтана Гидрохлорид

Clinical profile: Prolintane hydrochloride is a mild central stimulant. It has been used mainly in tonic preparations and also in narcolepsy.

WADA Status: Banned in competition

WADA Class: Stimulants

Includes prolintane and any optical isomers.

Propranolol Hydrochloride

Other names: AY-64043; Hidrocloruro de propranolol; ICI-45520; NSC-91523; Propanolol-hidroklorid; Propanololi Hydrochloridum; Propranolol, chlorhydrate de; Propranolol Hidroklorür; Propranolol-hydrochlorid; Propranololhydroklorid; Propranololi hydrochloridum; Propranololihydrokloridi; Propranololio hidrochloridas; Propranololu chlorowodorek.

Пропранолола Гидрохлорид

Clinical profile: Propranolol is a non-cardioselective beta blocker used in the management of hypertension, phaeochromocytoma, angina pectoris, myocardial infarction, cardiac arrhythmias, and hypertrophic cardiomyopathy. It is also used to control symptoms of sympathetic overactivity in the management of hyperthyroidism, anxiety, and tremor, and in the prophylaxis of migraine and of upper gastrointestinal bleeding in patients with portal hypertension.

WADA Status: Banned in and out of competition as specified below

WADA Class: Beta-Blockers

Unless otherwise specified, beta-blockers are prohibited *In-Competition* only in the following sports.

- Aeronautics (FAI)
- Archery (FITA, IPC) (also prohibited *Out-of-Competition*)
- Automobile (FIA)
- Billiards (WCBS)
- Bobsleigh (FIBT)
- Boules (CMSB, IPC bowls)
- Bridge (FMB)
- Curling (WCF)
- Gymnastics (FIG)
- Motorcycling (FIM)
- Modern Pentathlon (UIPM) for disciplines involving shooting
- Nine-pin bowling (FIQ)
- Powerboating (UIM)
- Sailing (ISAF) for match race helms only
- Shooting (ISSF, IPC) (also prohibited *Out-of-Competition*)
- Skiing/Snowboarding (FIS) in ski jumping, freestyle aerials/halfpipe and snowboard halfpipe/big air
- Wrestling (FILA)

WADA Class: Specified Substances

Also listed as a specified substance.

"*The prohibited List may identify specified substances which are particularly susceptible to unintentional anti-doping rule violations because of their general availability in medicinal products or which are less likely to be successfully abused as doping agents.*"

A doping violation involving such substances may result in a reduced sanction provided that the "*...Athlete can establish that the Use of such a specfied substance was not intended to enhance sport performance...*"

Preparations

Single ingredient: ***Arg.:*** Inderal; Pirimetan; Propaneitor; ***Austral.:*** Deralin; Inderal; ***Austria:*** Inderal; Proprahexal; ***Belg.:*** Inderal; ***Braz.:*** Antitensin; Cardiopranol; Inderal; Neo Propranol; Polol; Pradinolol; Pranolal; Propacor; Propalol; Propanox; Croparil; Propranol; Propranolil; Propranolum; Rebaten; Sanpronol; Uni Propralol; ***Canad.:*** Inderal; Novo-Pranol; ***Chile:*** Coriodal; ***Denm.:*** Propal; ***Fin.:*** Propral; Ranoprin; ***Fr.:*** Avlocardyl; Hemipralon; ***Ger.:*** Beta-Tablinen; Dociton; Elbrol; Obsidan; Prophylux; Propra-ratiopharm; propra; Propranur; ***Gr.:*** Inderal; ***Hong Kong:*** Inderal; Inpanol; ***Hung.:*** Huma-Pronol; ***India:*** Betabloc; Betaspan; Ciplar; Corbeta; Inderal; Propal; ***Indon.:*** Farmadral; Inderal; ***Irl.:*** Half Inderal; Inderal; ***Israel:*** Deralin; Inderal; Prolol; Slow Deralin; ***Ital.:*** Inderal; ***Malaysia:*** Inderal; ***Mex.:*** Inderalici; Propalem; Sintaser; ***Norw.:*** Inderal; Pranolol; ***NZ:*** Angilol; Cardinol; Inderal; ***Philipp.:*** Duranol; Inderal; Phanerol; ***Port.:*** Corpendol; Inderal; ***Rus.:*** Anaprilin (Анаприлин); Obsidan (Обзидан); ***S.Afr.:*** Cardiblok; Inderal; Prodorol; Pur-Bloka; ***Singapore:*** Inderal; Inpanol; ***Spain:*** Sumial; ***Swed.:*** Inderal; ***Switz.:*** Inderal; ***Thai.:*** Alperol; Betalol; Betapress; Cardenol; Emforal; Inderal; Normpress; Palon; Perlol; Pralol; Prolol; Syntonol; ***Turk.:*** Dideral; ***UAE:*** Cardilol; ***UK:*** Angilol; Bedranol; Beta-Prograne;

Half Beta-Prograne; Half Inderal; Inderal; Slo-Pro; Syprol; ***USA:*** Inderal; InnoPran; ***Venez.:*** Algoren; Docitral; Inderal.

Multi-ingredient: ***Braz.:*** Polol-H; Tenadren; ***Ger.:*** Beta-Turfa; Dociretic; Dociteren; Pertenso N; Propra comp; Triamteren tri-comp; ***India:*** Beptazine-H; Beptazine; Ciplar-H; Corbetazine; Zopax Plus; ***Neth.:*** Inderetic.

Propylhexedrine

P

Other names: Hexahydrodesoxyephedrine; Propilhexedrina; Propylhexed; Propylhexédrine; Propylhexedrinum.

Пропилгекседрин

Propylhexedrine Hydrochloride

Other names: Hidrocloruro de propilhexedrina; Propylhexédrine, Chlorhydrate de; Propylhexedrini Hydrochloridum.

Пропилгекседрина Гидрохлорид

Clinical profile: Propylhexedrine is a central stimulant and indirect-acting sympathomimetic. It has been used for nasal decongestion and as an anorectic in the treatment of obesity.

WADA Status: Banned in competition

WADA Class: Stimulants

Includes propylhexedrine and any optical isomers.

WADA Class: Specified Substances

Also listed as a specified substance.

"The prohibited List may identify specified substances which are particularly susceptible to unintentional anti-doping rule violations because of their general availability in medicinal products or which are less likely to be successfully abused as doping agents."

A doping violation involving such substances may result in a reduced sanction provided that the "*...Athlete can establish that the Use of such a specfied substance was not intended to enhance sport performance...*"

Preparations
Single ingredient: ***USA:*** Benzedrex.

Protheobromine

Other names: Proteobromina; Prothéobromine; Protheobrominum.

Протеобромин

Clinical profile: Protheobromine is a derivative of theobromine formerly used for its diuretic and vasodilating properties.

WADA Status: Banned in and out of competition

WADA Class: Diuretics and Other Masking Agents

Includes diuretics or substances with a similar chemical structure or similar biological effect(s).

Protokylol Hydrochloride

P

Other names: Hidrocloruro de protoquilol; JB-251; Protochylol Hydrochloride; Protokylol, Chlorhydrate de; Protokyloli Hydrochloridum.

Протокилола Гидрохлорид

Clinical profile: Protokylol hydrochloride is a sympathomimetic with predominantly beta-adrenergic activity. It has been given as a bronchodilator in the management of reversible airways obstruction.

WADA Status: Banned in competition

WADA Class: Stimulants

Includes stimulants or substances with a similar chemical structure or similar biological effect(s).

WADA Class: Specified Substances

Also listed as a specified substance.

"*The prohibited List may identify specified substances which are particularly susceptible to unintentional anti-doping rule violations because of their general availability in medicinal products or which are less likely to be successfully abused as doping agents.*"

A doping violation involving such substances may result in a reduced sanction provided that the "*...Athlete can establish that the Use of such a specfied substance was not intended to enhance sport performance...*"

Pyrovalerone

Other names: F-1983 (pyrovalerone hydrochloride); Pirovalerona; Pyrovalérone; Pyrovaleronum.

Пировалерон

Clinical profile: Pyrovalerone was formerly used as a central stimulant; it has been subject to abuse.

WADA Status: Banned in competition

WADA Class: Stimulants

Includes stimulants or substances with a similar chemical structure or similar biological effect(s).

WADA Class: Specified Substances

Also listed as a specified substance.

"*The prohibited List may identify specified substances which are particularly susceptible to unintentional anti-doping rule violations because of their general availability in medicinal products or which are less likely to be successfully abused as doping agents.*"

A doping violation involving such substances may result in a reduced sanction provided that the "*...Athlete can establish that the Use of such a specfied substance was not intended to enhance sport performance...*"

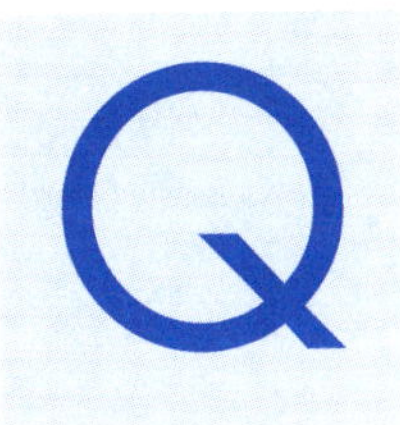

Quinbolone

Other names: Quinbolona; Quinbolonum.
Кинболон

Clinical profile: Quinbolone has been used for its anabolic properties.

WADA Status: Banned in and out of competition

WADA Class: Anabolic; Androgenic Steroids (exogenous)
Includes exogenous anabolic androgenic steroids or other substances with a similar chemical structure or similar biological effect(s).

Quinethazone

Other names: Chinethazonum; Kinetatsoni; Kinetazon; Quinetazona; Quinethazone; Quinethazonum.
Кинетазон

Clinical profile: Quinethazone is a diuretic similar to the thiazide diuretics. It has been used for oedema, including that associated with heart failure, and for hypertension.

WADA Status: Banned in and out of competition

WADA Class: Diuretics and Other Masking Agents
Includes diuretics or substances with a similar chemical structure or similar biological effect(s).

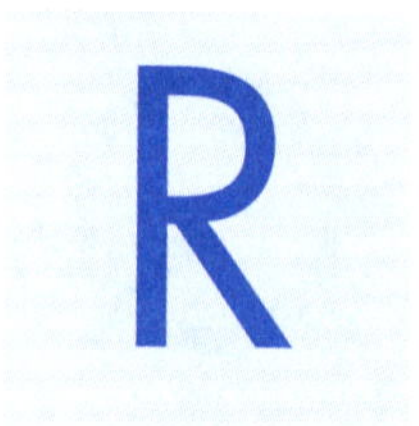

Raloxifene Hydrochloride

Other names: Hidrocloruro de raloxifeno; Keoxifene Hydrochloride; LY-15675€ LY-139481 (raloxifene); Raloksifen Hidroklorür; Raloxifène, chlorhydrate de Raloxifeni hydrochloridum.

Ралоксифена Гидрохлорид

Clinical profile: Raloxifene is a nonsteroidal anti-oestrogen related to tamoxifen that i used for treatment and prevention of postmenopausal osteoporosis.

WADA Status: Banned in and out of competition

WADA Class: Hormone Antagonists and Modulators
Includes selective estrogen receptor modulators.

Preparations
Single ingredient: ***Arg.:*** Evista; Ketidin; Oseofem; Raxeto; ***Austral.:*** Evista; ***Austria:*** Evista ***Belg.:*** Evista; ***Braz.:*** Evista; ***Canad.:*** Evista; ***Chile:*** Evista; ***Cz.:*** Evista; ***Denm.:*** Evista; ***Fin.*** Evista; ***Fr.:*** Evista; Optruma; ***Ger.:*** Evista; Optruma; ***Gr.:*** Evista; ***Hong Kong:*** Evista; ***Hung.*** Evista; ***India:*** Bonmax; Estroact; Ralista; ***Indon.:*** Evista; ***Irl.:*** Evista; ***Israel:*** Evista; ***Ital.:*** Evista Optruma; ***Jpn:*** Evista; ***Malaysia:*** Evista; ***Mex.:*** Evista; ***Neth.:*** Evista; Optruma; ***Norw.:*** Evista ***NZ:*** Evista; ***Philipp.:*** Evista; ***Pol.:*** Evista; ***Port.:*** Evista; Optruma; ***S.Afr.:*** Evista; ***Singapore*** Evista; ***Spain:*** Evista; Optruma; ***Swed.:*** Evista; ***Switz.:*** Evista; ***Thai.:*** Celvista; ***Turk.:*** Evista; ***UK*** Evista; ***USA:*** Evista; ***Venez.:*** Evista.

Red Blood Cells

Other names: Eritrocitos.

Clinical profile: Transfusions of red blood cells are given for the treatment of severe anaemia without hypovolaemia and for exchange transfusion in babies with haemolytic disease of the newborn. Red cells may be used with volume expanders for acute blood loss if less than half of the blood volume has been lost.

WADA Status: Banned in and out of competition

WADA Class: Enhancement of Oxygen Transfer: Blood Doping

Includes blood or red blood cell products that may be used to enhance the uptake, transport or delivery of oxygen.

Remifentanil Hydrochloride

Other names: GI-87084B; Hidrocloruro de remifentanilo; Rémifentanil, Chlorhydrate de; Remifentanili Hydrochloridum.

Ремифентанила Гидрохлорид

Clinical profile: Remifentanil, an anilidopiperidine derivative, is a short-acting μ-receptor opioid agonist used for analgesia during induction and/or maintenance of general anaesthesia. It is also used to provide analgesia in the immediate postoperative period.

WADA Status: Banned in competition

WADA Class: Narcotics

Includes specified narcotics.

Preparations

Single ingredient: ***Arg.:*** Remicit; Ultiva; ***Austral.:*** Ultiva; ***Austria:*** Ultiva; ***Belg.:*** Ultiva; ***Braz.:*** Ultiva; ***Canad.:*** Ultiva; ***Chile:*** Ultiva; ***Cz.:*** Ultiva; ***Denm.:*** Ultiva; ***Fin.:*** Ultiva; ***Fr.:*** Ultiva; ***Ger.:*** Ultiva; ***Gr.:*** Ultiva; ***Hong Kong:*** Ultiva; ***Israel:*** Ultiva; ***Ital.:*** Ultiva; ***Mex.:*** Ultiva; ***Neth.:*** Ultiva; ***Norw.:*** Ultiva; ***NZ:*** Ultiva; ***Pol.:*** Ultiva; ***Port.:*** Ultiva; ***S.Afr.:*** Ultiva; ***Singapore:*** Ultiva; ***Spain:*** Ultiva; ***Swed.:*** Ultiva; ***Switz.:*** Ultiva; ***Turk.:*** Ultiva; ***UK:*** Ultiva; ***USA:*** Ultiva; ***Venez.:*** Ultiva.

Reproterol Hydrochloride

Other names: D-1959 (reproterol); Hidrocloruro de reproterol; Réprotérol, Chlorhydrate de; Reproteroli Hydrochloridum; W-2946M.

Репротерола Гидрохлорид

Clinical profile: Reproterol hydrochloride is a direct-acting sympathomimetic with a selective action on beta$_2$ adrenoceptors. It has been given as a bronchodilator in respiratory disorders such as asthma and chronic obstructive pulmonary disease.

WADA Status: Banned in and out of competition

WADA Class: Beta-2 Agonists

Includes beta-2 agonists or their isomers.

WADA Class: Specified Substances

Also listed as a specified substance.

"The prohibited List may identify specified substances which are particularly susceptible to unintentional anti-doping rule violations because of their general availability in medicinal products or which are less likely to be successfully abused as doping agents."

A doping violation involving such substances may result in a reduced sanction provided that the "*...Athlete can establish that the Use of such a specfied substance was not intended to enhance sport performance...*"

Resocortol Butyrate

Preparations
Single ingredient: ***Ger.:*** Bronchospasmin.
Multi-ingredient: ***Ger.:*** Aarane N; Allergospasmin.

Resocortol Butyrate

Other names: ALO-2184; Butirato de resocortol; Org-7417; Résocortol, Butyrate de; Resocortoli Butiras; Resocortoli Butyras; Resokortolbutyrat; Resokortolibutyraatti.

Резокортола Бутират

Clinical profile: Resocortol butyrate is a corticosteroid that is used topically in veterinary medicine.

WADA Status: Banned in competition

WADA Class: Glucocorticosteroids

All glucocorticosteroids are prohibited when administered orally, rectally, intravenously or intramuscularly. Their use requires a Therapeutic Use Exemption approval. Other routes of administration (intraarticular / periarticular / peritendinous / epidural / intradermal injections and inhalation) require an Abbreviated Therapeutic Use Exemption except as noted below.

Topical preparations when used for dermatological (including iontophoresis / phonophoresis), auricular, nasal, ophthalmic, buccal, gingival and perianal disorders are not prohibited and do not require any form of Therapeutic Use Exemption.

WADA Class: Specified Substances

Also listed as a specified substance.

"*The prohibited List may identify specified substances which are particularly susceptible to unintentional anti-doping rule violations because of their general availability in medicinal products or which are less likely to be successfully abused as doping agents.*"

A doping violation involving such substances may result in a reduced sanction provided that the "*...Athlete can establish that the Use of such a specfied substance was not intended to enhance sport performance...*"

Rimexolone

Other names: Org-6216; Rimeksolon; Rimeksoloni; Rimexolon; Rimexolona; Rimexolonum; Trimexolone.

Римексолон

Clinical profile: Rimexolone is a corticosteroid that is applied topically to the eye in the treatment of inflammatory eye disorders including uveitis, and following ophthalmic surgery.

WADA Status: Banned in competition

WADA Class: Glucocorticosteroids

All glucocorticosteroids are prohibited when administered orally, rectally, intravenously or intramuscularly. Their use requires a Therapeutic Use Exemption approval. Other routes of administration (intraarticular / periarticular / peritendinous / epidural / intradermal injections and inhalation) require an Abbreviated Therapeutic Use Exemption except as noted below.

Topical preparations when used for dermatological (including iontophoresis / pho-

nophoresis), auricular, nasal, ophthalmic, buccal, gingival and perianal disorders are not prohibited and do not require any form of Therapeutic Use Exemption.

WADA Class: Specified Substances

Also listed as a specified substance.

"The prohibited List may identify specified substances which are particularly susceptible to unintentional anti-doping rule violations because of their general availability in medicinal products or which are less likely to be successfully abused as doping agents."

A doping violation involving such substances may result in a reduced sanction provided that the "*...Athlete can establish that the Use of such a specfied substance was not intended to enhance sport performance...*"

Preparations

Single ingredient: ***Austria:*** Vexol; ***Belg.:*** Vexolon; ***Braz.:*** Vexol; ***Canad.:*** Vexol; ***Cz.:*** Vexol; ***Denm.:*** Vexol; ***Fin.:*** Vexol; ***Fr.:*** Vexol; ***Ger.:*** Rimexel; Vexol; ***Gr.:*** Vexol; ***Hong Kong:*** Vexol; ***Irl.:*** Vexol; ***Ital.:*** Vexol; ***Mex.:*** Vexol; ***Neth.:*** Vexol; ***Norw.:*** Vexol; ***Port.:*** Vexol; ***Spain:*** Vexol; ***Swed.:*** Vexol; ***Switz.:*** Vexol; ***Turk.:*** Vexol; ***UK:*** Vexol; ***USA:*** Vexol.

R

Rimiterol Hydrobromide

Other names: Hidrobromuro de rimiterol; R-798; Rimitérol, Bromhydrate de; Rimiteroli Hydrobromidum; WG-253.

Римитерола Гидробромид

Clinical profile: Rimiterol hydrobromide is a direct-acting sympathomimetic with a selective action on $beta_2$ adrenoceptors. It has been used as a bronchodilator in the management of respiratory disorders such as asthma and chronic obstructive pulmonary disease.

WADA Status: Banned in and out of competition

WADA Class: Beta-2 Agonists

Includes beta-2 agonists or their isomers.

WADA Class: Specified Substances

Also listed as a specified substance.

"The prohibited List may identify specified substances which are particularly susceptible to unintentional anti-doping rule violations because of their general availability in medicinal products or which are less likely to be successfully abused as doping agents."

A doping violation involving such substances may result in a reduced sanction provided that the "*...Athlete can establish that the Use of such a specfied substance was not intended to enhance sport performance...*"

Ritodrine Hydrochloride

Other names: DU-21220 (ritodrine); Hidrocloruro de ritodrina; Ritodrin Hidroklorür; Ritodrine, Chlorhydrate de; Ritodrini Hydrochloridum.

Ритодрина Гидрохлорид

Clinical profile: Ritodrine hydrochloride is a direct-acting sympathomimetic with a selective action on $beta_2$ adrenoceptors. It is given to arrest premature labour.

WADA Status: Banned in and out of competition

WADA Class: Beta-2 Agonists

Includes beta-2 agonists or their isomers.

Preparations

Single ingredient: ***Arg.:*** Ritopar; ***Belg.:*** Pre-Par; ***Braz.:*** Miodrina; ***Cz.:*** Pre-Par; ***Gr.:*** Yutopar;

India: Yutopar; ***Indon.:*** Yutopar; ***Israel:*** Ritopar; ***Ital.:*** Miolene; ***Port.:*** Pre-Par; ***Spain:*** Pre-Par; ***Turk.:*** Pre-Par; ***UK:*** Yutopar.

Rogletimide

Other names: Pyridoglutethimide; Rogletimida; Roglétimide; Rogletimidum. Роглетимид

Clinical profile: Rogletimide is an aromatase inhibitor that has been investigated in the treatment of breast cancer.

WADA Status: Banned in and out of competition

WADA Class: Hormone Antagonists and Modulators
Includes aromatase inhibitors.

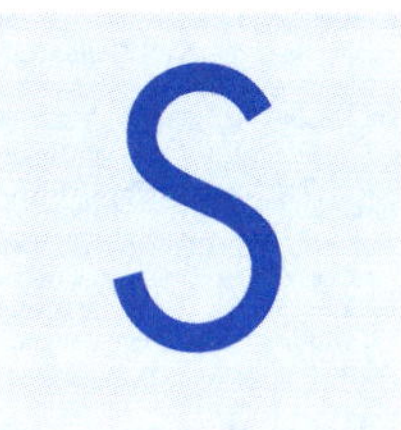

Salbutamol

Other names: AH-3365; Albuterol; Salbutamoli; Salbutamolis; Salbutamolum; Sch-13949W; Szalbutamol.

Сальбутамол

Salbutamol Sulfate

Other names: Albuterol Sulfate; Salbutamol Hemisulphate; Salbutamol, sulfate de; Salbutamol Sulphate; Salbutamoli sulfas; Salbutamolio sulfatas; Salbutamolisulfaatti; Salbutamolsulfat; Salbutamol-sulfát; Salbutamolu siarczan; Sulfato de salbutamol; Szalbutamol-szulfát.

Сальбутамола Сульфат

Clinical profile: Salbutamol is a direct-acting sympathomimetic with a relatively selective action on beta$_2$-adrenoceptors. It is used as a bronchodilator in the management of respiratory disorders such as asthma and chronic obstructive pulmonary disease. It is also given to arrest premature labour.

WADA Status: Banned in and out of competition

WADA Class: Beta-2 Agonists

Includes beta-2 agonists or their isomers. Salbutamol when administered by inhalation requires an abbreviated Therapeutic Use Exemption. Despite the granting of any form of Therapeutic Use Exemption, a concentration of salbutamol (free plus glucuronide) greater than 1000 ng/mL will be considered an *Adverse Analytical Finding* unless the Athlete proves that the abnormal result was the consequence of the therapeutic use of inhaled salbutamol.

WADA Class: Specified Substances

Also listed as a specified substance.

"*The prohibited List may identify specified substances which are particularly susceptible to unintentional anti-doping rule violations because of their general availability in medicinal products or which are less likely to be successfully abused as doping agents.*"

A doping violation involving such substances may result in a reduced sanction provided that the "*...Athlete can establish that the Use of such a specfied substance was not intended to enhance sport performance...*"

Preparations

Single ingredient: ***Arg.:*** Airsalbu; Amocasin; Asmatol; Butamol; Duopack; Microterol; Nebutrax; Respiret; Salbulin; Salbutol; Salbutral + Aeromed; Salbutral; Ventolin; Yontal; Zoom; ***Austral.:*** Airomir; Asmol; Butamol; Epaq; Respax; Ventolin; ***Austria:*** Buventol; Sultanol; ***Belg.:*** Airomir; Docsalbuta; Ventolin; ***Braz.:*** Aerobelin; Aero-Ped; Aerodini; Aerogreen; Aerojet; Aerolin; Aerotamol; Aerotrat; Asmakil; Asmaliv; Bronconal; Bronquil; Butovent; Dilamol; Oxiterol; Prodotamol; Pulmoflux; Salburin; Salbutalin; Salbutam; Salbutamax; Salbutib; Salrolin; Teoden; Tussiliv; ***Canad.:*** Airomir; Apo-Salvent; Ventodisk; Ventolin; ***Chile:*** Aerolin; Airomir; Asmavent; Bropil; Butotal; Fesema; Respolin; Salbutral; Sinasmal; ***Cz.:*** Apo-Salvent; Asthalin; Broncovaleas; Butovent; Buventol; Ecosal; Etinoline; Salamol; Steri-Neb Salamol; Ventodisks; Ventolin; Volmax; ***Denm.:*** Airomir; Buventol; Salbuvent; Ventoline; Volmax; ***Fin.:*** Airomir; Buventol; Ventoline; ***Fr.:*** Airomir; Asmasal; Buventol; Salbumol; Ventilastin; Ventoline; ***Ger.:*** Apsomol; Asthmalitan; Broncho Fertiginhalat; Broncho Inhalat; Bronchospray; Epaq; Loftan; Padiamol; Pentamol; Salbu; Salbubreathe; Salbuhexal; Salbulair; Salbulind; Sultanol; Ventilastin; Volmac; ***Gr.:*** Aerolin; Asthmotrat; Normobron; Salbunova; ***Hong Kong:*** Airomir; Azmacon; Cybutol; Respolin; Salamol; Salmol; Ventodisks; Ventolin; Ventomol; Volmax; Zenmolin; ***Hung.:*** Buventol; Ecosal; Ventolin; ***India:*** Asthalin; Derihaler; Salbetol; Salmaplon; Salsol; ***Indon.:*** Asmacare; Azmacon; Buventol; Fartolin; Glisend; Hivent; Lasal; Librentin; Pritasma; Salbron; Salbuven; Suprasma; Ventolin; Volmax; ***Irl.:*** Aerolin; Airomir; Asmasal; Gerivent; Salamol; Steri-Neb Salamol; Ventamol; Ventolin; ***Israel:*** Ventolin; ***Ital.:*** Broncovaleas; Ventmax; Ventolin; Volmax; ***Malaysia:*** Airomir; Beatolin; Butahale; Buventol; Salmax; Salmol; Ventamol; Ventolin; Volmax; ***Mex.:*** Apo-Salvent; Assal; Avedox-FC; Azyrol; Biorenyn; Bonair; Capacit; Cobamol; Dicoterol; Exafil; Oladin; Salamol; Salbutalan; Salcomed; Unibron; Ventolin; Volmax; Zibil; ***Neth.:*** Airomir; Butovent; Ventolin; ***Norw.:*** Airomir; Buventol; Ventoline; ***NZ:*** Airomir; Apo-Salvent; Asmigen; Buventol; Respigen; Respolin; Salamol; Salapin; Ventolin; Volmax; ***Philipp.:*** Activent; Airomir; Amoltex; Asbunyl; Asfrenon; Asmacaire; Asmalin; Astagen; Asvimol; Axmaxolv; Cletal; Emplusal; Hivent; Librentin; Provexel NS; Prox-S; Resdil; Rhinol; Salbumed; Salvex; Sedalin; Venalax; Ventar; Vento-Broncho; Ventolin; Ventosal; ***Pol.:*** Steri-Neb Salamol; Velaspir; Ventodisk; Ventolin; ***Port.:*** Ventilan; ***Rus.:*** Salamol (Саламол); Salben (Сальбен); Salgim (Сальгим); Saltos (Сальтос); Ventolin (Вентолин); ***S.Afr.:*** Airomir; Asthavent; Venteze; Ventolin; Volmax; ***Singapore:*** Azmasol; Butahale; Buventol; Medolin; Salbuair; Salmol; Venderol; Ventolin; Volmax; ***Spain:*** Aldobronquial; Buto Air; Buto Asma; Respiroma; Ventadur; Ventilastin; Ventolin; ***Swed.:*** Airomir; Buventol; Ventoline; ***Switz.:*** Ecovent; Ventodisk; Ventolin; Volmax; ***Thai.:*** Asmasal; Butamol; Buto Asma; Butovent; Buventol; Salbusian; Salbutac; Salda; Salmol; Solia; Venterol; Ventolin; Violin; Zebu; ***Turk.:*** Asthavent; Salbulin; Salbutam; Salbutol; Ven-o-sal; Ventodisks; Ventolin; Volmax; ***UAE:*** Butalin; ***UK:*** Airomir; Asmasal; Pulvinal Salbutamol; Salamol; Salapin; Ventmax; Ventolin; Volmax; ***USA:*** Accuneb; ProAir; Proventil; Ventolin; VoSpire; ***Venez.:*** Asthalin; Butoas; Salbulis; Salbumed; Salburol; Salbutan.

S

Multi-ingredient: ***Arg.:*** Beclasma; Butocort; Butosol; Combivent; Iprasalb; Salbutol Beclo; Salbutral AC; Ventide; ***Austral.:*** Combivent; ***Austria:*** Combivent; Di-Promal; Ventide; ***Belg.:*** Combivent; ***Braz.:*** Aeroflux; Aerotide; Clenil Compositum; Combivent; ***Canad.:*** Combivent; ratio-Ipra Sal UDV; ***Chile:*** Aero-Plus; Aerosoma; Asmavent-B; Belomet; Butotal B; Combivent; Herolan Aerosol; Salbutral AC; Ventide; ***Cz.:*** Combivent; Intal Plus; ***Denm.:*** Combivent; ***Fin.:*** Atrodual; Redol Comp; ***Fr.:*** Combivent; ***Gr.:*** Berovent; ***Hong Kong:*** Combivent; Ventide; Ventolin Expectorant; ***India:*** Aerocort; Albutamol; Ambrodil-S; Amcof; Asthacrom; Asthalin AX; Asthalin Expectorant; Axalin-AX; Duolin; Kofarest; Mucolinc; Okaril; Pulmo-Rest Expectorant; Pulmo-Rest; Suprivent-A; Suprivent; Theo-Asthalin; Ventorlin; ***Indon.:*** Combivent; Fartolin Expectorant; Lasal Expectorant; Proventol Expectorant; Salbron Expectorant; Salbuven Expectorant; Teosal; Ventide; Ventolin Expectorant; ***Irl.:*** Combivent; Ipramol; ***Ital.:*** Breva; Clenil Compositum; Plenaer; ***Malaysia:*** Combivent; Salbutamol Expectorant; Ventamol Expectorant; Ventolin Expectorant; ***Mex.:*** Aeroflux; Broxol Air; Combivent; Flamebin; Fluvicil; Fluxol; Fultac; Mucoflux; Musaldox; Neumyn-AS; Removil; Salamflux; Sibilex; Ulax-C; Ventide; ***Neth.:*** Combivent; ***NZ:*** Combivent; Duolin; ***Philipp.:*** Asbunyl Plus; Asfrenon GF; Asmalin Broncho; Broncaire Expectorant; Clarituss Plus; Combipul; Combivent; Duavent; Hicaryl; Histaril; Neovent; Pecof; Pulmovent; Salvex XP; SGX; Solmux-Broncho (Reformulated); Ventar EXP; Vento-Broncho G; Ventolin Expectorant; Venzadril; ***Port.:*** Combivent; Propavente; ***Rus.:*** Ascoril Expectorant (Аскорил Экспекторант); Biasten (Биастен); ***S.Afr.:*** Combivent; Duolin; Sabax Combineb; ***Singapore:*** Combivent; ***Spain:*** Butosol; Combivent; ***Swed.:*** Combivent; ***Switz.:*** Dospir; ***Thai.:*** Almasal; Biovent; Clenil Compositum; Combivent; Royalin; Salmol Expectorant; Ventolin Expectorant; ***Turk.:*** Combivent; Ventide; ***UK:*** Combivent; Ipramol; ***USA:*** Combivent; DuoNeb; ***Venez.:*** Aerocort; Aeroflux; Beclosal; Broxodin; Butosol; Combivent; Duolin; Ipralin; Venticort; Ventide.

Salmeterol Xinafoate

Other names: GR-33343G; Salmaterol Xinafoate; Salmeterol 1-Hydroxy-2-naphthoate; Salmeterol Ksinafoat; Salmétérol, xinafoate de; Salmeteroli xinafoas; Salmeteroliksinafoaatti; Salmeterolio ksinafoatas; Salmeterol-xinafoát; Sameterolxinafoat; Xinafoato de Salmeterol.

Салметерола Ксинафоат

Clinical profile: Salmeterol xinafoate is a direct-acting sympathomimetic with beta-adrenoceptor stimulant activity and a selective action on beta$_2$ receptors. It is used as a bronchodilator in the management of respiratory disorders such as chronic asthma and chronic obstructive pulmonary disease, although its onset of action is too slow to provide acute symptomatic relief.

WADA Status: Banned in and out of competition

WADA Class: Beta-2 Agonists

Includes beta-2 agonists or their isomers. Salmeterol when administered by inhalation requires an abbreviated Therapeutic Use Exemption.

WADA Class: Specified Substances

Also listed as a specified substance.

"The prohibited List may identify specified substances which are particularly susceptible to unintentional anti-doping rule violations because of their general availability in medicinal products or which are less likely to be successfully abused as doping agents."

A doping violation involving such substances may result in a reduced sanction provided that the "*...Athlete can establish that the Use of such a specfied substance was not intended to enhance sport performance...*"

Preparations

Single ingredient: ***Arg.:*** Serevent; ***Austral.:*** Serevent; ***Austria:*** Serevent; ***Belg.:*** Serevent; ***Braz.:*** Serevent; ***Canad.:*** Serevent; ***Chile:*** Serevent; Xemos; ***Cz.:*** Serevent; ***Denm.:*** Serevent; ***Fin.:*** Serevent; ***Fr.:*** Serevent; ***Ger.:*** Aeromax; Serevent; ***Gr.:*** Serevent; ***Hong Kong:*** Serevent; ***Hung.:*** Serevent; ***India:*** Salmeter; Serobid; ***Indon.:*** Serevent; ***Irl.:*** Serevent; ***Israel:*** Serevent; ***Ital.:*** Arial; Salmetedur; Serevent; ***Jpn:*** Serevent; ***Malaysia:*** Serevent; ***Mex.:*** Serevent; ***Neth.:*** Serevent; ***Norw.:*** Serevent; ***NZ:*** Serevent; ***Philipp.:*** Serevent; ***Pol.:*** Serevent; ***Port.:*** Dilamax; Serevent; Ultrabeta; ***Rus.:*** Seretide (Серетид); Serevent (Серевент); ***S.Afr.:*** Serevent; ***Singapore:*** Serevent; ***Spain:*** Beglan; Betamican; Inaspir; Serevent; ***Swed.:*** Serevent; ***Switz.:*** Serevent; ***Thai.:*** Serevent; ***Turk.:*** Astmerole; Serevent; ***UK:*** Serevent; ***USA:*** Serevent; ***Venez.:*** Salspray; Serevent.

Multi-ingredient: ***Arg.:*** Flutivent; Neumotide; Seretide; ***Austral.:*** Seretide; ***Austria:*** Seretide; Viani; ***Belg.:*** Seretide; ***Braz.:*** Seretide; ***Canad.:*** Advair; ***Chile:*** Aerometrol Plus; Aurituss; Brexotide; Seretide; ***Cz.:*** Seretide; ***Denm.:*** Seretide; ***Fin.:*** Seretide; ***Fr.:*** Seretide; ***Ger.:*** Atmadisc; Viani; ***Gr.:*** Seretide; ***Hong Kong:*** Seretide; ***Hung.:*** Seretide; Thoreus; ***India:*** Forair; Seretide; Seroflo; ***Indon.:*** Seretide; ***Irl.:*** Seretide; ***Israel:*** Seretide; ***Ital.:*** Aliflus; Seretide; ***Malaysia:*** Seretide; ***Mex.:*** Seretide; ***Neth.:*** Seretide; Viani; ***Norw.:*** Seretide; ***NZ:*** Seretide; ***Philipp.:*** Seretide; ***Pol.:*** Seretide; ***Port.:*** Brisomax; Maizar; Seretaide; Veraspir; ***S.Afr.:*** Seretide; ***Singapore:*** Seretide; ***Spain:*** Anasma; Brisair; Inaladuo; Plusvent; Seretide; ***Swed.:*** Seretide; ***Switz.:*** Seretide; ***Thai.:*** Seretide; ***Turk.:*** Seretide; ***UK:*** Seretide; ***USA:*** Advair; ***Venez.:*** Seretide.

S

Selegiline Hydrochloride

Other names: Deprenyl; L-Deprenyl; Hidrocloruro de selegilina; Selegiliinihydrokloridi; Selegilin Hidroklorür; Selegilin hydrochlorid; Sélégiline, chlorhydrate de; Selegilinhydroklorid; Selegilini hydrochloridum; Selegilino hidrochloridas; Szelegilin-hidroklorid.

Селегилина Гидрохлорид

Clinical profile: Selegiline is an irreversible selective inhibitor of monoamine oxidase type B that enhances the effects of levodopa. It is used in the treatment of Parkinson's disease and in depression, and has also been tried in dementia.

WADA Status: Banned in competition

WADA Class: Stimulants

Includes selegiline and any optical isomers

WADA Class: Specified Substances

Also listed as a specified substance.

"The prohibited List may identify specified substances which are particularly susceptible to unintentional anti-doping rule violations because of their general availability in medicinal products or which are less likely to be successfully abused as doping agents."

A doping violation involving such substances may result in a reduced sanction pro-

vided that the "*...Athlete can establish that the Use of such a specfied substance was not intended to enhance sport performance...*"

Preparations
Single ingredient: ***Arg.:*** Brintenal; Jumex; Zelapar; ***Austral.:*** Eldepryl; Selgene; ***Austria:*** Amboneural; Cognitiv; Jumex; Regepar; Xilopar; ***Belg.:*** Eldepryl; ***Braz.:*** Deprilan; Elepril; Jumexil; Niar; Parkexin; ***Chile:*** Selgina; ***Cz.:*** Apo-Seleg; Cognitiv; Jumex; Niar; Segalin; Sepatrem; ***Denm.:*** Eldepryl; ***Fin.:*** Eldepryl; ***Fr.:*** Deprenyl; Otrasel; ***Ger.:*** Antiparkin; Jutagilin; Movergan; Selemerck; Selepark; Selgimed; Xilopar; ***Gr.:*** Cosmopril; Ermolax; Feliselin; Krautin; Legil; Procythol; Resostyl; ***Hong Kong:*** Julab; Jumex; Sefmex; Selegos; ***Hung.:*** Cognitiv; Jumex; ***India:*** Selerin; Selgin; ***Indon.:*** Jumex; ***Irl.:*** Eldepryl; ***Israel:*** Jumex; ***Ital.:*** Egibren; Jumex; Selecom; Seledat; Xilopar; ***Jpn:*** FP Tab; ***Malaysia:*** Jumex; Selegos; ***Mex.:*** Niar; ***Neth.:*** Eldepryl; ***Norw.:*** Eldepryl; ***NZ:*** Eldepryl; ***Philipp.:*** Jumex; ***Pol.:*** Apo-Selin; Jumex; Segan; Selerin; Selgin; Selgres; ***Port.:*** Jumex; Xilopar; ***Rus.:*** Cognitiv (Когнитив); Segan (Сеган); Selegos (Селегос); ***S.Afr.:*** Eldepryl; Parkilyne; ***Singapore:*** Jumex; Selegos; ***Spain:*** Plurimen; ***Swed.:*** Eldepryl; ***Switz.:*** Jumexal; ***Thai.:*** Julab; Jumex; Sefmex; ***Turk.:*** Moverdin; Seldepar; ***UK:*** Eldepryl; Zelapar; ***USA:*** Atapryl; Carbex; Eldepryl; Emsam; Zelapar; ***Venez.:*** Jumex.

Sibutramine Hydrochloride

Other names: BTS-54524; Hidrocloruro de sibutramina; Sibutramin Hidroklorür; Sibutramine, Chlorhydrate de; Sibutramini Hydrochloridum.

Сибутрамина Гидрохлорид

Clinical profile: Sibutramine hydrochloride is a serotonin and noradrenaline reuptake inhibitor used in the management of obesity.

WADA Status: Banned in competition

WADA Class: Stimulants

Includes sibutramine and any optical isomers.

WADA Class: Specified Substances

Also listed as a specified substance.

"*The prohibited List may identify specified substances which are particularly susceptible to unintentional anti-doping rule violations because of their general availability in medicinal products or which are less likely to be successfully abused as doping agents.*"

A doping violation involving such substances may result in a reduced sanction provided that the "*...Athlete can establish that the Use of such a specfied substance was not intended to enhance sport performance...*"

Preparations
Single ingredient: ***Arg.:*** Aderan; Downtrat; Ipomex; Sacietyl; Sertinal; Sibu-Estirol; Sibu-Tratobes; ***Austral.:*** Reductil; ***Austria:*** Meridia; Reductil; ***Belg.:*** Reductil; ***Braz.:*** Plenty; Reductil; ***Canad.:*** Meridia; ***Chile:*** Adisar; Atenix; Ipogras; Medixil; Mesura; Milical; Mintagras; Noducil; Reductil; Reduten; Saton; ***Cz.:*** Meridia; ***Denm.:*** Reductil; ***Fin.:*** Reductil; ***Fr.:*** Sibutral; ***Ger.:*** Reductil; ***Gr.:*** Reductil; ***Hong Kong:*** Reductil; ***Hung.:*** Reductil; ***India:*** Obestat; ***Indon.:*** Reductil; ***Irl.:*** Reductil; ***Israel:*** Reductil; ***Ital.:*** Ectiva; Reductil; ***Malaysia:*** Reductil; ***Mex.:*** Ectiva; Ifa-Certez; Raductil; Serotramin; ***Neth.:*** Reductil; ***Norw.:*** Reductil; ***NZ:*** Reductil; ***Philipp.:*** Reductil; ***Pol.:*** Meridia; Zelixa; ***Port.:*** Reductil; ***Rus.:*** Meridia (Меридиа); ***S.Afr.:*** Reductil; ***Singapore:*** Reductil; ***Spain:*** Reductil; ***Swed.:*** Reductil; ***Switz.:*** Reductil; ***Thai.:*** Reductil; ***Turk.:*** Reductil; ***UK:*** Reductil; ***USA:*** Meridia; ***Venez.:*** Milical; Reductil; Repentil; Vintix.
Multi-ingredient: ***Mex.:*** Redumed.

Somatomedins

Other names: IGFs; Insulin-like Growth Factors; Somatomedinas; Sulphation Factors.

Clinical profile: The somatomedins are a group of polypeptide hormones, some of which are involved in mediating the effects of growth hormone in the body. Somatomedin C (Insulin-like growth factor 1, IGF-1) is believed to be responsible for many of the anabolic effects of growth hormone; a biosynthetic form, mecasermin, is used clinically. Mecasermin rinfabate, a complex of IGF-I with IGF binding protein-3, is also under investigation.

Mecasermin

Other names: CEP-151; FK-780; IGF-I; Insulin-like growth factor I (human); Mecasermina; Mécasermine; Mecaserminum; rhIGF-1; Somatomedin C.

Меказермин

Clinical profile: Mecasermin is a biosynthetic form of insulin-like growth factor I (IGF-I), the somatomedin believed to be responsible for many of the anabolic effects of growth hormone. Mecasermin is used in the treatment of growth failure in children with severe primary IGF-I deficiency and in those with growth hormone gene deletion who have developed neutralising antibodies to growth hormone. It is also being investigated in diabetes mellitus and insulin resistance, motor neurone disease, and osteoporosis.

Mecasermin Rinfabate

Other names: Mecasermina rinfabato; Mécasermine Rinfabate; Mecaserminum Rinfabas; rhIGF-I/rhIGFBP-3.

Меказермин Ринфабат

Clinical profile: Mecasermin is a biosynthetic form of insulin-like growth factor I (IGF-I), the somatomedin believed to be responsible for many of the anabolic effects of growth hormone. Mecasermin rinfabate is a complex of mecasermin with IGF binding protein-3 that is used in the treatment of growth failure in children with severe primary IGF-I deficiency and in those with growth hormone gene deletion who have developed neutralising antibodies to growth hormone. They are also under investigation in the treatment of conditions such as diabetes mellitus and severe insulin resistance, osteoporosis, and severe burns.

WADA Status: Banned in and out of competition

WADA Class: Hormones and Related Substances: Growth Hormone, Insulin-like Growth Factors, Mechano Growth Factors
Includes growth hormone or insulin-like growth factors or mechano growth factor or substances with a similar chemical structure or similar biological effect(s), or one of their releasing factors.

Preparations
Single ingredient: ***UK:*** Increlex; ***USA:*** Increlex; Iplex.

Somatorelin

Other names: GHRF; GHRH; GRF; GRF-44; Growth Hormone-releasing Factor (Human); Growth Hormone-releasing Hormone; Somatoliberin; Somatoreliini; Somatorelina; Somatoréline; Somatorelinum.

Соматорелин

Clinical profile: Somatorelin is a peptide secreted by the hypothalamus which promotes the release of growth hormone from the anterior pituitary. Synthetic somatorelin has been used in the diagnosis and treatment of growth hormone deficiency.

Sermorelin Acetate

Other names: Acetato de sermorelina; GRF(1-29)NH_2 (sermorelin); Growth Hormone-releasing Factor (Human)-(1-29)-peptide Amide (sermorelin); Serméline, Acétate de; Sermorelini Acetas.

Серморелина Ацетат

Clinical profile: Sermorelin is a synthetic peptide corresponding to the 1–29 amino acid sequence of human growth hormone-releasing hormone (somatorelin). It is used for the diagnosis of growth hormone deficiency and has been used for its treatment. It has also been investigated as an adjunct to gonadotrophin in ovulation induction, and in the treatment of HIV-related wasting.

WADA Status: Banned in and out of competition

WADA Class: Hormones and Related Substances: Growth Hormone, Insulin-like Growth Factors, Mechano Growth Factors

Includes growth hormone or insulin-like growth factors or mechano growth factor or substances with a similar chemical structure or similar biological effect(s), or one of their releasing factors.

Preparations

Single ingredient: ***Austria:*** Geref; ***Belg.:*** GHRH; ***Fin.:*** Geref; ***Fr.:*** Stimu-GH; ***Ger.:*** GHRH; ***Gr.:*** Geref; ***Irl.:*** Geref; ***Ital.:*** Geref; GHRH; ***Neth.:*** GHRH; ***Norw.:*** Geref; ***Port.:*** Geref; ***Spain:*** Geref; ***Switz.:*** GHRH; ***UK:*** GHRH; ***USA:*** Geref.

Sotalol Hydrochloride

S

Other names: Hidrocloruro de sotalol; MJ-1999; Sotalol, chlorhydrate de; Sotalol Hidroklorür; *d,l*-Sotalol Hydrochloride; Sotalol-hydrochlorid; Sotalolhydroklorid; Sotaloli hydrochloridum; Sotalolihydrokloridi; Sotalolio hidrochloridas; Szotalol-hidroklorid.

Соталола Гидрохлорид

Clinical profile: Sotalol is a non-cardioselective beta blocker that also has class III antiarrhythmic activity. It is used in the management of cardiac arrhythmias. It was also formerly used in the management of angina pectoris, hypertension, and myocardial infarction but, because of its proarrhythmic effect, it is no longer recommended for these indications.

WADA Status: Banned in and out of competition as specified below

WADA Class: Beta-Blockers

Unless otherwise specified, beta-blockers are prohibited *In-Competition* only in the following sports.

- Aeronautics (FAI)
- Archery (FITA, IPC) (also prohibited *Out-of-Competition*)
- Automobile (FIA)
- Billiards (WCBS)
- Bobsleigh (FIBT)
- Boules (CMSB, IPC bowls)
- Bridge (FMB)
- Curling (WCF)
- Gymnastics (FIG)
- Motorcycling (FIM)
- Modern Pentathlon (UIPM) for disciplines involving shooting
- Nine-pin bowling (FIQ)
- Powerboating (UIM)
- Sailing (ISAF) for match race helms only
- Shooting (ISSF, IPC) (also prohibited *Out-of-Competition*)
- Skiing/Snowboarding (FIS) in ski jumping, freestyle aerials/halfpipe and snowboard halfpipe/big air
- Wrestling (FILA)

WADA Class: Specified Substances

Also listed as a specified substance.

"The prohibited List may identify specified substances which are particularly susceptible to unintentional anti-doping rule violations because of their general availability in medicinal products or which are less likely to be successfully abused as doping agents."

A doping violation involving such substances may result in a reduced sanction provided that the "*...Athlete can establish that the Use of such a specfied substance was not intended to enhance sport performance...*"

Preparations
Single ingredient: ***Arg.:*** Sotacor; ***Austral.:*** Cardol; Solavert; Sotacor; Sotahexal; ***Austria:*** Darob; Sotacor; Sotahexal; Sotamed; Sotanorm; Sotastad; ***Belg.:*** Sotalex; ***Braz.:*** Sotacor; ***Chile:*** Hipecor; ***Cz.:*** Darob; Rentibloc; Sotahexal; Sotalex; ***Denm.:*** Dutacor; Sotacor; ***Fin.:*** Sotacor; Sotalin; ***Fr.:*** Sotalex; ***Ger.:*** Darob; Favorex; Gilucor; Jutalex; Rentibloc; Sota Lich; Sota-Puren; Sota-saar; Sota; Sotabeta; Sotagamma; Sotahexal; Sotalex; Sotalodoc; Sotastad; ***Hong Kong:*** Sotacor; ***Hung.:*** Sotahexal; Sotalex; ***Irl.:*** Sotacor; Sotoger; ***Ital.:*** Rytmobeta; Sotalex; ***Malaysia:*** Sotacor; ***Mex.:*** Sotaper; ***Neth.:*** Sotacor; ***Norw.:*** Sotacor; ***NZ:*** Sotacor; Sotahexal; ***Philipp.:*** Sotalex; ***Pol.:*** Biosotal; Darob; Sotahexal; ***Port.:*** Darob; ***Rus.:*** Sotahexal (Сотагексал); Sotalex (Соталекс); ***S.Afr.:*** Sotacor; Sotahexal; ***Singapore:*** Sotacor; ***Spain:*** Sotapor; ***Swed.:*** Sotacor; ***Switz.:*** Sotalex; ***Turk.:*** Darob; Sotarit; Talozin; ***UK:*** Beta-Cardone; Sotacor; ***USA:*** Betapace.

Multi-ingredient: ***S.Afr.:*** Sotazide.

Spironolactone

Other names: Espironolactona; SC-9420; Spirolactone; Spironolactonum; Spironolakton; Spironolaktonas; Spironolaktoni.

Спиронолактон

Clinical profile: Spironolactone is a potassium-sparing diuretic and an aldosterone antagonist. It is used mainly in the treatment of refractory oedema in patients with heart failure, nephrotic syndrome, or hepatic cirrhosis. Its effects on the endocrine system are utilised in the treatment of hirsutism and in primary hyperaldosteronism.

WADA Status: Banned in and out of competition

WADA Class: Diuretics and Other Masking Agents

Includes diuretics or substances with a similar chemical structure or similar biological effect(s).

Preparations
Single ingredient: ***Arg.:*** Aldactone; Drimux A; Espimax; Expal; Lanx; Modulactone; Normital; Rediun-E; ***Austral.:*** Aldactone; Spiractin; ***Austria:*** Aldactone; Spirobene; Spirohexal; Spirono; ***Belg.:*** Aldactone; Docspirono; Spirotop; ***Braz.:*** Aldactone; Aldosterin; Espirolona; Spiroctan; ***Canad.:*** Aldactone; Novo-Spiroton; ***Chile:*** Alizar; Cardactona; ***Cz.:*** Spirolone; Uractone; Verospiron; Xenalon; ***Denm.:*** Hexalacton; Spirix; Spiron; ***Fin.:*** Aldactone; Spiresis; Spirix; ***Fr.:*** Aldactone; Flumach; Practon; Spiroctan; Spironone; ***Ger.:*** Aldactone; Jenaspiron; Osyrol; Spiro; Spirobeta; Spirogamma; Spirono; Verospiron; ***Gr.:*** Aldactone; ***Hong Kong:*** Aldactone; ***Hung.:*** Huma-Spiroton; Spiron; Verospiron; ***India:*** Aldactone; ***Indon.:*** Aldactone; Carpiaton; Letonal; Spirola; ***Irl.:*** Aldactone; ***Israel:*** Aldactone; Aldospirone; Spironol; ***Ital.:*** Aldactone; Spirolang; Uractone; ***Mex.:*** Aldactone; Biolactona; Vivitar; ***Neth.:*** Aldactone; ***Norw.:*** Aldactone; Spirix; ***NZ:*** Spirotone; ***Philipp.:*** Aldactone; ***Pol.:*** Spironol; Verospiron; ***Port.:*** Aldactone; Aldonar; Nefrolactona; ***Rus.:*** Verospiron (Верошпирон); ***S.Afr.:*** Aldactone; Spiractin; ***Singapore:*** Aldactone; Uractonum; ***Spain:*** Aldactone; ***Swed.:*** Aldactone; Spirix; ***Switz.:*** Aldactone; Primacton; Xenalon; ***Thai.:*** Aldactone; Altone; Hyles; Pondactone; ***Turk.:*** Aldacton; ***UK:*** Aldactone; ***USA:*** Aldactone; ***Venez.:*** Aldactone.

Multi-ingredient: ***Arg.:*** Aldactone-D; Aldazida; Lasilacton; ***Austria:*** Aldactone Saltucin; Buti-Spirobene; Deverol mit Thiazid; Digi-Aldopur; Furo-Aldopur; Furo-Spirobene; Furolacton; Lasilacton; Sali-Aldopur; Spirono comp; Supracid; ***Belg.:*** Aldactazine; Docspirochlor; ***Braz.:*** Aldazida; Lasilactona; ***Canad.:*** Aldactazide; Novo-Spirozine; ***Cz.:*** Spiro Compositum; ***Fr.:*** Aldactazine; Aldalix; Practazin; Spiroctazine; ***Ger.:*** Furo-Aldopur; Furorese Comp; Osyrol Lasix; Spiro comp; Spiro-D; Spironothiazid; ***India:*** Lasilactone; Spiromide; ***Indon.:*** Aldazide; ***Irl.:*** Aldactide; ***Ital.:*** Aldactazide; Lasitone; Spiridazide; Spirofur; ***Mex.:*** Aldazida; Lasilacton; ***Philipp.:*** Aldazide; ***Port.:*** Aldactazine; Ondolen; ***S.Afr.:*** Aldazide; ***Spain:*** Aldactacine; Aldoleo; Spirometon; ***Switz.:***

S

Aldozone; Furocombin; Furospir; Lasilactone; ***Turk.:*** Aldactazide; ***UK:*** Aldactide; Lasilactone; ***USA:*** Aldactazide; ***Venez.:*** Aldactazida.

Stanozolol

Other names: Androstanazol; Androstanazole; Estanazol; Estanozolol; Methylstanazole; Metistanazol; NSC-43193; Stanotsololi; Stanozololis; Stanozololum; Stanozolum; Sztanozolol; Win-14833.

Станозолол

Clinical profile: Stanozolol is an anabolic steroid that has been used in the management of hereditary angioedema. It has also been used in breast cancer in postmenopausal women, and for anaemias, osteoporosis, and catabolic disorders.

WADA Status: Banned in and out of competition

WADA Class: Anabolic; Androgenic Steroids (exogenous)

Includes exogenous anabolic androgenic steroids or other substances with a similar chemical structure or similar biological effect(s).

Preparations
Single ingredient: ***Gr.:*** Stromba; ***India:*** Menabol; Neurabol; ***Spain:*** Winstrol; ***USA:*** Winstrol.
Multi-ingredient: ***Thai.:*** Cetabon.

S

Strychnine

Other names: Estricnina; Strychnina.

Strychnine Hydrochloride

Other names: Estricnina, hidrocloruro de; Strych. Hydrochlor.; Strychninae Hydrochloridum.

Strychnine Nitrate

Other names: Azotato de Estricnina; Estricnina, nitrato de; Nitrato de Estricnina; Strychninae Nitras; Strychnini Nitras; Strychninum Nitricum; Strykniininitraatti; Stryknninitrat.

Strychnine Sulfate

Other names: Estricnina, sulfato de; Strychninae Sulphas; Strychnine Sulphate; Strychninum Sulfuricum; Sulfato de Estricnina.

Clinical profile: Strychnine is an alkaloid obtained from the seeds of nux vomica (*Strychnos nux-vomica* (Loganiaceae)) and other species of *Strychnos*. Strychnine competes with glycine which is an inhibitory neurotransmitter; it thus exerts a central stimulant effect through blocking an inhibitory activity. Strychnine was formerly used as a bitter and analeptic but is now mainly used under strict control as a rodenticide, or as a mole poison. It has been used in multi-ingredient preparations for the treatment of ophthalmic and urinary-tract disorders. It has also been tried in the treatment of nonketotic hyperglycinaemia.

WADA Status: Banned in competition

WADA Class: Stimulants

Includes strychnine and any optical isomers.

Preparations
Multi-ingredient: ***Chile:*** Vigofortal; ***Israel:*** Tesopalmed Forte cum Yohimbine; ***Pol.:*** Cardiamid-Coffein; ***Thai.:*** Hemo-Cyto-Serum.

Sufentanil

Other names: R-30730; Sufentaniili; Sufentanilis; Sufentanilo; Sufentanilum; Szufentanil.

Суфентанил

Sufentanil Citrate

Other names: Citrato de sufentanilo; R-33800; Sufentaniilisitraatti; Sufentanil citrát; Sufentanil, citrate de; Sufentanil Sitrat; Sufentanilcitrat; Sufentanili citras; Sufentanilio citratas; Szufentanil-citrát.

Суфентанила Цитрат

Clinical profile: Sufentanil, a phenylpiperidine derivative, is a short-acting opioid analgesic related to fentanyl. It is used as an analgesic adjunct in anaesthesia and as a primary anaesthetic agent.

WADA Status: Banned in competition

WADA Class: Narcotics

Includes specified narcotics.

Preparations
Single ingredient: ***Arg.:*** Sufenta; ***Austria:*** Sufenta; ***Belg.:*** Sufenta; ***Braz.:*** Fastfen; Sufenta; ***Canad.:*** Sufenta; ***Chile:*** Sufenta; ***Cz.:*** Sufenta; ***Denm.:*** Sufenta; ***Fin.:*** Sufenta; ***Fr.:*** Sufenta; ***Ger.:*** Sufenta; ***Indon.:*** Sufenta; ***Ital.:*** Disufen; Fentatienil; ***Malaysia:*** Sufenta; ***Neth.:*** Sufenta; ***Norw.:*** Sufenta; ***S.Afr.:*** Sufenta; ***Swed.:*** Sufenta; ***Switz.:*** Sufenta; ***Turk.:*** Sufenta.

Suprarenal Cortex

Other names: Corteza suprarrenal.

Clinical profile: Suprarenal cortex was formerly used for the treatment of Addison's disease. It has largely been superseded by hydrocortisone and other corticosteroids. Suprarenal cortex is an ingredient of a wide range of preparations, often with other organ extracts or vitamins, promoted for indications ranging from asthenia to liver disorders.

WADA Status: Banned in competition

WADA Class: Glucocorticosteroids

All glucocorticosteroids are prohibited when administered orally, rectally, intravenously or intramuscularly. Their use requires a Therapeutic Use Exemption approval. Other routes of administration (intraarticular / periarticular / peritendinous / epidural / intradermal injections and inhalation) require an Abbreviated Therapeutic Use Exemption except as noted below.

Topical preparations when used for dermatological (including iontophoresis / phonophoresis), auricular, nasal, ophthalmic, buccal, gingival and perianal disorders are not prohibited and do not require any form of Therapeutic Use Exemption.

WADA Class: Specified Substances

Also listed as a specified substance.

"The prohibited List may identify specified substances which are particularly susceptible to unintentional anti-doping rule violations because of their general availability in medicinal products or which are less likely to be successfully abused as doping agents."

A doping violation involving such substances may result in a reduced sanction provided that the "*...Athlete can establish that the Use of such a specfied substance was not intended to enhance sport performance...*"

Preparations

Multi-ingredient: ***Austria:*** Mobilat; ***Belg.:*** Mobilat; ***Braz.:*** Mobilat; ***Canad.:*** ratio-Heracline; ***Chile:*** Mobilat; ***Cz.:*** Mobilat; ***Fin.:*** Mobilat; ***Philipp.:*** Mobilat; ***Pol.:*** Mobilat; ***Thai.:*** Mobilat.

Sympathomimetics

Clinical profile: Sympathomimetics are direct or indirect agonists at postganglionic (adrenergic) receptors and have actions that mimic stimulation of the sympathetic nervous system. Alpha agonists and $beta_1$ agonists are used in cardiovascular medicine, for example to maintain the blood pressure and provide inotropic support in shock and acute heart failure. Alpha agonists are also used in nasal congestion and eye disorders. $Beta_2$ agonists are used as bronchodilators and uterine relaxants. Sympathomimetics with CNS effects are used as central stimulants.

WADA Status: Banned in competition

WADA Class: Stimulants

Includes stimulants or substances with a similar chemical structure or similar biological effect(s).

S

WADA Class: Specified Substances

Also listed as a specified substance.

"*The prohibited List may identify specified substances which are particularly susceptible to unintentional anti-doping rule violations because of their general availability in medicinal products or which are less likely to be successfully abused as doping agents.*"

A doping violation involving such substances may result in a reduced sanction provided that the "*...Athlete can establish that the Use of such a specfied substance was not intended to enhance sport performance...*"

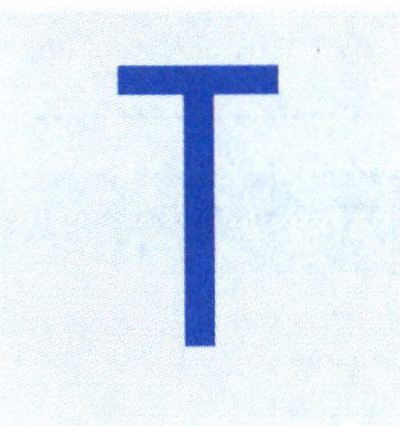

Talinolol

Other names: Talinololum.

Талинолол

Clinical profile: Talinolol is a cardioselective beta blocker used in the management of hypertension and other cardiovascular disorders.

WADA Status: Banned in and out of competition as specified below

WADA Class: Beta-Blockers

Unless otherwise specified, beta-blockers are prohibited *In-Competition* only in the following sports.

- Aeronautics (FAI)
- Archery (FITA, IPC) (also prohibited *Out-of-Competition*)
- Automobile (FIA)
- Billiards (WCBS)
- Bobsleigh (FIBT)
- Boules (CMSB, IPC bowls)
- Bridge (FMB)
- Curling (WCF)
- Gymnastics (FIG)
- Motorcycling (FIM)
- Modern Pentathlon (UIPM) for disciplines involving shooting
- Nine-pin bowling (FIQ)
- Powerboating (UIM)
- Sailing (ISAF) for match race helms only
- Shooting (ISSF, IPC) (also prohibited *Out-of-Competition*)
- Skiing/Snowboarding (FIS) in ski jumping, freestyle aerials/halfpipe and snowboard halfpipe/big air
- Wrestling (FILA)

WADA Class: Specified Substances

Also listed as a specified substance.

"*The prohibited List may identify specified substances which are particularly susceptible to unintentional anti-doping rule violations because of their general availability in medicinal products or which are less likely to be successfully abused as doping agents.*"

A doping violation involving such substances may result in a reduced sanction provided that the "*...Athlete can establish that the Use of such a specfied substance was not intended to enhance sport performance...*"

Preparations
Single ingredient: ***Cz.:*** Cordanum; ***Ger.:*** Cordanum; ***Rus.:*** Cordanum (Корданум).

Tamoxifen Citrate

Other names: Citrato de tamoxifeno; ICI-46474; Tamoksifeenisitraatti; Tamoksifen Sitrat; Tamoksifeno citratas; Tamoxifen citrát; Tamoxifencitrat; Tamoxifén-citrát; Tamoxifène, citrate de; Tamoxifeni citras.

Тамоксифена Цитрат

Clinical profile: Tamoxifen is an anti-oestrogen which is given in the treatment of advanced breast cancer and the adjuvant treatment of early breast cancer as well as for prophylaxis in women at high risk. It has been tried in some other malignancies. It is also used in the treatment of anovulatory infertility.

WADA Status: Banned in and out of competition

WADA Class: Hormone Antagonists and Modulators
Includes selective estrogen receptor modulators.

Preparations
Single ingredient: ***Arg.:*** Crisafeno; Diemon; Ginarsan; Nolvadex; Rolap; Tamoxis; Taxfeno; Trimetrox; ***Austral.:*** Genox; Nolvadex; Tamosin; Tamoxen; ***Austria:*** Ebefen; Kessar; Nolvadex; Tamax; Tamoplex; ***Belg.:*** Doctamoxifene; Nolvadex; Tamizam; Tamoplex; ***Braz.:*** Bioxifeno; Estrocur; Kessar; Nolvadex; Tamoplex; Tamox; Tamoxin; Taxofen; Tecnotax; ***Canad.:*** Apo-Tamox; Nolvadex; Tamofen; ***Chile:*** Kessar; Nolvadex; Oncotamox; Taxus; ***Cz.:*** Nolvadex; Tamifen; Zitazonium; ***Fin.:*** Tadex; Tamexin; Tamofen; ***Fr.:*** Kessar; Nolvadex; ***Ger.:*** Jenoxifen; Mandofen; Nolvadex; Nourytam; Tamokadin; Tamox; Tamoximerck; Tamoxistad; ***Gr.:*** Adifen; Kessar; Nolvadex; Puretam; Tamoplex; Zymoplex; ***Hong Kong:*** Apo-Tamox; Nolvadex; Novofen; Zitazonium; ***Hung.:*** Zitazonium; ***India:*** Caditam; Cytotam; Mamofen; Nolvadex; ***Indon.:*** Nolvadex; Tamofen; Tamoplex; Taxen; ***Irl.:*** Nolvadex; Tamox; ***Israel:*** Nolvadex; Tamofen; Tamoxen; Tamoxi; ***Ital.:*** Kessar; Nolvadex; Nomafen; Tamoxene; ***Malaysia:*** Genox; Nolvadex; Novofen; Tamoplex; Zitazonium; ***Mex.:*** Bilem; Cryoxifeno; Fenobest; Nolvadex; Ralsifen-X; Taxus; Tecnofen; ***Neth.:*** Nolvadex; ***Norw.:*** Nolvadex; ***NZ:*** Genox; Nolvadex; Tamofen; ***Philipp.:*** Fenahex; Gynatam; Gyraxen; Kessar; Nolvadex; Tamoplex; Tamoxsta; Zitazonium; ***Pol.:*** Nolvadex; ***Port.:*** Nolvadex; Tamoxan; ***Rus.:*** Tamifen (Тамифен); Zitazonium (Зитазониум); ***S.Afr.:*** Kessar; Neophedan; Nolvadex; Tamoplex; ***Singapore:*** Apo-Tamox; Nolvadex; Tamofen; ***Spain:*** Nolvadex; Yacesal; ***Swed.:*** Nolvadex; ***Switz.:*** Nolvadex; Tamec; ***Thai.:*** Bilem; Gynatam; Nolvadex; Novofen; Tamoplex; Tuosomin; Zitazonium; ***Turk.:*** Nolvadex; Tadex; Tamofen; ***UAE:*** Tamophar; ***UK:*** Nolvadex; Soltamox; ***USA:*** Soltamox; ***Venez.:*** Gynatam; Nolvadex; Taxus.

Teclothiazide Potassium

Other names: Kalii Teclothiazidum; Téclothiazide Potassique; Teclotiazida potásica; Tetrachlormethiazide Potassium.

Калия Теклотиазид

Clinical profile: Teclothiazide potassium is a thiazide diuretic used in the treatment of oedema.

WADA Status: Banned in and out of competition

WADA Class: Diuretics and Other Masking Agents
Includes diuretics or substances with a similar chemical structure or similar biological effect(s)

Preparations
Multi-ingredient: ***Spain:*** Quimodril.

Tefazoline

Other names: Tefazolina; Téfazoline; Tefazolinum; Tenaphtoxaline.

Тефазолин

Clinical profile: Tefazoline is a sympathomimetic agent related to naphazoline that has been used as a nasal decongestant.

WADA Status: Banned in competition

WADA Class: Stimulants

Includes stimulants or substances with a similar chemical structure or similar biological effect(s). Tefazoline is an imidazole derivative. Imidazole derivatives for topical use are exempt.

Tenamfetamine

Other names: MDA; Methylenedioxyamphetamine; 3,4-Methylenedioxyamphetamine; SKF-5; Ténamfétamine; Tenamfetaminum; Tenanfetamina.

Тенамфетамин

Clinical profile: Tenamfetamine is a phenylethylamine compound, structurally related to amfetamine and mescaline, with hallucinogenic effects. It has been subject to abuse and dependence.

WADA Status: Banned in competition

WADA Class: Stimulants

Includes tenamfetamine and any optical isomers.

T

Terbutaline Sulfate

Other names: KWD-2019; Sulfato de terbutalina; Terbutaliinisulfaatti; Terbutalin Sülfat; Terbutaline, sulfate de; Terbutaline Sulphate; Terbutalini sulfas; Terbutalino sulfatas; Terbutalinsulfat; Terbutalin-sulfát; Terbutalin-szulfát.

Тербуталина Сульфат

Clinical profile: Terbutaline sulfate is a direct-acting sympathomimetic with a selective action on beta$_2$ adrenoceptors, used as a bronchodilator in the management of respiratory disorders such as asthma and chronic obstructive pulmonary disease. It is also given to arrest premature labour.

WADA Status: Banned in and out of competition

WADA Class: Beta-2 Agonists

Includes beta-2 agonists or their isomers. Terbutaline when administered by inhalation requires an abbreviated Therapeutic Use Exemption.

WADA Class: Specified Substances

Also listed as a specified substance.

"The prohibited List may identify specified substances which are particularly susceptible to

unintentional anti-doping rule violations because of their general availability in medicinal products or which are less likely to be successfully abused as doping agents."

A doping violation involving such substances may result in a reduced sanction provided that the "*...Athlete can establish that the Use of such a specfied substance was not intended to enhance sport performance...*"

Preparations

Single ingredient: ***Arg.:*** Bricanyl; ***Austral.:*** Bricanyl; ***Austria:*** Bricanyl; ***Belg.:*** Bricanyl; ***Braz.:*** Bricanyl; ***Canad.:*** Bricanyl; ***Cz.:*** Bricanyl; ***Denm.:*** Bricanyl; ***Fin.:*** Bricanyl; ***Fr.:*** Bricanyl; ***Ger.:*** Aerodur; Bricanyl; Contimit; Terbul; ***Gr.:*** Bricanyl; Dracanyl; ***Hong Kong:*** Ataline; Bricanyl; Dhatalin; Lanterbine; Terbron; Terbuta; Vida-Butaline; ***Hung.:*** Bricanyl; ***India:*** Bricanyl; ***Indon.:*** Astherin; Brasmatic; Bricasma; Forasma; Lasmalin; Nairet; Pulmobron; Relivan; Sedakter; Tabas; Terasma; Tismalin; Yarisma; ***Irl.:*** Bricanyl; ***Israel:*** Bricalin; Terbulin; ***Ital.:*** Bricanyl; ***Malaysia:*** Ataline; Bricanyl; Bucanil; Butaline; ***Mex.:*** Terbuken; ***Neth.:*** Bricanyl; Terbasmin; ***Norw.:*** Bricanyl; ***NZ:*** Bricanyl; ***Philipp.:*** Alloxygen; Astebron; Bricanyl; Bronchodam; Pulmonyl; Pulmoxcel; Terbulin; ***Port.:*** Bricanyl; ***S.Afr.:*** Bricanyl; ***Singapore:*** Ataline; Bricanyl; ***Spain:*** Tedipulmo; Terbasmin; ***Swed.:*** Bricanyl; ***Switz.:*** Bricanyl; ***Thai.:*** Asmaline; Asthmasian; Bricanyl; Broncholine; Bronchonyl; Bronco Asmo; Bucaril; Cencanyl; Proasma-T; Sulterline; Terbulin; Terbuno; Tolbin; ***Turk.:*** Bricanyl; ***UK:*** Bricanyl; ***USA:*** Brethine.

Multi-ingredient: ***Austria:*** Bricanyl comp; ***Braz.:*** Bricanyl Composto; ***India:*** Ascoril +; Ascoril +; Asmotone Plus; Bricarex; Bro-Zedex; Bronchosolvin; Cof QX; Grilinctus-BM; Mucosol; Okaril Plus; Tergil-T; Tergil; Terpect; Terpect; Terphylate; Terphylin; Theobric; Toscof; Tuspel Plus; ***Indon.:*** Bricasma Expectorant; Terasma Expectorant; ***Irl.:*** Bricanyl Expectorant; ***Mex.:*** Bricanyl EX; ***Philipp.:*** Bricanyl Expectorant; ***S.Afr.:*** Benylin Bronchospect; Bronchoped; ***Spain:*** Terbasmin Expectorante; ***Thai.:*** Cofbron; Tolbin.

Tertatolol Hydrochloride

T

Other names: Hidrocloruro de tertatolol; S-2395 (tertatolol or tertatolol hydrochloride); SE-2395 (tertatolol or tertatolol hydrochloride); Tertatolol, Chlorhydrate de; Tertatololi Hydrochloridum.

Тертатолола Гидрохлорид

Clinical profile: Tertatolol is a non-cardioselective beta blocker used in the management of hypertension.

WADA Status: Banned in and out of competition as specified below

WADA Class: Beta-Blockers

Unless otherwise specified, beta-blockers are prohibited *In-Competition* only in the following sports.

- Aeronautics (FAI)
- Archery (FITA, IPC) (also prohibited *Out-of-Competition*)
- Automobile (FIA)
- Billiards (WCBS)
- Bobsleigh (FIBT)
- Boules (CMSB, IPC bowls)
- Bridge (FMB)
- Curling (WCF)
- Gymnastics (FIG)
- Motorcycling (FIM)
- Modern Pentathlon (UIPM) for disciplines involving shooting
- Nine-pin bowling (FIQ)
- Powerboating (UIM)
- Sailing (ISAF) for match race helms only
- Shooting (ISSF, IPC) (also prohibited *Out-of-Competition*)
- Skiing/Snowboarding (FIS) in ski jumping, freestyle aerials/halfpipe and snowboard halfpipe/big air
- Wrestling (FILA)

WADA Class: Specified Substances

Also listed as a specified substance.

"*The prohibited List may identify specified substances which are particularly susceptible to unintentional anti-doping rule violations because of their general availability in medicinal*

products or which are less likely to be successfully abused as doping agents."

A doping violation involving such substances may result in a reduced sanction provided that the "...*Athlete can establish that the Use of such a specfied substance was not intended to enhance sport performance...*"

Preparations
Single ingredient: ***Denm.:*** Artexal; ***Fr.:*** Artex; ***Irl.:*** Artexal; ***Neth.:*** Artex; ***Port.:*** Artex.

Testis Extracts

Other names: Extractos testiculares; Testicular Extracts.

Тестикулярный Экстракт

Clinical profile: Testis extracts are usually of bovine origin and have been used in a variety of disorders. They have been given to elderly men as androgenic supplements. They have also been used topically, often in preparations containing other mammalian tissue extracts, in the treatment of peripheral circulatory or musculoskeletal disorders.

WADA Status: Banned in and out of competition

WADA Class: Anabolic; Androgenic Steroids (endogenous)

Includes endogenous anabolic androgenic steroids or specified metabolites or isomers.

Preparations
Multi-ingredient: ***Canad.:*** ratio-Heracline; ***Hong Kong:*** Wari-Procomil.

Testolactone

T

Other names: 1-Dehydrotestololactone; NSC-23759; SQ-9538; Testolactona; Testolactonum; Testolakton; Testolaktoni.

Тестолактон

Clinical profile: Testolactone is a derivative of testosterone and it has been used in the palliative treatment of breast cancer in postmenopausal women. It is reported to be an aromatase inhibitor but has no significant androgenic activity.

WADA Status: Banned in and out of competition

WADA Class: Hormone Antagonists and Modulators

Includes aromatase inhibitors.

Testosterone

Other names: Testosteron; Testosterona; Testosteronas; Testostérone; Testosteroni; Testosteronum; Tesztoszteron.

Тестостерон

Testosterone Cipionate

Other names: Cipionato de testosterona; Testostérone, Cipionate de; Testosterone Cyclopentylpropionate; Testosterone Cypionate; Testosteroni Cipionas.

Тестостерона Ципионат

Testosterone Decanoate

Other names: Decanoato de testosterona; Testosteron Dekanoat; Testostérone, décanoate de; Testosteroni decanoas.

Тестостерона Деканоат

Testosterone Enantate

Other names: Enantato de testosterona; NSC-17591; Testosteron enantát; Testostérone, enantate de; Testosterone Enanthate; Testosterone Heptanoate; Testosterone Heptylate; Testosteronenantat; Testosteroni enantas; Testosteronienantaatti; Testosterono enantatas; Testosteronu enantan; Tesztoszteronönantát.

Тестостерона Энантат

Testosterone Isocaproate

Other names: Isocaproato de testosterona; Testosteron Isokaproat; Testostérone, isocaproate de; Testosterone Isohexanoate; Testosteroni isocaproas.

Тестостерона Изокапронат

Testosterone Phenylpropionate

Other names: Fenilpropionato de testosterona; Testosteron Fenilpropiyonat; Téstosterone, Phénylpropionate de; Testosteroni Phenylpropionas.

Тестостерона Фенилпропионат

Testosterone Propionate

Other names: NSC-9166; Propionato de testosterona; Testosteron Propiyonat; Testostérone, propionate de; Testosteroni propionas; Testosteronipropionaatti; Testosterono propionatas; Testosteronpropionat; Testosteron-propionát; Testosteronu propionian; Tesztoszteronpropionát.

Тестостерона Пропионат

Testosterone Undecylate

Other names: Org-538; Testosteron Undekanoat; Testosterone Undecanoate; Testostérone, Undécylate de; Testosteroni Undecylas; Undecilato de testosterona.

Тестостерона Ундесилат

Clinical profile: Testosterone is the main androgenic hormone formed in the testes. It is administered as testosterone or one of its esters in replacement therapy for the treatment of male hypogonadism. It has also been used in boys with delayed puberty, in some postmenopausal disorders, and in the management of breast cancer in postmenopausal women.

WADA Status: Banned in and out of competition

WADA Class: Anabolic; Androgenic Steroids (endogenous)

Includes endogenous anabolic androgenic steroids or specified metabolites or isomers.

Preparations

Single ingredient: ***Arg.:*** Androlone; Androtag; Nebido; Sustanon 250; Testoviron Depot 100; Testoviron Depot 250; Undestor; ***Austral.:*** Andriol; Androderm; Primoteston Depot; Reandron; Sustanon 100; Sustanon 250; Testogel; ***Austria:*** Andriol; Nebido; Reandron; Testoderm; Testoviron 250; ***Belg.:*** AndroGel; Sustanon 250; Testim; Testocaps; ***Braz.:*** Androxon; Deposteron; ***Canad.:*** Andriol; Androderm; AndroGel; Delatestryl; ***Chile:*** Actiser-T; Nebido; Primoniat Depot; Sustenan 250; Sustenan; Testocaps; ***Cz.:*** Agovirin; Sustanon; Undestor; ***Denm.:*** Andriol; Nebido; Restandol; Testogel; Testoviron Depot 135; Testoviron Depot 250; ***Fin.:*** Atmos; Nebido; Panteston; Sustanon 250; Testim; Testogel; ***Fr.:*** AndroGel; Androtardyl; Intrinsa; Nebido; Pantestone; Testopatch; ***Ger.:*** Andriol; Androtop; Nebido; Striant; Testim; Testogel; Testoviron Depot 250; ***Gr.:*** Androderm; Andropatch; Nebido; Restandol; Testim; Testoviron; ***Hong Kong:*** Andriol; Sustanon; Testoviron Depot; ***Hung.:*** Andriol; Nebido; ***India:*** Aquaviron; Nuvir; Sustanon 100; Sustanon 250; Testanon 25; Testanon 50; Testoviron Depot; ***Indon.:*** Andriol Testocaps; Nebido;

Sustanon 250; ***Irl.:*** Andropatch; Nebido; Restandol; Striant; Sustanon 100; Sustanon 250; Testim; Testogel; ***Israel:*** AndroGel; Androxon; Sustanon 250; Testoviron Depot; ***Ital.:*** Andriol; AndroGel; Sustanon; Testim; Testo-Enant; Testogel; Testovis; ***Malaysia:*** Andriol; Jenasteron; ***Mex.:*** Andriol; Nebido; Primoteston Depot; Sostenon; Testoprim-D; ***Neth.:*** Andriol; AndroGel; Nebido; Striant; Sustanon 100; Sustanon 250; Testim; Testogel; ***Norw.:*** Andriol; Atmos; Nebido; Testogel; ***NZ:*** Androderm; Panteston; Primoteston Depot; Sustanon; ***Philipp.:*** Andriol; Nebido; ***Pol.:*** Nebido; Omnadren; Testosteronum Prolongatum; Undestor; ***Port.:*** Andriol; Testogel; Testoviron Depot; ***Rus.:*** Andriol (Андриол); AndroGel (Андрогель); Nebido (Небидо); Omnadren (Омнадрен); ***S.Afr.:*** Androxon; Depotrone; Sustanon 250; ***Singapore:*** Andriol; Sustanon 250; ***Spain:*** Androderm; Numanis; Reandron; Testex; Testim; Testogel; Testoviron Depot 250; ***Swed.:*** Atmos; Nebido; Testim; Testogel; Testoviron Depot; Tostrex; Undestor; ***Switz.:*** Andriol; Androderm; Nebido; Testogel; Testoviron Depot; ***Thai.:*** Andriol; Testoviron Depot; ***Turk.:*** Afro; Sustanon 250; Virigen; ***UK:*** Andropatch; Intrinsa; Nebido; Restandol; Striant; Sustanon 100; Sustanon 250; Testim; Testogel; Testosterone Implants; Tostran; Virormone; ***USA:*** Androderm; AndroGel; Delatestryl; Striant; Testim; Testopel; ***Venez.:*** Andriol; AndroGel; Polysteron 250; Proviron Depot.

Multi-ingredient: ***Braz.:*** Durateston; Estandron P; Trinestril; ***Canad.:*** Climacteron; ***Chile:*** Estandron Prolongado; ***Cz.:*** Folivirin; ***India:*** Mixogen; ***Ital.:*** Facovit; Testoviron; ***Malaysia:*** Sustanon 250; ***Mex.:*** Despamen; Sten; ***Neth.:*** Estandron Prolongatum; ***Norw.:*** Primoteston Depot; ***Port.:*** Sustenon 250; ***S.Afr.:*** Mixogen; Primodian Depot; ***Spain:*** Testoviron Depot 100; ***Thai.:*** Metharmon-F; Primodian Depot; ***Turk.:*** Estandron Prolongatum; ***USA:*** Depo-Testadiol; Depotestogen.

Tetracosactide

Other names: α^{1-24}-Corticotrophin; β^{1-24}-Corticotrophin; Cosyntropin; Tetracosactida; Tétracosactide; Tetracosactido; Tetracosactidum; Tetracosactrin; Tetrakosaktid; Tetrakosaktidi; Tetrakosaktrin; Tetrakozaktidas.

Тетракозактид

Clinical profile: Tetracosactide is a synthetic polypeptide similar to corticotropin. Tetracosactide is used diagnostically to investigate adrenocortical insufficiency. It has also been used for many of the indications for which systemic corticosteroid therapy is indicated, but is now rarely employed for such purposes.

WADA Status: Banned in and out of competition

WADA Class: Hormones and Related Substances: Corticotrophins

Includes corticotrophin or substances with a similar chemical structure or similar biological effect(s), or one of their releasing factors.

Preparations

Single ingredient: ***Austral.:*** Synacthen; ***Austria:*** Synacthen; ***Belg.:*** Synacthen; ***Canad.:*** Cortrosyn; Synacthen Depot; ***Chile:*** Synacthen; ***Cz.:*** Synacthen; ***Denm.:*** Synacthen; ***Fr.:*** Synacthene; ***Ger.:*** Synacthen Depot; Synacthen; ***Gr.:*** Cortrosyn; Nuvacthen; Synacthene; ***Hong Kong:*** Cortrosyn; ***Irl.:*** Synacthen; ***Israel:*** Synacthen; ***Ital.:*** Synacthen; ***Neth.:*** Synacthen; ***NZ:*** Synacthen; ***Port.:*** Synacthen; ***Rus.:*** Synacthen (Синактен); Synacthen Depot (Синактен Депо); ***S.Afr.:*** Synacthen Depot; ***Spain:*** Nuvacthen Depot; ***Swed.:*** Synacthen; ***Switz.:*** Synacthen Depot; Synacthen; ***Thai.:*** Cortrosyn; ***Turk.:*** Synacthen Depot; ***UK:*** Synacthen Depot; Synacthen; ***USA:*** Cortrosyn; ***Venez.:*** Synacthen.

Tetrahydrogestrinone

Other names: THG.

Clinical profile: Tetrahydrogestrinone is a synthetic anabolic steroid that has been subject to abuse in sport.

WADA Status: Banned in and out of competition

WADA Class: Anabolic; Androgenic Steroids (exogenous)

Includes exogenous anabolic androgenic steroids or other substances with a similar chemical structure or similar biological effect(s).

Tetryzoline Hydrochloride

Other names: Hidrocloruro de tetrizolina; Tetrahydrozoline Hydrochloride; Tetrazolin Hidroklorür; Tetrizolino hidrochloridas; Tetrytsoliinihydrokloridi; Tétryzoline, chlorhydrate de; Tetryzolin-hydrochlorid; Tetryzolinhydroklorid; Tetryzolini hydrochloridum.

Тетризолина Гидрохлорид

Clinical profile: Tetryzoline is a sympathomimetic with alpha-adrenergic activity. It is used as a nasal and conjunctival decongestant.

WADA Status: Banned in competition

WADA Class: Stimulants

Includes stimulants or substances with a similar chemical structure or similar biological effect(s). Tetryzoline is an imidazole derivative. Imidazole derivatives for topical use are exempt.

Preparations

Single ingredient: ***Arg.:*** Bano Ocular; Chiosan; Piam; ***Austral.:*** Murine Sore Eyes; Visine Original; ***Belg.:*** Visine; ***Canad.:*** Visine Original; ***Chile:*** Visional Gotas; ***Cz.:*** Rhinal; Tyzine; Vasopos N; Visine; ***Denm.:*** Tyzine; ***Fin.:*** Oftan Starine; Visine; ***Fr.:*** Constrilia; ***Ger.:*** Ophtalmin N; Rhinex mit Tetryzolin; Tetrilin; Vasopos N; Visine Yxin; ***Gr.:*** Ursa-Fin; Visine; ***Hong Kong:*** Optizoline; Visine Original; ***Hung.:*** Tyzine; Visine; ***India:*** Visine; ***Indon.:*** Braito; Insto; Isotic Clearin; Visine; Visolin; Visto; ***Israel:*** Azoline; Stilla; V-Zoline; Visine; ***Ital.:*** Demetil; Octilia; Stilla Decongestionante; Vasorinil; Visine; ***Malaysia:*** Visine; ***Mex.:*** Eye-Mo; Tetrazol; ***NZ:*** Visine; ***Philipp.:*** Eye-Mo; Sinutab NS; Visine Advanced Relief; Visine Cool; Visine; ***Pol.:*** Berberil; Starazolin; Tetryvil; Visine; ***Port.:*** Visine; ***Rus.:*** Octilia (Октилия); Tyzine (Тизин); Visine (Визин); ***S.Afr.:*** Visine; ***Singapore:*** Visine; ***Spain:*** Azulina; Vispring; ***Switz.:*** Rhinopront Top; Visine; ***Thai.:*** Visine; ***Turk.:*** Burnil; Eye-Visol; Visine; Zenkain; ***USA:*** Eye Drops; Eye-Zine; Optigene 3; Tyzine; Visine Original.

Multi-ingredient: ***Arg.:*** Antiflogol; Efemolina; Larsimal; Provisual Compuesto; Toflam; Visine Plus; Visubril; ***Austral.:*** In A Wink Allergy; Visine Advanced Relief; Visine Allergy; Visine Revive; ***Braz.:*** Fenidex; Mirabel; Vislin; Visodin; Visolux; ***Canad.:*** Visine Advance Triple Action; Visine Allergy; Visine Cool; ***Chile:*** Spersallerg; ***Cz.:*** Spersallerg; ***Ger.:*** Allergopos N; Berberil N; Efemolin; Spersallerg; ***Gr.:*** Spersallerg; ***Hong Kong:*** Efemoline; Spersallerg; Visine AC; Visine Moisturizing; ***Hung.:*** Spersallerg; ***Indon.:*** Visine Extra; ***Israel:*** Visine AC; ***Ital.:*** Biorinil; Cromozil; Dexoline; Efemoline; Eta Biocortilen VC; Flumezina; Ischemol A; Stillergy; Tetramil; Vasosterone Antibiotico; Vasosterone Collirio; Vasosterone; Visublefarite; Visucloben Decongestionante; Visumetazone Antibiotico; Visumetazone Decongestionante; Visustrin; ***Malaysia:*** Efemoline; Gentadexa; Spersadexoline; Spersallerg; ***Mex.:*** Fluorometil; Visine Extra; ***Norw.:*** Spersallerg; ***NZ:*** Visine Advanced Relief; ***Philipp.:*** Efemoline; Spersallerg; ***Pol.:*** Spersallerg; ***Port.:*** Gentadexa; Medrivas Antibiotico; ***Rus.:*** Spersallerg (Сперсаллерг); ***S.Afr.:*** Efemoline; Gemini; Oculerge; Spersadexoline; Spersallerg; ***Singapore:*** Efemoline; Spersallerg; ***Spain:*** Fluorvas; Gentadexa; Medrivas Antib; Medrivas; Tivitis; Vasodexa; ***Switz.:*** Collypan; Efemoline; Spersallerg; ***Thai.:*** Antazallerge; Efemoline; Histaoph; Mano; Opsil-A; Spersadexoline; Spersallerg; ***Turk.:*** Efemoline; Flumetol; ***USA:*** Advanced Relief Visine; Murine Plus; Visine Allergy Relief; ***Venez.:*** Gentidexa.

Theodrenaline Hydrochloride

Other names: H-8352; Hidrocloruro de teodrenalina; Noradrenaline Theophylline Hydrochloride; Théodrénaline, Chlorhydrate de; Theodrenalini Hydrochloridum.

Теодреналина Гидрохлорид

Clinical profile: Theodrenaline is mainly used in preparations with cafedrine promoted for the treatment of hypotension.

WADA Status: Banned in competition

WADA Class: Stimulants

Includes stimulants or substances with a similar chemical structure or similar biological effect(s).

WADA Class: Specified Substances

Also listed as a specified substance.

"The prohibited List may identify specified substances which are particularly susceptible to unintentional anti-doping rule violations because of their general availability in medicinal products or which are less likely to be successfully abused as doping agents."

A doping violation involving such substances may result in a reduced sanction provided that the "*...Athlete can establish that the Use of such a specfied substance was not intended to enhance sport performance...*"

Preparations
Multi-ingredient: ***Austria:*** Akrinor; ***Fr.:*** Praxinor; ***S.Afr.:*** Akrinor.

Tibolone

Other names: 7α-Methylnorethynodrel; Org-OD-14; Tibolon; Tibolona; Tiboloni; Tibolonum.

Тиболон

Clinical profile: Tibolone is a steroid derived from noretynodrel that has oestrogenic, progestogenic, and weak androgenic properties. It is used in the treatment of menopausal symptoms and for osteoporosis prophylaxis.

T

WADA Status: Banned in and out of competition

WADA Class: Other Anabolic Agents

Includes other anabolic agents not listed elsewhere.

Preparations
Single ingredient: ***Arg.:*** Climatix; Discretal; Paraclim; Senalina; Tiboclim; Tibofem; Tirovarina; Tocline; ***Austral.:*** Livial; ***Austria:*** Liviel; ***Belg.:*** Livial; ***Braz.:*** Libiam; Livial; Livolon; Reduclim; Tibial; ***Chile:*** Climafen; Lirex; Livial; Plenovid; Tinox; Tobe; ***Cz.:*** Livial; ***Denm.:*** Livial; ***Fin.:*** Livial; ***Fr.:*** Livial; ***Ger.:*** Liviella; ***Gr.:*** Livial; ***Hong Kong:*** Livial; ***Hung.:*** Livial; ***India:*** Livial; Tibofem; Tibomax; ***Indon.:*** Livial; ***Irl.:*** Livial; ***Israel:*** Livial; ***Ital.:*** Livial; ***Malaysia:*** Livial; ***Mex.:*** Livial; ***Neth.:*** Livial; ***Norw.:*** Livial; ***NZ:*** Livial; ***Philipp.:*** Livial; ***Pol.:*** Livial; ***Rus.:*** Livial (Ливиал); ***S.Afr.:*** Livifem; ***Singapore:*** Livial; ***Spain:*** Boltin; ***Swed.:*** Livial; ***Switz.:*** Livial; ***Thai.:*** Livial; ***Turk.:*** Livial; ***UK:*** Livial; ***Venez.:*** Femsel; Fomene; Livial; Tinox.

Tienilic Acid

Other names: Acide Tiénilique; Ácido tienílico; Acidum Tienilicum; SKF-62698; Ticrynafen; Tieniilihappo; Tienilsyra.

Тиениловая Кислота

Clinical profile: Tienilic acid is a diuretic that was formerly used in the treatment of oedema and hypertension. It was withdrawn from the market because of reports of severe, sometimes fatal, liver damage.

WADA Status: Banned in and out of competition

WADA Class: Diuretics and Other Masking Agents

Includes diuretics or substances with a similar chemical structure or similar biological effect(s).

Tilisolol Hydrochloride

Other names: Hidrocloruro de tilisolol; N-696; Tilisolol, Chlorhydrate de; Tilisololi Hydrochloridum.

Тилизолола Гидрохлорид

Clinical profile: Tilisolol is a non-cardioselective beta blocker with direct vasodilator activity and has been used in the management of angina pectoris and hypertension.

WADA Status: Banned in and out of competition as specified below

WADA Class: Beta-Blockers

Unless otherwise specified, beta-blockers are prohibited *In-Competition* only in the following sports.

- Aeronautics (FAI)
- Archery (FITA, IPC) (also prohibited *Out-of-Competition*)
- Automobile (FIA)
- Billiards (WCBS)
- Bobsleigh (FIBT)
- Boules (CMSB, IPC bowls)
- Bridge (FMB)
- Curling (WCF)
- Gymnastics (FIG)
- Motorcycling (FIM)
- Modern Pentathlon (UIPM) for disciplines involving shooting
- Nine-pin bowling (FIQ)
- Powerboating (UIM)
- Sailing (ISAF) for match race helms only
- Shooting (ISSF, IPC) (also prohibited *Out-of-Competition*)
- Skiing/Snowboarding (FIS) in ski jumping, freestyle aerials/halfpipe and snowboard halfpipe/big air
- Wrestling (FILA)

WADA Class: Specified Substances

Also listed as a specified substance.

"The prohibited List may identify specified substances which are particularly susceptible to unintentional anti-doping rule violations because of their general availability in medicinal products or which are less likely to be successfully abused as doping agents."

A doping violation involving such substances may result in a reduced sanction provided that the "*...Athlete can establish that the Use of such a specfied substance was not intended to enhance sport performance...*"

Preparations
Single ingredient: ***Jpn:*** Selecal.

Timolol Maleate

Other names: Maleato de timolol; MK-950; Timolol Maleat; Timolol, maléate de; Timolol maleinát; Timololi maleas; Timololimaleaatti; Timololio maleatas; Timolol-maleat; Timolol-maleát.

Тимолола Малеат

Clinical profile: Timolol is a non-cardioselective beta blocker used in the management of glaucoma, hypertension, angina pectoris, and myocardial infarction, and in the prophylaxis of migraine.

WADA Status: Banned in and out of competition as specified below

WADA Class: Beta-Blockers

Unless otherwise specified, beta-blockers are prohibited *In-Competition* only in the following sports.

- Aeronautics (FAI)
- Archery (FITA, IPC) (also prohibited *Out-of-Competition*)
- Automobile (FIA)
- Billiards (WCBS)
- Bobsleigh (FIBT)
- Boules (CMSB, IPC bowls)
- Bridge (FMB)
- Curling (WCF)
- Gymnastics (FIG)
- Motorcycling (FIM)
- Modern Pentathlon (UIPM) for disciplines involving shooting
- Nine-pin bowling (FIQ)
- Powerboating (UIM)
- Sailing (ISAF) for match race helms only
- Shooting (ISSF, IPC) (also prohibited *Out-of-Competition*)
- Skiing/Snowboarding (FIS) in ski jumping, freestyle aerials/halfpipe and snowboard halfpipe/big air
- Wrestling (FILA)

WADA Class: Specified Substances

Also listed as a specified substance.

"*The prohibited List may identify specified substances which are particularly susceptible to unintentional anti-doping rule violations because of their general availability in medicinal products or which are less likely to be successfully abused as doping agents.*"

A doping violation involving such substances may result in a reduced sanction provided that the "*...Athlete can establish that the Use of such a specfied substance was not intended to enhance sport performance...*"

Preparations

Single ingredient: ***Arg.:*** Glatim; Ingetim; Klonalol; Ofal; Plostim; Poentimol; Proflax; Protevis; Timed; Timoler; Timolpres; Timoptic; Zopirol; ***Austral.:*** Nyogel; Tenopt; Timoptol-XE; Timoptol; ***Austria:*** Blocadren; Dispatim; Tim-Ophtal; Timabak; Timax; Timo-COMOD; Timoftal; Timohexal; Timoptic; ***Belg.:*** Blocadren; Nyogel; Nyolol; Timabak; Timo-POS; Timoptol; Timoptolgel; ***Braz.:*** Glautimol; Nyolol; Timabak; Timoptol; ***Canad.:*** Apo-Timol; Apo-Timop; Novo-Timol; Timoptic; ***Chile:*** Glausolets; Nyolol; Timabak; Timop; Timoptol-XE; Tiof; ***Cz.:*** Arutimol; Oftensin; Timo-COMOD; Timogal; Timohexal; Timoptol; ***Denm.:*** Aquanil; Oftamolol; Optimol; Timacar; Timosan; ***Fin.:*** Blocanol; Timosan; ***Fr.:*** Digaol; Nyogel; Ophtim; Timabak; Timacor; Timo-COMOD; Timoptol; ***Ger.:*** Arutimol; Chibro-Timoptol; Dispatim; Nyogel; Tim-Ophtal; Timo-COMOD; Timo-Stulln; TimoEDO; Timohexal; Timomann; ***Gr.:*** Glafemak; Lithimole; Noval; Nyogel; Nyolol; Temserin; Thilotim; Timabak; Yesan; ***Hong Kong:*** Apo-Timop; Nyolol; Oftan; Optimol; Timabak; Timoptol; ***Hung.:*** Arutimol; Cusimolol; Nyolol; Oftan Timolol; ***India:*** Glucomol; Glucotim; Ocupres; Ocutim; Timolo; ***Indon.:*** Isotic Adretor; Kentimol; Nyolol; Tim-Ophtal; Ximex Opticom; ***Irl.:*** Nyogel; Timoptol; ***Israel:*** Nyolol; Tiloptic; V-Optic; ***Ital.:*** Blocadren; Cusimolol; Droptimol; Ialutim; Nyogel; Oftimolo; Timolabak; Timolux; Timoptol; Timosoft; ***Jpn:*** Timoptol; ***Malaysia:*** Cusimolol; Nyolol; Timo-COMOD; Timoptol; ***Mex.:*** Blocadren; Horex; Imot; Jertz; Nyolol; Shemol; Timoptol; Timozzard; ***Mon.:*** Nyolol; ***Neth.:*** Nyogel; Timo-COMOD; Timoptol; ***Norw.:*** Aquanil; Blocadren; Oftamolol; Oftan; Timosan; ***NZ:*** Apo-Timol; Apo-Timop; Hypermol; Tilmat; Timolux; Timoptol; ***Philipp.:*** Elevex; Glocure-Opta; Nyolol; Oftan; Timabak; Timoptol; ***Pol.:*** Cusimolol; Nyolol; Oftan; Oftensin; Timo-Comod; Timohexal; Timoptic; ***Port.:*** Blocadren; Cusimolol; Nyogel; Nyolol; Timoglau; Timolen; Timoptol; ***Rus.:*** Arutimol (Арутимол); Glymol (Глимол); Nyolol (Ниолол); Ocumed (Окумед); Ocupres-E (Окупрес-Е); Oftan Timolol (Офтан Тимолол); Optimol (Оптимол); Timohexal (Тимогексал); ***S.Afr.:*** Glaucosan; Nyogel; Timoptol; ***Singapore:*** Nyolol; Timabak; Timoptol; ***Spain:*** Cusimolol; Nyolol; Timabak; Timoftol; Timogel; ***Swed.:*** Blocadren; Optimol; Timosan; ***Switz.:*** Nyolol; Timisol; Timo-COMOD; Timoptic; ***Thai.:*** Glauco-Oph; Nyolol; Timo-Optal; Timodrop; Timoptol; Timosil; ***Turk.:*** Cusimolol; Nyolol; Timo-COMOD; Timoftal; Timoptic; Timosol; ***UK:*** Betim; Nyogel; Timoptol; ***USA:*** Betimol; Blocadren; Isatol; Istalol; Timoptic; ***Venez.:*** Globitan; Matigel; Matilol; Nyolol; Timoptol.

Multi-ingredient: ***Arg.:*** Combigan; Cosopt; Dorlamida T; Glaucotensil TD; Glaucotensil; Louten T; Ocuprostim; Pilotim; Timed 0.5; Timed D; Xalacom; ***Austral.:*** Cosopt; Timpilo; Xalacom; ***Austria:*** Cosopt; Fotil; Moducrin; Timpilo; Timsopt; Xalacom; ***Belg.:*** Cosopt; Xalacom;

Braz.: Cosopt; Xalacom; ***Canad.:*** Combigan; Cosopt; Xalacom; ***Chile:*** Combigan; Cosopt; Dorsof T; Gaax T; Glaucotensil T; Glausolets Plus; Latof-T; Tiof Plus; Xalacom; ***Cz.:*** Cosopt; Fotil; Timpilo; Xalacom; ***Denm.:*** Cosopt; Fotil; Xalcom; ***Fin.:*** Cosopt; Fotil; Xalcom; ***Fr.:*** Cosopt; Moducren; Pilobloq; Xalacom; ***Ger.:*** Cosopt; Fotil; Moducrin; TP-Ophtal; Xalacom; ***Gr.:*** Combigan; Cosopt; Dropiltim; DuoTrav; Ganfort; T+P; Timpilo; Xalacom; Yvano; ***Hong Kong:*** Cosopt; Moducren; Timpilo; Xalacom; ***Hung.:*** Combigan; Cosopt; DuoTrav; Fotil; Xalacom; ***Indon.:*** Xalacom; ***Irl.:*** Combigan; Cosopt; Moducren; Xalacom; ***Israel:*** Cosopt; Timpilo; Xalacom; ***Ital.:*** Cosopt; Equiton; Glautimol; Pilobloc; Timicon; Xalacom; ***Malaysia:*** Xalacom; ***Mex.:*** Combigan-D; Cosopt; Xalacom; ***Neth.:*** Cosopt; Fotil; Xalacom; ***Norw.:*** Cosopt; Fotil; Xalcom; ***NZ:*** Combigan; Cosopt; DuoTrav; Timpilo; Xalacom; ***Philipp.:*** Cosopt; Fotil; Xalacom; ***Pol.:*** Cosopt; DuoTrav; Fotil; Xalacom; ***Port.:*** Cosopt; Moducren; Timoglau Plus; Xalacom; ***Rus.:*** Fotil (Фотил); Xalacom (Ксалаком); ***S.Afr.:*** Cosopt; Moducren; Servatrin; Xalacom; ***Singapore:*** Cosopt; Xalacom; ***Spain:*** Xalacom; ***Swed.:*** Cosopt; Fotil; Xalcom; ***Switz.:*** Combigan; Cosopt; Moducren; Xalacom; ***Thai.:*** Cosopt; Xalacom; ***Turk.:*** Cosopt; ***UK:*** Combigan; Cosopt; DuoTrav; Ganfort; Moducren; Prestim; Xalacom; ***USA:*** Cosopt; Timolide; ***Venez.:*** Cosopt; Dobet; Glaucotensil T; Xalacom.

Tixocortol Pivalate

Other names: JO-1016; Pivalato de tixocortol; Tixocortol, Pivalate de; Tixocortoli Pivalas.

Тиксокортола Пивалат

Clinical profile: Tixocortol pivalate is a glucocorticoid corticosteroid. It is used as buccal, nasal, throat, and rectal preparations.

WADA Status: Banned in competition

WADA Class: Glucocorticosteroids

All glucocorticosteroids are prohibited when administered orally, rectally, intravenously or intramuscularly. Their use requires a Therapeutic Use Exemption approval. Other routes of administration (intraarticular / periarticular / peritendinous / epidural / intradermal injections and inhalation) require an Abbreviated Therapeutic Use Exemption except as noted below.

Topical preparations when used for dermatological (including iontophoresis / phonophoresis), auricular, nasal, ophthalmic, buccal, gingival and perianal disorders are not prohibited and do not require any form of Therapeutic Use Exemption.

WADA Class: Specified Substances

Also listed as a specified substance.

"*The prohibited List may identify specified substances which are particularly susceptible to unintentional anti-doping rule violations because of their general availability in medicinal products or which are less likely to be successfully abused as doping agents.*"

A doping violation involving such substances may result in a reduced sanction provided that the "*...Athlete can establish that the Use of such a specfied substance was not intended to enhance sport performance...*"

Preparations

Single ingredient: ***Fr.:*** Pivalone; ***Singapore:*** Pivalone; ***Switz.:*** Pivalone.

Multi-ingredient: ***Fr.:*** Thiovalone; ***Switz.:*** Oro-Pivalone; Pivalone compositum.

Torasemide

Other names: AC-4464; BM-02015; Torasemid; Torasemid bezvodý; Torasemid, vattenfri; Torasemida; Torasémide; Torasémide anhydre; Torasemidi; Torasemidi, vedetön; Torasemidum; Torasemidum anhydricum; Torazemidas, bevandenis; Torsemide.

Торасемид

Clinical profile: Torasemide is a loop diuretic used in the treatment of oedema, including that associated with heart failure and with renal and hepatic disorders, and for hypertension.

WADA Status: Banned in and out of competition

WADA Class: Diuretics and Other Masking Agents

Includes diuretics or substances with a similar chemical structure or similar biological effect(s).

Preparations

Single ingredient: ***Arg.:*** Torem; ***Austria:*** Unat; ***Belg.:*** Torrem; ***Cz.:*** Trifas; ***Ger.:*** Toracard; Toragamma; Torasid; Torem; Unat; ***Hong Kong:*** Unat; ***India:*** Dytor; ***Ital.:*** Diuremid; Diuresix; Toradiur; ***Jpn:*** Luprac; ***Pol.:*** Diuver; Trifas; ***Rus.:*** Diuver (Диувер); ***S.Afr.:*** Unat; ***Spain:*** Dilutol; Isodiur; Sutril; Tadegan; ***Swed.:*** Torem; ***Switz.:*** Toramide; Torasem; Torasis; Torem; ***Thai.:*** Unat; ***UK:*** Torem; ***USA:*** Demadex.

Toremifene Citrate

Other names: Citrato de toremifeno; FC-1157a; Toremifen Sitrat; Torémifène, Citrate de; Toremifeni Citras.

Торемифена Цитрат

Clinical profile: Toremifene is an anti-oestrogen that is used in the treatment of breast cancer and is being investigated for lung tumours.

WADA Status: Banned in and out of competition

WADA Class: Hormone Antagonists and Modulators

Includes selective estrogen receptor modulators.

Preparations

Single ingredient: ***Austral.:*** Fareston; ***Austria:*** Fareston; ***Belg.:*** Fareston; ***Cz.:*** Fareston; ***Fin.:*** Fareston; ***Fr.:*** Fareston; ***Ger.:*** Fareston; ***Gr.:*** Fareston; ***Hung.:*** Fareston; ***Irl.:*** Fareston; ***Ital.:*** Fareston; ***Mex.:*** Fareston; ***Neth.:*** Fareston; ***NZ:*** Fareston; ***Port.:*** Fareston; ***Rus.:*** Fareston (Фарестон); ***S.Afr.:*** Fareston; ***Spain:*** Fareston; ***Swed.:*** Fareston; ***Switz.:*** Fareston; ***Thai.:*** Fareston; ***Turk.:*** Fareston; ***UK:*** Fareston; ***USA:*** Fareston.

T

Tosactide

Other names: α^{1-28}-Corticotrophin (human); Octacosactrin; Tosactida; Tosactidum.

Тозактид

Clinical profile: Tosactide is a synthetic polypeptide representing the first 28 amino-acid residues of human corticotropin.

WADA Status: Banned in and out of competition

WADA Class: Hormones and Related Substances: Corticotrophins

Includes corticotrophin or substances with a similar chemical structure or similar biological effect(s), or one of their releasing factors.

Tramazoline Hydrochloride

Other names: Hidrocloruro de tramazolina; Tramazoline, chlorhydrate de; Tramazolin-hidroklorid; Tramazolin-hydrochlorid; Tramazolini hydrochloridum; Tramazolino hidrochloridas; Tramazoliny chlorowodorek.

Трамазолина Гидрохлорид

Clinical profile: Tramazoline hydrochloride is a sympathomimetic used as a nasal and conjunctival decongestant.

WADA Status: Banned in competition

WADA Class: Stimulants

Includes stimulants or substances with a similar chemical structure or similar biological effect(s). Tramazoline is an imidazole derivative. Imidazole derivatives for topical use are exempt.

Preparations

Single ingredient: ***Austral.:*** Spray-Tish; ***Austria:*** Rinorix; ***Belg.:*** Rhinospray; ***Cz.:*** Muconasal Plus; ***Ger.:*** Biciron; Ellatun; Rhinospray; ***Ital.:*** Rinogutt Spray-Fher; ***Neth.:*** Bisolnasal; ***Port.:*** Rhinospray; ***Spain:*** Rhinospray.

Multi-ingredient: ***Arg.:*** Dexa-Rhinospray N; ***Austral.:*** Spray-Tish Menthol; ***Austria:*** Rhinospray Plus; ***Belg.:*** Dexa-Rhinospray; ***Ger.:*** Dexa Biciron; Oxy Biciron; Rhinospray Plus; Rhinospray sensitiv; ***Gr.:*** Dexa-Rhinaspray-N; ***Hung.:*** Rhinospray Plus; ***Irl.:*** Dexa-Rhinaspray Duo; ***Ital.:*** Rinogutt Antiallergico Spray; Rinogutt Eucalipto-Fher; ***Neth.:*** Rhinospray met menthol; ***Rus.:*** Adrianol (Адрианол); ***Spain:*** Rhinospray Antialergico.

Trefentanil

Other names: Tréfentanil; Trefentanilo; Trefentanilum.

Трефентанил

Clinical profile: Trefentanil is an opioid analgesic.

WADA Status: Banned in competition

WADA Class: Narcotics

Includes specified narcotics.

Trenbolone Acetate

Other names: Acetato de trenbolona; RU-1697; Trenbolone, Acétate de; Trenboloni Acetas; Trienbolone Acetate.

Тренболона Ацетат

Clinical profile: Trenbolone acetate has been used as an anabolic agent in veterinary practice.

WADA Status: Banned in and out of competition

WADA Class: Anabolic; Androgenic Steroids (exogenous)

Includes exogenous anabolic androgenic steroids or other substances with a similar chemical structure or similar biological effect(s).

Tretoquinol Hydrochloride

Other names: AQ-110 (tretoquinol); Hidrocloruro de tretoquinol; Ro-07-5965; Trétoquinol, Chlorhydrate de; Tretoquinoli Hydrochloridum; Trimethoquinol Hydrochloride; Trimetoquinol Hydrochloride.

Третоквинола Гидрохлорид

Clinical profile: Tretoquinol is a direct-acting sympathomimetic with a selective action on $beta_2$ adrenoceptors. It has been given as a bronchodilator in the management of respiratory disorders such as asthma and chronic obstructive pulmonary disease.

WADA Status: Banned in and out of competition

WADA Class: Beta-2 Agonists

Includes beta-2 agonists or their isomers.

WADA Class: Specified Substances

Also listed as a specified substance.

"The prohibited List may identify specified substances which are particularly susceptible to unintentional anti-doping rule violations because of their general availability in medicinal products or which are less likely to be successfully abused as doping agents."

A doping violation involving such substances may result in a reduced sanction provided that the "*...Athlete can establish that the Use of such a specfied substance was not intended to enhance sport performance...*"

Preparations
Single ingredient: ***Indon.:*** Inolin.

Triamcinolone

Other names: 9α-Fluoro-16α-hydroxyprednisolone; Fluoxiprednisolonum; Triamcinolon; Triamcinolona; Triamcinolonas; Triamcinolonum; Triamcynolon; Triamsinoloni.

Триамцинолон

Triamcinolone Acetonide

Other names: Acetónido de triamcinolona; Triamcinolon acetonid; Triamcinolonacetonid; Triamcinolone, acétonide de; Triamcinoloni acetonidum; Triamcinolono acetonidas; Triamcynolonu acetonid; Triamsinolon Asetonid; Triamsinoloniasetonidi.

Триамцинолона Ацетонид

Triamcinolone Acetonide Sodium Phosphate

Other names: CL-61965; CL-106359; Fosfato de sodio del acetónido de triamcinolona; Triamcinolone Acétonide, Phosphate Sodique de; Triamcinoloni Acetonidi Natrici Phosphas.

Триамцинолона Ацетонида Натрия Фосфат

Triamcinolone Diacetate

Other names: Diacetato de triamcinolona; Triamcinolone, Diacetate de; Triamcinoloni Diacetas.

Триамцинолона Диацетат

Triamcinolone Hexacetonide

Other names: CL-34433; Hexacetónido de triamcinolona; TATBA; Triamcinolone Acetonide 21-(3,3-Dimethylbutyrate); Triamcinolone, hexacétonide de; Triamcinolonhexacetonid; Triamcinolon-hexacetonid; Triamcinoloni hexacetonidum; Triamcinolono heksacetonidas; Triamsinoloniheksasetonidi.

Триамцинолона Гексасетонид

Clinical profile: Triamcinolone is a glucocorticoid corticosteroid. It has been used, either in the form of the free alcohol or in one of the esterified forms, in the treatment of a wide range of conditions that respond to the anti-inflammatory and immunosuppressant effects of corticosteroid therapy.

WADA Status: Banned in competition

WADA Class: Glucocorticosteroids

All glucocorticosteroids are prohibited when administered orally, rectally, intravenously or intramuscularly. Their use requires a Therapeutic Use Exemption approval. Other routes of administration (intraarticular / periarticular / peritendinous / epidural / intradermal injections and inhalation) require an Abbreviated Therapeutic Use Exemption except as noted below.

Topical preparations when used for dermatological (including iontophoresis / phonophoresis), auricular, nasal, ophthalmic, buccal, gingival and perianal disorders are not prohibited and do not require any form of Therapeutic Use Exemption.

WADA Class: Specified Substances

Also listed as a specified substance.

"The prohibited List may identify specified substances which are particularly susceptible to unintentional anti-doping rule violations because of their general availability in medicinal products or which are less likely to be successfully abused as doping agents."

A doping violation involving such substances may result in a reduced sanction provided that the "*...Athlete can establish that the Use of such a specfied substance was not intended to enhance sport performance...*"

Preparations

Single ingredient: ***Arg.:*** Fortcinolona; Glytop; Kenacort-A; Kenacort; Ledercort; Nasacort; Triamciterap; Triampoen; ***Austral.:*** Aristocort; Kenacort-A; Kenalog in Orabase; Telnase; Tricortone; ***Austria:*** Delphicort; Nasacort; Solu-Volon A; Triamhexal; Volon A; Volon; ***Belg.:*** Albicort; Delphi; Kenacort-A; ***Braz.:*** Airclin; Azmacort; Nasacort; Omcilon A Orabase; Theracort; Triancil; ***Canad.:*** Aristocort; Aristospan; Kenalog in Orabase; Kenalog; Nasacort; Oracort; Triaderm; ***Chile:*** Kenacort-A; Nasacort; ***Cz.:*** Azmacort; Kenalog; Nasacort; Triamcinolon-Galena; ***Denm.:*** Kenalog; Lederspan; Nasacort; ***Fin.:*** Aftab; Kenacort-T; Lederspan; Nasacort; ***Fr.:*** Hexatrione; Kenacort; Nasacort; ***Ger.:*** Aftab; Delphicort; Kortikoid-ratiopharm; Lederlon; Linola Cort Triam; Nasacort; Rhinisan; Triam; TriamCreme; Triamgalen; Triamhexal; TriamSalbe; Volon A; Volon; Volonimat N; Volonimat; ***Gr.:*** Forlion; Kenacort-A; Nasacort; Nasatrim; Triamcinal; ***Hong Kong:*** Aftach; Aristo; Dermacort; Kenacort-A; Kenalog in Orabase; Nasacort; Triam; ***Hung.:*** Ftorocort; Kenalog; Polcortolone; ***India:*** Kenacort; Ledercort; Tess; Tricort; ***Indon.:*** Flamicort; Kenacort-A; Kenacort; Kenalog in Orabase; Ketricin; Nasacort; Triamcort; Tridez; Trilac; Trinolon; ***Irl.:*** Adcortyl in Orabase; Adcortyl; Kenalog; Nasacort; ***Israel:*** Oracort; Sterocort; Steronase Aq; ***Ital.:*** Aftab; Ipercortis; Kenacort; Nasacort; Triacort; Triamvirgi; ***Jpn:*** Aftach; ***Malaysia:*** Dermacort; Kenacort-A; Kenalog in Orabase; Nasacort AQ; Orrepaste; Shincort; ***Mex.:*** Azucort; Intralon; Kenacort; Kenalog Dental; Nasacort; Triamsicort; Zamacort; ***Neth.:*** Kenacort-A; Nasacort; ***Norw.:*** Kenacort-T; Lederspan; Nasacort; ***NZ:*** Aristocort; Kenacort-A; Kenalog in Orabase; Oracort; Telnase; ***Philipp.:*** Kenacort-A; Kenacort; ***Pol.:*** Polcortolon; ***Port.:*** Aftach; ***Rus.:*** Berlicort (Берликорт); Ftorocort (Фторокорт); Kenalog (Кеналог); Polcortolon (Полькортолон); Polcortolon (Полькортолон); Polcortolon TC (Полькортолон TC); Triacort (Триакорт); ***S.Afr.:*** Kenalog in Orabase; Nasacor; ***Singapore:*** Dermacort; Kenacort-A; Kenalog in Orabase; Nasacort; Oramedy; Orrepaste; Shincort; Trinolone; ***Spain:*** Flutenal; Kenalog in Orabase; Nasacort; Proctosteroid; Trigon Depot; ***Swed.:*** Kenacort-T; Lederspan; Nasacort; ***Switz.:*** Kenacort-A Solubile; Kenacort-A; Kenacort; Nasacort; Triamcort; ***Thai.:*** Aristocort; Centocort; Facort; Ftorocort; Generlog; Kanolone; Kela; Kemzid; Kena-Lite; Kenacort; Kenalog in Orabase; Keno; Laver; Manolone; Metoral; Milanolone; Nasacort; Oral-T; Oralog; Orcilone; Risto; Shincort; Simacort; T-1; TA Osoth; Tacinol; Topilone; Tramsilone; Trim; Unif; V-Nolone; Vacinolone; Zyno; ***Turk.:*** Kenacort-A; Nasacort; Sinakort-A; ***UK:*** Adcortyl in Orabase; Adcortyl; Kenalog; Nasacort; ***USA:*** Aristospan; Atolone; Azmacort; Flutex; Kenalog in Orabase; Kenalog; Kenonel; Nasacort; Oralone Dental; Tac; Tri-Kort; Tri-Nasal; Triacet; Triam-A; Triamonide; Triderm; Trilog; ***Venez.:*** Kenacort; Nasacort.

Multi-ingredient: ***Arg.:*** Bagovit A Plus; Biotaer Nasal; Kenacomb; Mantus; Sorsis; ***Austral.:*** Kenacomb; Otocomb Otic; ***Austria:*** Aureocort; Ledermix; Mycostatin V; Neo-Delphicort; Pevisone; Steros-Anal; Volon A antibiotikahaltig; Volon A Tinktur; Volon A-Zinklotion; ***Belg.:*** Mycolog; Pevisone; Trianal; ***Braz.:*** Londerm-N; Neolon-D; Omcilon A M; Onciplus; ***Canad.:*** ratio-Triacomb; Viaderm-KC; ***Cz.:*** Triamcinolon Compositum; Triamcinolon E; Triamcinolon S; Triamcinolon-Galena; Triamcinolon-Galena; ***Denm.:*** Kenacutan; Kenalog Comp med Mycostatin; Kenalog med Salicylsyre; Pevisone; ***Fin.:*** Pevisone; ***Fr.:*** Cidermex; Kenalcol; Localone; Pevisone; ***Ger.:*** Epipevisone; Ledermix; Moronal V; Mykoproct sine; Polcortolon TC; Volon A Tinktur N; Volon A-Schuttelmix; Volonimat Plus N; ***Gr.:*** Kenacomb; Olamyc; Pevison; ***Hong Kong:*** Anso; Clotrinolon; Kenacomb; Oragesic; Pevisone; Tri-Gel; Triacomb; Triconazole; Triditol-G; ***Hung.:*** Alkcema; Polcortolon TC; ***India:*** Kenacomb; Kenalog-S; Ledercort-N; ***Indon.:*** Kenantist; New Kenacomb; ***Irl.:*** Kenacomb; ***Israel:*** Dermacombin; Ledermix; Oracort E; Pevisone; ***Ital.:*** Assocort; Aureocort; Dirahist; Kataval; Pevisone; ***Malaysia:*** Ecocort; Econazine; Kenacomb; Oral-Aid; Pevisone;

Mex.: Bidrozil; Biotriamin; Kenacomb; ***Neth.:*** Mycolog; Trianal; Will-Anal; ***Norw.:*** Kenacort-T comp; Kenacutan; Pevisone; ***NZ:*** Kenacomb; Viaderm-KC; ***Philipp.:*** Kenacomb; Nizolex; Pevisone; ***Pol.:*** Pevisone; Polcortolon TC; Triacomb; ***Port.:*** Kenacomb; Localone; Pevisone; ***S.Afr.:*** Kenacomb; Pevisone; Trialone; ***Singapore:*** Ecocort; Econazine; Oral-Aid; ***Spain:*** Aldoderma; Anasilpiel; Anso; Cemalyt; Cremsol; Flutenal Gentamicina; Flutenal Sali; Interderm; Nesfare; Positon; Trigon Rectal; Trigon Topico; ***Swed.:*** Kenacombin Novum; Kenacort-T comp; Kenacutan; Pevisone; ***Switz.:*** Kenacort-A; Ledermix; Pevisone; ***Thai.:*** Dermacombin; Ecocort; Ecoderm; Fungisil-T; KA-Cilone; Kelaplus; Kenacomb; Tara-Plus; Timi; Tricozole; Trimicon; ***UAE:*** Panderm; ***UK:*** Aureocort; Ledermix; Tri-Adcortyl; ***USA:*** Myco-Biotic II; Myco-Triacet II; Mycogen II; Mycolog-II; Myconel; NGT; Tri-Statin II; ***Venez.:*** Kenacomb; Kenalog.

Triamterene

Other names: NSC-77625; SKF-8542; Triamtereeni; Triamterén; Triamteren; Triamterenas; Triamtérène; Triamtereno; Triamterenum; Triantereno.

Триамтерен

Clinical profile: Triamterene is a weak diuretic with potassium-sparing properties. It is used mainly as an adjunct to thiazide and loop diuretics in the treatment of oedema and hypertension.

WADA Status: Banned in and out of competition

WADA Class: Diuretics and Other Masking Agents

Includes diuretics or substances with a similar chemical structure or similar biological effect(s).

Preparations

Single ingredient: ***Belg.:*** Dytac; ***UK:*** Dytac; ***USA:*** Dyrenium.

Multi-ingredient: ***Austral.:*** Hydrene; ***Austria:*** Confit; Dytide H; Hydrotrix; Salodiur; Triamteren comp; Triastad HCT; Trioral/HCT; ***Belg.:*** Dyta-Urese; Dytenzide; ***Braz.:*** Diurana; Iguassina; ***Canad.:*** Apo-Triazide; Novo-Triamzide; Nu-Triazide; ***Chile:*** Drinamil; Hidroronol T; Uren; ***Fin.:*** Furesis comp; Uretren Comp; ***Fr.:*** Isobar; Prestole; ***Ger.:*** Beta-Turfa; dehydro sanol tri; Diu Venostasin; Diucomb; Diuretikum Verla; Dociteren; Dytide H; Hydrotrix; Neotri; Nephral; Propra comp; Thiazid-comp; Tri-Thiazid; Triampur Compositum; Triamteren comp; Triamteren HCT; Triamteren tri-comp; Triarese; Turfa; Veratide; ***Hong Kong:*** Apo-Triazide; Dyazide; ***India:*** Ditide; ***Irl.:*** Dyazide; ***Ital.:*** Fluss 40; ***Malaysia:*** Apo-Triazide; ***Mex.:*** Dyazide; ***Neth.:*** Dyta-Urese; Dytenzide; ***NZ:*** Triamizide; ***Port.:*** Dyazide; Triam-Tiazida R; ***Rus.:*** Apo-Triazide (Апо-триазид); Triam-Co (Триам-ко); Triampur Compositum (Триампур Композитум); ***S.Afr.:*** Dyazide; Renezide; ***Singapore:*** Apo-Triazide; ***Spain:*** Salidur; ***Switz.:*** Dyazide; Dyrenium compositum; t/hbasan; ***Thai.:*** Dinazide; Dyazide; ***Turk.:*** Triamteril; ***UK:*** Dyazide; Dytide; Frusene; Kalspare; Triamco; ***USA:*** Dyazide; Maxzide.

Trichlormethiazide

Other names: Trichlorméthiazide; Trichlormethiazidum; Triclormetiazida; Trikloorimetiatsidi; Triklormetiazid.

Трихлорметиазид

Clinical profile: Trichlormethiazide is a thiazide diuretic used for oedema, including that associated with heart failure, and for hypertension.

WADA Status: Banned in and out of competition

WADA Class: Diuretics and Other Masking Agents

Includes diuretics or substances with a similar chemical structure or similar biological effect(s).

Preparations
Multi-ingredient: ***Fin.:*** Uretren Comp; ***Spain:*** Rulun.

Tripamide

Other names: ADR-033; E-614; Tripamida; Tripamidum.

Трипамид

Clinical profile: Tripamide is a diuretic structurally related to indapamide and is used in the treatment of hypertension.

WADA Status: Banned in and out of competition

WADA Class: Diuretics and Other Masking Agents

Includes diuretics or substances with a similar chemical structure or similar biological effect(s).

Preparations
Single ingredient: ***Thai.:*** Normonal.

Triptorelin

Other names: AY-25650; BIM-21003; BN-52014; CL-118532; Triptorelina; Triptoréline; Triptoreline; Triptorelinum; D-Trp^{6}-LHRH; [6-D-Tryptophan] luteinising hormone-releasing factor.

Трипторелин

Triptorelin Acetate

Other names: Acetato de triptorelina; Triptoreliiniasetaatti; Triptorelin Asetat; Triptorelinacetat; Triptoréline, Acétate de; Triptorelini Acetas.

Трипторелина Ацетат

Triptorelin Diacetate

Other names: Diacetato de triptorelina; Triptoréline, Diacetate de; Triptorelini Diacetas.

Трипторелина Диацетат

Triptorelin Embonate

Other names: Embonato de triptorelina; Triptorelin Pamoate; Triptoréline, Embonate de; Triptorelini Embonas.

Трипторелина Эмбонат

Clinical profile: Triptorelin is an analogue of gonadorelin used for the suppression of testosterone in the treatment of malignant neoplasms of the prostate, in precocious puberty, and in the management of endometriosis, female infertility, and uterine fibroids.

WADA Status: Banned in and out of competition

WADA Class: Hormones and Related Substances: Gonadotrophins

Includes gonadotrophin or a substance with a similar chemical structure or similar biological effect(s), or one of their releasing factors. Prohibited in males only.

Preparations
Single ingredient: ***Arg.:*** Decapeptyl; Gonapeptyl; ***Austria:*** Decapeptyl; Pamorelin; ***Belg.:*** Decapeptyl; ***Braz.:*** Neo Decapeptyl; ***Chile:*** Decapeptyl; ***Cz.:*** Decapeptyl; Diphereline; ***Denm.:*** Decapeptyl; Pamorelin; ***Fin.:*** Decapeptyl; ***Fr.:*** Decapeptyl; Gonapeptyl; ***Ger.:*** Decapeptyl; Pamorelin; ***Gr.:*** Arvekap; Gonapeptyl; ***Hong Kong:*** Decapeptyl; Diphereline; ***Hung.:*** De-

capeptyl; Diphereline; ***India:*** Decapeptyl; ***Irl.:*** Decapeptyl; Gonapeptyl; ***Israel:*** Decapeptyl; Diphereline; ***Ital.:*** Decapeptyl; Gonapeptyl; ***Malaysia:*** Decapeptyl; ***Neth.:*** Decapeptyl; Gonapeptyl; Pamorelin; ***Pol.:*** Decapeptyl; Diphereline; ***Port.:*** Decapeptyl; ***Rus.:*** Decapeptyl (Декапептил); Diphereline (Диферелин); ***S.Afr.:*** Decapeptyl; ***Singapore:*** Decapeptyl; ***Spain:*** Decapeptyl; Gonapeptyl; ***Swed.:*** Decapeptyl; ***Switz.:*** Decapeptyl; ***Thai.:*** Decapeptyl; Diphereline; ***Turk.:*** Decapeptyl; ***UK:*** Decapeptyl; Gonapeptyl; ***USA:*** Trelstar; ***Venez.:*** Decapeptyl.

Trometamol

Other names: NSC-6365; THAM; Trihydroxymethylaminomethane; TRIS; Tris(hydroksymetylo)aminometan; Tris(hydroxymethyl)aminomethane; Trométamol; Trometamoli; Trometamolis; Trometamolum; Tromethamine.

Трометамол

Clinical profile: Trometamol is an organic amine proton acceptor which is used as an alkalinising agent in the treatment of metabolic acidosis. It also acts as a weak osmotic diuretic. Trometamol is mainly used during cardiac bypass surgery and during cardiac arrest. It may also be used to reduce the acidity of citrated blood for use in bypass surgery. Trometamol citrate is given by mouth for the management of urinary calculi and acidosis.

WADA Status: Banned in and out of competition

WADA Class: Diuretics and Other Masking Agents

Includes diuretics or substances with a similar chemical structure or similar biological effect(s).

Preparations

Single ingredient: ***Austral.:*** Tham; ***Austria:*** Tris; ***Ger.:*** Tham; Tris; ***Ital.:*** Thamesol; ***Swed.:*** Addex-THAM.

Multi-ingredient: ***Arg.:*** Solocalm Plus; ***Fr.:*** Alcaphor; ***Norw.:*** Tribonat; ***Swed.:*** Tribonat.

T

Tuaminoheptane Sulfate

Other names: Sulfato de tuaminoheptano; Tuaminoheptane, Sulfate de; Tuaminoheptane Sulphate; Tuaminoheptani Sulfas.

Туаминогептана Сульфат

Clinical profile: Tuaminoheptane is a volatile sympathomimetic that has been used for the symptomatic relief of nasal congestion.

WADA Status: Banned in competition

WADA Class: Stimulants

Includes tuaminoheptane and any optical isomers.

WADA Class: Specified Substances

Also listed as a specified substance.

"The prohibited List may identify specified substances which are particularly susceptible to unintentional anti-doping rule violations because of their general availability in medicinal products or which are less likely to be successfully abused as doping agents."

A doping violation involving such substances may result in a reduced sanction provided that the "*...Athlete can establish that the Use of such a specfied substance was not intended to enhance sport performance...*"

Preparations

Multi-ingredient: ***Braz.:*** Rinofluimucil; ***Fr.:*** Rhinofluimucil; ***Hong Kong:*** Rinofluimucil; ***Hung.:***

Rinofluimucil; ***Ital.:*** Rinofluimucil; ***Rus.:*** Rinofluimucil (Ринофлуимуцил); ***Spain:*** Rinoflumil; ***Switz.:*** Rinofluimucil; ***Thai.:*** Rinofluimucil.

Tucaresol

Other names: BW-589C; 589C; 589C80; Tucarésol; Tucaresolum.

Тукарезол

Clinical profile: Tucaresol is reported to interact with haemoglobin to increase oxygen affinity and has been investigated for the treatment of sickle-cell disease. It is also reported to have immunostimulant properties.

WADA Status: Banned in and out of competition

WADA Class: Enhancement of Oxygen Transfer: Artificial Enhancers

Includes products that may be used to artificially enhance the uptake, transport, or delivery of oxygen.

Tulobuterol Hydrochloride

Other names: C-78; Hidrocloruro de tulobuterol; HN-078 (tulobuterol); Tulobutérol, Chlorhydrate de; Tulobuterolhydroklorid; Tulobuteroli Hydrochloridum; Tulobuterolihydrokloridi.

Тулобутерола Гидрохлорид

Clinical profile: Tulobuterol is a direct-acting sympathomimetic with a selective action on $beta_2$ adrenoceptors. It is used as a bronchodilator in the management of respiratory disorders such as asthma and chronic obstructive pulmonary disease.

WADA Status: Banned in and out of competition

WADA Class: Beta-2 Agonists

Includes beta-2 agonists or their isomers.

WADA Class: Specified Substances

Also listed as a specified substance.

"The prohibited List may identify specified substances which are particularly susceptible to unintentional anti-doping rule violations because of their general availability in medicinal products or which are less likely to be successfully abused as doping agents."

A doping violation involving such substances may result in a reduced sanction provided that the "*...Athlete can establish that the Use of such a specfied substance was not intended to enhance sport performance...*"

Preparations

Single ingredient: ***Austria:*** Bremax; ***Ger.:*** Atenos; Brelomax; ***Jpn:*** Hokunalin; ***Mex.:*** Bremax; ***Philipp.:*** Bremax; ***Port.:*** Atenos; ***Venez.:*** Bretol.

Tymazoline Hydrochloride

Other names: 2-Thymyloxymethyl-2-imidazoline Hydrochloride; Timazolina, hidrocloruro de; Tymazolini Hydrochloridum; Tymazoliny chlorowodorek.

Clinical profile: Tymazoline hydrochloride is a sympathomimetic with alpha-adrenergic activity that has been used as a nasal decongestant.

WADA Status: Banned in competition

WADA Class: Stimulants

Includes stimulants or substances with a similar chemical structure or similar biological effect(s). Tymazoline is an imidazole derivative. Imidazole derivatives for topical use are exempt.

Preparations
Single ingredient: ***Pol.:*** Thymazen; ***Thai.:*** Pernazene.

Tyramine Hydrochloride

Other names: Tiramina, hidrocloruro de; *p*-Tyramine Hydrochloride; Tyrosamine Hydrochloride.

Clinical profile: Tyramine hydrochloride is a sympathomimetic with indirect effects on adrenergic receptors. It has been given in the tyramine pressor test in the investigation of monoamine oxidase inhibitory activity or of amine uptake blocking activity. It has also been used in studies of physiological and disease states, and in the diagnosis of migraine and phaeochromocytoma.

WADA Status: Banned in competition

WADA Class: Stimulants

Includes stimulants or substances with a similar chemical structure or similar biological effect(s).

WADA Class: Specified Substances

Also listed as a specified substance.
"The prohibited List may identify specified substances which are particularly susceptible to unintentional anti-doping rule violations because of their general availability in medicinal products or which are less likely to be successfully abused as doping agents."
A doping violation involving such substances may result in a reduced sanction provided that the "*...Athlete can establish that the Use of such a specfied substance was not intended to enhance sport performance...*"

T

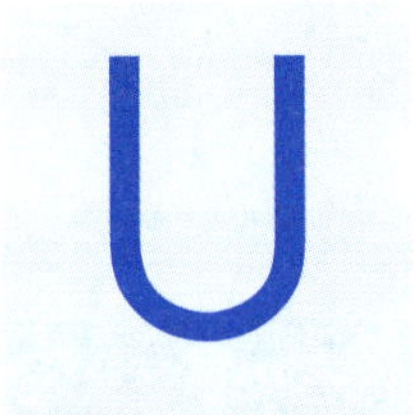

Ulobetasol Propionate

Other names: BMY-30056; CGP-14458; 6-α-Fluoroclobetasol Propionate; Halobetasol Propionate; Propionato de ulobetasol; Ulobétasol, Propionate d'; Ulobetasoli Propionas.

Улобетазола Пропионат

Clinical profile: Ulobetasol propionate is a corticosteroid used topically in the treatment of various skin disorders.

WADA Status: Banned in competition

WADA Class: Glucocorticosteroids

All glucocorticosteroids are prohibited when administered orally, rectally, intravenously or intramuscularly. Their use requires a Therapeutic Use Exemption approval. Other routes of administration (intraarticular / periarticular / peritendinous / epidural / intradermal injections and inhalation) require an Abbreviated Therapeutic Use Exemption except as noted below.

Topical preparations when used for dermatological (including iontophoresis / phonophoresis), auricular, nasal, ophthalmic, buccal, gingival and perianal disorders are not prohibited and do not require any form of Therapeutic Use Exemption.

WADA Class: Specified Substances

Also listed as a specified substance.

"*The prohibited List may identify specified substances which are particularly susceptible to unintentional anti-doping rule violations because of their general availability in medicinal products or which are less likely to be successfully abused as doping agents.*"

A doping violation involving such substances may result in a reduced sanction provided that the "...*Athlete can establish that the Use of such a specfied substance was not intended to enhance sport performance...*"

Preparations
Single ingredient: ***Canad.:*** Ultravate; ***USA:*** Ultravate.

Urea

Other names: Carbamida; Carbamide; E927b; Karbamid; Karbamidi; Močovina; Mocznik; Üre; Urée; Ureia; Urėja; Ureum.

Карбамид; Мочевина

Clinical profile: Urea is an osmotic agent applied topically in the treatment of ichthyosis and hyperkeratotic skin disorders. It has osmotic diuretic properties and is also used intravenously to reduce raised intracranial pressure due to cerebral oedema and raised intraocular pressure in acute glaucoma. Urea has also been given intra-amniotically for the termination of pregnancy. Urea labelled with carbon-13 or carbon-14 is used in breath tests in the diagnosis of *Helicobacter pylori* infection.

WADA Status: Banned in and out of competition

WADA Class: Diuretics and Other Masking Agents

Includes diuretics or substances with a similar chemical structure or similar biological effect(s).

Preparations

Single ingredient: ***Arg.:*** Hidroplus; Keratopic; Lociherp; Nutralcon; Ureadin; Urecrem; Uremol; Xerobase; ***Austral.:*** Aquacare; Hamilton Dry Skin; Nutraplus; Urecare; Urederm; ***Austria:*** Nubral; ***Braz.:*** Emoderm; Hidrapel; Nutraplus; Ureadin; ***Canad.:*** Dermaflex; Ultra Mide; Uree; Uremol; Urisec; ***Chile:*** Ayr con urea; Ayr-5; Hyderm; Uramol; Ureadin 10 and 20; ***Cz.:*** Excipial U; ***Fin.:*** Fenuril; ***Fr.:*** Anti-Dessechement; Nutraplus; Sedagel; ***Ger.:*** Balisa; Basodexan; Elacutan; Hyanit N; Linola Urea; Nubral; Onychomal; Sebexol cum urea; Ureotop; ***Hong Kong:*** Balneum Intensiv; Carmol; Caruderma; Euderm; Urecare; Urederm; ***Hung.:*** Linola Urea; ***Indon.:*** Calmuderm; Carmed; Moisderm; Soft U Derm; Urederm; ***Irl.:*** Aquadrate; Nutraplus; ***Ital.:*** Dermal Care; ***Jpn:*** Keratinamin; ***Malaysia:*** Balneum Intensiv; Nutraplus; UO; ***Mex.:*** Derma-Keri; Dermoplast; Karmosan; Nutraplus; Uramol; ***NZ:*** Aquacare; Nutraplus; ***Philipp.:*** Nutraplus; ***Port.:*** Eucerin Pele Seca; Rebladerm; Ureadin 10 and 20; ***Singapore:*** Aqurea; Balneum Intensiv; Excipial U; Nutraplus; UO; ***Swed.:*** Calmuril; Canoderm; Caress; Fenuril; Karbasal; Monilen; ***Switz.:*** Carbamide Emulsion; Eucerin peau seche; Excipial U; Linola Uree; Nutraplus; ***Thai.:*** Nutraplus; ***Turk.:*** Excipial; Nutraplus; Urederm; ***UK:*** Aquadrate; Nutraplus; ***USA:*** Aquacare; Carmol; Gormel; Hydro 40; Kerafoam; Keralac; Lanaphilic; Nutraplus; Ultra Mide; Umecta; Ureacin; Ureaphil; Vanamide; ***Venez.:*** Aquaphar; Dermisol; Uricrim.

Multi-ingredient: ***Arg.:*** Acilac; Akerat; Aloebel; Cremsor N; Hidrolac; Lactiderm; Lactocrem; Masivol Urea; Oxidermos; Turgent Colageno; Turgent Emulsion; Ureadin Facial; Urecrem Hidro; Vansame; ***Austral.:*** Aussie Tan Skin Moisturiser; Calmurid; Dermadrate; Psor-Asist; ***Austria:*** Aleot; Calmurid HC; Calmurid; Canesten Bifonazol comp; Ichth-Oestren; Keratosis forte; Keratosis; Mirfulan; Optiderm; ***Braz.:*** Donnagel; Oticerim; Oto-Biotic; Tricolpex; Tricomax; Vagi Biotic; Vagi-Sulfa; ***Canad.:*** Amino-Cerv; Hydrophil; Kerasal; Uremol-HC; ***Chile:*** Akerat; Ureadin 30; Ureadin Facial; Ureadin Forte; Ureadin Pediatrics; Ureadin Rx DB; Ureadin Rx PS; Ureadin Rx RD; ***Cz.:*** Betacorton U; Mycospor Sada na Nehty; ***Fin.:*** Calmuril; Wicaran; Wicarba; Wicnecarb; Wicnevit; ***Fr.:*** Akerat; Amycor Onychoset; Body Peel; Charlieu Topicrem; Day Peel; Liperol; Night Peel; PSO; PSO; Topic 10; ***Ger.:*** Balisa VAS; Brand- u. Wundgel-Medice N; Canesten Extra Nagelset; Carbamid + VAS; Fungidexan; Hydrodexan; Mirfulan; Optiderm; Psoradexan; Remederm; Ureotop + VAS; ***Gr.:*** Lyoderm; Urecortin; ***Hong Kong:*** Balneum Intensiv Plus; Dermadrate; ***Hung.:*** Reseptyl-Urea; Squa-med; ***India:*** Cotaryl; ***Indon.:*** Foothy; ***Irl.:*** Alphaderm; Calmurid HC; Calmurid; ***Israel:*** Agispor Onychoset; Calmurid; Derma-Care; Keratospor; U-Lactin Foot Cream; U-Lactin Forte; ***Ital.:*** Altadrine; Ipso Urea; Keraflex; Optiderm; Verunec; Xerial; ***Malaysia:*** Balneum Intensiv Plus; Ucort; ***Mex.:*** Lowila; Mycospor Onicoset; Suavene; Urader Lactato; Ureaderm Lactato; ***Neth.:*** Calmurid HC; Calmurid; Symbial; ***NZ:*** Dermadrate; ***Philipp.:*** Remederm; ***Pol.:*** Hasceral; Keratolit; Mycospor Onychoset; Optiderm; SolcoKerasal; Sterovag; ***Port.:*** Calmurid; Carmitol; Creme Laser Hidrante; Hidratoderme; U Lactin; Ureadin 10 Plus; Ureadin 30; Ureadin Facial; Ureadin Forte; Ureadin Maos; ***Rus.:*** Mycospor (Микоспор); ***S.Afr.:*** Covancaine; Mycospor Onycho-set; ***Singapore:*** Balneum Intensiv Plus; Dermadrate; Topicrem; U-Lactin; ***Spain:*** Cortisdin Urea; Kanapomada; Mycospor Onicoset; ***Swed.:*** Fenuril-Hydrokortison; ***Switz.:*** Acne Gel; Antikeloides Creme; Betacortone; Calmurid; Carbamide + VAS; Carbamide Creme; Kerasal; Klyx Magnum; Optiderm; Sebo Creme; Sebo-Psor; Turexan Capilla; Turexan Lotion; ***Thai.:*** Gynestin; ***Turk.:*** Betacorton; Kerasal; Mycospor; Ureacort; ***UK:*** Alphaderm; Antipeol; Balneum Plus; Calmurid HC; Calmurid; Cymex; E45 Itch Relief; St James Balm; Vesagex Heelbalm; ***USA:*** Accuzyme; AllanEnzyme; AllanEnzyme; AllanfillEnzyme; Amino-Cerv; Ethezyme; Gladase-C; Gladase; Hydrocerin Plus; Kovia; Panafil-White; Panafil; Pap-Urea; Rosula NS; Rosula; Ziox; ***Venez.:*** Akerat; Caduril; Hidribet 5/5; Hidribet; Mycospor Onicoset; Pantonic; Pelset Plus; Ureaderm Lactato.

Urofollitropin

Other names: Ürofolitropin; Urofolitropin; Urofolitropina; Urofolitropinas; Urofollitrophin; Urofollitropiini; Urofollitropine; Urofollitropinum.

Урофоллитропин

Urofollitropin

Clinical profile: Urofollitropin is a gonadotrophin, obtained from the urine of postmenopausal women, possessing follicle-stimulating hormone (FSH) activity, but virtually no luteinising activity. Urofollitropin is used in the treatment of female infertility where an increase in luteinising hormone activity is not required, as in polycystic ovarian disease. It is also used with other drugs as part of *in-vitro* fertilisation procedures.

WADA Status: Banned in and out of competition

WADA Class: Hormones and Related Substances: Gonadotrophins

Includes gonadotrophin or a substance with a similar chemical structure or similar biological effect(s), or one of their releasing factors. Prohibited in males only.

Preparations

Single ingredient: ***Arg.:*** Follitrin; Fostimon; ***Austral.:*** Metrodin; ***Braz.:*** Metrodin; ***Canad.:*** Bravelle; ***Chile:*** Follitrin; ***Cz.:*** Fostimon; Metrodin; ***Fr.:*** Fostimon; ***Gr.:*** Bravelle; ***Hong Kong:*** Fostimon; ***Hung.:*** Fostimon; ***India:*** Gonotrop F; Metrodin; Neogentin; ***Ital.:*** Fostimon; ***Mex.:*** Fostimon; ***Neth.:*** Bravelle; ***Port.:*** Metrodin; ***Rus.:*** Metrodin (Метродин); ***Switz.:*** Fostimon; ***Thai.:*** Follimon; ***Turk.:*** Metrodin; ***USA:*** Bravelle; Fertinex; Metrodin.

U

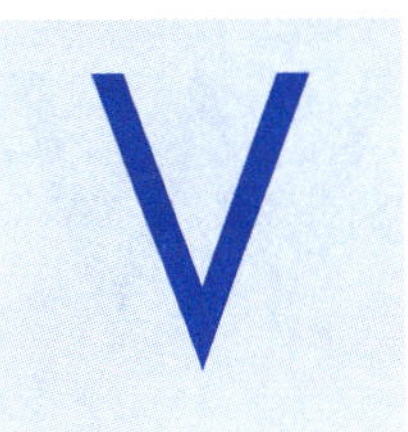

Vorozole

Other names: R-83842; Vorozol; Vorozolum.

Ворозол

Clinical profile: Vorozole is a selective nonsteroidal aromatase inhibitor that has been investigated in the treatment of breast cancer.

WADA Status: Banned in and out of competition

WADA Class: Hormone Antagonists and Modulators

Includes aromatase inhibitors.

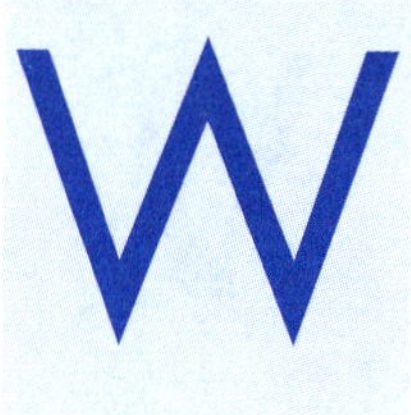

No monographs have been included for drugs beginning with the letter W.

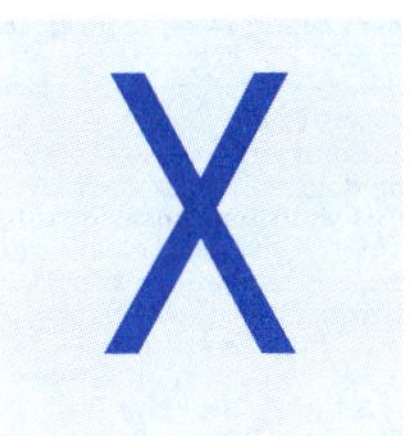

Xipamide

Other names: Be-1293; Ksipamidi; MJF-10938; Xipamid; Xipamida; Xipamidum.

Ксипамид

Clinical profile: Xipamide is a diuretic used for hypertension, and for oedema, including that associated with heart failure.

WADA Status: Banned in and out of competition

WADA Class: Diuretics and Other Masking Agents

Includes diuretics or substances with a similar chemical structure or similar biological effect(s).

Preparations

Single ingredient: ***Austria:*** Aquaphoril; ***Ger.:*** Aquaphor; Aquex; Xipa-Isis; Xipa; Xipagamma; ***India:*** Xipamid; ***Port.:*** Diurexan; ***Spain:*** Diurex; ***UK:*** Diurexan.

Multi-ingredient: ***Ger.:*** Neotri.

Xylometazoline Hydrochloride

Other names: Hidrocloruro de xilometazolina; Ksilometazolin Hidroklorür; Ksilometazolino hidrochloridas; Ksylometatsoliinihydrokloridi; Ksylometazoliny chlorowodorek; Xilometazolinhidroklorid; Xylométazoline, chlorhydrate de; Xylometazolinhydro; Xylometazolin-hydrochlorid; Xylometazolini hydrochloridum.

Ксилометазолина Гидрохлорид

Clinical profile: Xylometazoline hydrochloride is a sympathomimetic with marked alpha-adrenergic activity and vasoconstrictor properties. It is used for the relief of nasal and conjunctival congestion.

WADA Status: Banned in competition

WADA Class: Stimulants

Includes stimulants or substances with a similar chemical structure or similar biological effect(s). Xylometazoline is an imidazole derivative. Imidazole derivatives for topical use are exempt.

Preparations

Single ingredient: ***Arg.:*** Nastizol; Otrivina; ***Austral.:*** Otrivin; ***Austria:*** Olynth; Otrivin; Rati-oSoft; Xylo-COMOD; ***Belg.:*** Nasa Rhinathiol; Nasasinutab; Nuso-San; Otrivine Anti-Rhinitis; ***Braz.:*** Otrivina; ***Canad.:*** Balminil Nasal Decongestant; Certified Decongestant; Decongestant Nasal Spray; Decongestant Nose Drops; Nasal Decongestant; Otrivin; ***Cz.:*** Dr Rentschler Snupfenspray; Dr Rentschler Snupfentropfen; Nasenspray AL; Nasentropfen AL; Olynth; Otrivin; Rhino-Stas; Xylo-COMOD; ***Denm.:*** Otrivin; Passagen; Zymelin; ***Fin.:*** Naso-Ratiopharm; Nasolin; Otrivin; ***Ger.:*** Balkis; Gelonasal; Imidin N; Nasan; Nasengel AL; Nasengel; Nasenspray AL; Nasenspray E; Nasenspray K; Nasenspray-CT; Nasenspray; Nasentropfen AL; Nasentropfen E; Nasentropfen K; Nasentropfen Stada; Olynth; Otriven gegen Schnupfen; Otriven; Rapako xylo; Rhinex mit Xylometazolin; schnupfen endrine; Snup; Tussamag Nasenspray; Xylo-POS; Xylo; ***Gr.:*** Otrivin-Menthol; Otrivin; ***Hong Kong:*** Decongestant Nasal Spray; Otrivin; Xyloma; ***Hung.:*** Nasan; Novorin; Otrivin; Rhinathiol; Rhino-Stas; ***India:*** Decon; Nazalin; Otrivin; ***Indon.:*** Otrivin; ***Irl.:*** Otrivine; ***Israel:*** Nazalet; Otrivin; Xylovit; ***Ital.:*** Neo Rinoleina; Otrivin; Respiro; ***Malaysia:*** Otrivin; ***Neth.:*** Kruidvat Neusdruppels; Kruidvat Neusspray; Mucorhinyl; Otrivin; Xylo-COMOD; ***Norw.:*** Naso; Nazaren; Otrivin; Xolin; Zymelin; ***NZ:*** Otrivine; ***Philipp.:*** Otrivin; ***Pol.:*** Otrivin; Xylogel; Xylorin; ***Port.:*** Otrivina; ***Rus.:*** Dlianos (Длянос); Grippostad Rhino (Гриппостад Рино); Halazolin (Галазолин); Olynth (Олинт); Otrivin (Отривин); Rhinonorm (Ринонорм); Rhinostop (Риностоп); Suprima-Nos (Суприма-Ноз); Tyzine Xylo (Тизин Ксило); Xymelin (Ксимелин); ***S.Afr.:*** Otrivin; ***Singapore:*** Otrivin; ***Spain:*** Amidrin; Idasal; Otrivin; Rinoblanco; ***Swed.:*** Nasoferm; Otrivin; Zymelin; ***Switz.:*** Nasben; Nasobol Xylo; Olynth; Otrivin; Rhinostop; Rinosedin; Xylo-Mepha; ***Thai.:*** Otrivin; ***Turk.:*** Naze; Otrivine; Rinizol; Xylo-COMOD; ***UAE:*** Xylolin; ***UK:*** Non-Drowsy Sudafed Decongestant Nasal Spray; Otradrops; Otraspray; Otrivine; Tixycolds Cold and Allergy; ***USA:*** Otrivin.

Multi-ingredient: ***Chile:*** Bacitopic Compuesto; Nasomin; Rinobanedif; ***Denm.:*** Otrivin Menthol; ***Fin.:*** Otrivin Menthol; ***Ger.:*** Nasic; ***Irl.:*** Otrivine-Antistin; ***Israel:*** Aforinol; ***Ital.:*** Inalar; ***Mex.:*** Rinadex Compuesto; ***Neth.:*** Otrivin Menthol; ***NZ:*** Otrivine Menthol; Otrivine-Antistin; ***Swed.:*** Otrivin Menthol; ***Switz.:*** Triofan; ***Turk.:*** Rynacrom Compound; ***UK:*** Otrivine-Antistin.

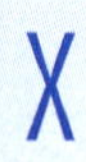

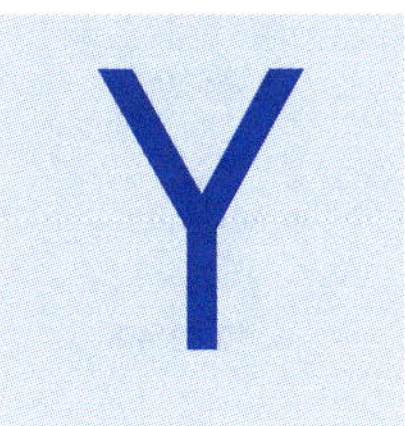

No monographs have been included for drugs beginning with the letter Y.

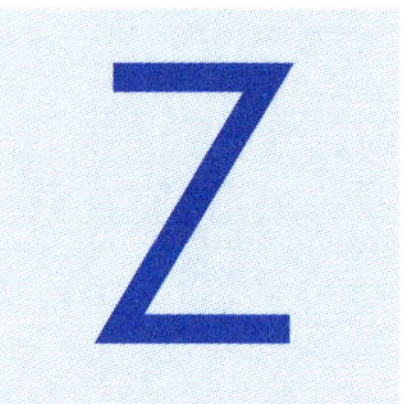

Zeranol

Other names: MK-188; P-1496; THFES (HM); Zearalanol; Zéranol; Zeranolum.

Зеранол

Clinical profile: Zeranol is a nonsteroidal oestrogen that has been used for the management of menopausal and menstrual disorders. It has also been used as a growth promotor in veterinary practice. Its anabolic properties may be subject to abuse in sport.

WADA Status: Banned in and out of competition

WADA Class: Other Anabolic Agents
Includes other anabolic agents not listed elsewhere.

Zilpaterol Hydrochloride

Other names: Hidrocloruro de zilpaterol; RU-42173 (base or hydrochloride); Zilpatérol, Chlorhydrate de; Zilpateroli Hydrochloridum.

Зилпатерола Гидрохлорид

Clinical profile: Zilpaterol hydrochloride is a beta2-agonist used in some countries as an animal-feed additive to promote weight gain. Its anabolic properties may be subject to abuse in sport.

WADA Status: Banned in and out of competition

WADA Class: Other Anabolic Agents
Includes other anabolic agents not listed elsewhere.

WADA Status: Banned in and out of competition

WADA Class: Beta-2 Agonists
Includes beta-2 agonists or their isomers.

Index

B

C

D

E

F

G

H

I

J

K

L

M

N

O

P

Q

R

T

U

V

Y

Z

Cyrillic Index

В

Г

Д

З

И

К

Н

О

П

У

Ф

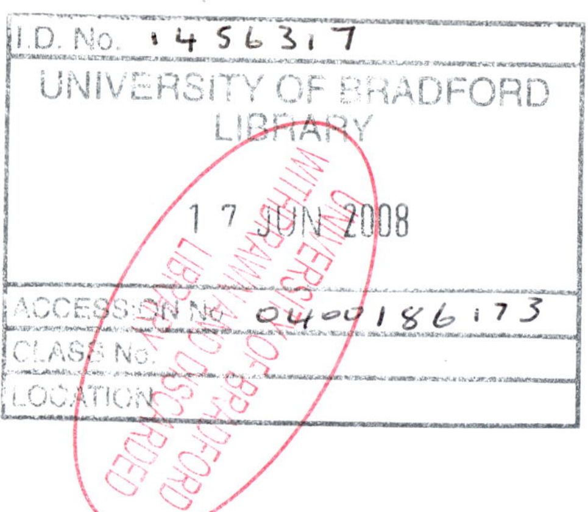